Mechanical Circulatory Support

Principles and Applications

Mechanical Circulatory Support

Principles and Applications

EDITORS

David L. Joyce, MD
Department of Cardiothoracic Surgery
Stanford University Hospitals and Clinics
Stanford, California

Lyle D. Joyce, MD, PhD
Professor of Surgery
Division of Cardiovascular Surgery
Mayo Clinic
Rochester, Minnesota

Matthias Loebe, MD, PhD
Division Chief
Transplant Surgery and Assist Devices
Methodist Hospital
Houston, Texas

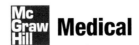 **Medical**

New York   Chicago   San Francisco   Lisbon   London   Madrid   Mexico City
Milan   New Delhi   San Juan   Seoul   Singapore   Sydney   Toronto

The McGraw·Hill Companies

Mechanical Circulatory Support: Principles and Applications

1 2 3 4 5 6 7 8 9 0 CTP/CTP 15 14 13 12 11

ISBN 978-0-07-175344-9
MHID 0-07-175344-3

This book was set in Minion by Cenveo Publisher Services.
The editors were James Shanahan, Christine Diedrich, and Christie Naglieri.
The production supervisor was Catherine Saggese.
Project management was provided by Manisha Singh, Cenveo Publisher Services.
The interior designer was Alan Barnett; the cover designer was Mary McKeon.
The cover image is from HeartWare, Inc. (HeartWare's HVAD is an investigational device.)
China Translation & Printing Services, Ltd. was printer and binder.

This book is printed on acid-free paper.

Library of Congress Cataloging-in-Publication Data

Mechanical Circulatory Support: Principles and Applications /[edited by] David L. Joyce, Lyle D. Joyce,
    Matthias Loebe. — 1st ed.
        p. ; cm.
    Includes bibliographical references and index.
    ISBN-13: 978-0-07-175344-9 (hbk. : alk. paper)
    ISBN-10: 0-07-175344-3 (hbk. : alk. paper)
    1. Blood, Circulation, Artificial—Instruments.   2. Heart failure—Treatment.   I. Joyce, David L.
II. Joyce, Lyle D.   III. Loebe, M. (Matthias)
    [DNLM: 1. Heart Failure—surgery.   2. Assisted Circulation.   3. Heart, Artificial. WG 370]
    RD598.35.A77H43 2011
    617.4'120645—dc22
                                                            2011007774

McGraw-Hill books are available at special quantity discounts to use as premiums and sales promotions, or for use in corporate training programs. To contact a representative please e-mail us at bulksales@mcgraw-hill.com.

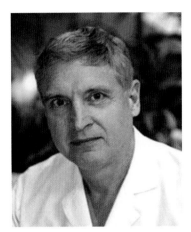

Dr George P. Noon

The history of mechanical circulatory support has been closely related to the group around Dr Michael E. DeBakey and the Texas Medical Center. As a medical student, Dr DeBakey developed the first continuous blood pump when he designed the roller pump. His mission was to actually build a pulsatile pump for his physics professor. However, the pump that became known as the first roller pump provided continuous blood flow and Dr. DeBakey traveled around New Orleans where he went to Tulane University providing blood transfusion services in the entire area. He continued to have an extensive interest in artificial heart and blood pump development, so it is no wonder that one of his closest associates, Dr George P. Noon, followed his footsteps and worked in the development of left ventricular assist devices. When cyclosporine became available for the aftercare of heart transplant patients and the heart transplant program at The Methodist Hospital in Houston, TX, resumed its activity, it was Dr Noon who led the program. Quite early on an engineer from the space agency NASA was one of the recipients of a heart transplant. In the aftermath of the transplantation, Dr Noon and Dr DeBakey began to confer with this NASA engineer about their interest in developing blood pumps. This was the beginning of a close cooperation between Baylor College of Medicine, The Methodist Hospital, and NASA space agency in developing and testing continuous blood flow pumps. The design of the fuel injection pumps of the space shuttle was adopted and the continuous-flow pump developed. This pump was tested by Dr Noon in animal experiments at Texas A&M University in College Station.

Over this extensive and very successful animal testing, the decision was made to take the concept into human use in a number of centers in Europe identified, where first implants may be performed.

Under the leadership of Dr Noon, the first MicroMed DeBakey VAD, as it was then called, was implanted on November 13, 1998 at the German Heart Institute in Berlin, Germany. A number of patients followed, first in Europe and then around the world, and finally this concept was taken to the United States. In 1998, it is fair to say that the majority of our colleagues did not believe in the concept of continuous blood flow as a means of long-term support in patients with heart failure. Currently, there is not a single left ventricular assist device in development or in testing that is not a continuous blood flow pump. This concept has taken over widely and the success of these miniaturized, no noise pumps with relatively good long-term reliability has totally changed the face of use of mechanical circulatory assist devices. This type of therapy can now be offered and is applied in hundreds and thousands of patients around the world with a great success rate. One-year survival of 80% to 90% is reported repeatedly from single centers or in clinical trials. There is no question that in the future more and more patients will receive this type of therapy and will be supported successfully.

In the pioneering days of applying this technology a lot of things had to be learned; how patients react to continuous blood flow and how a patient who does not exhibit any pulsatility can be monitored and managed. A very substantial part of this learning curve and this experience was accumulated under the leadership of Dr Noon, both in the European trials of the MicroMed DeBakey VAD as well as in the United States application of this device. Those pioneering days certainly were not easy and, as always, learning was hard and some patients did not do as well as one might have hoped for, but it became very clear that this technology was the right technology to be used in patients with severe end-stage heart failure. The wide application of this concept and the high safety of using those devices are in no small part based on those great efforts to successfully prove and apply the concept of continuous blood flow pumps as it was pioneered by Dr Noon.

This book is dedicated to Dr George P. Noon as a pioneer, leader, and great promoter of the idea of miniaturized blood pumps in patients with end-stage heart failure.

Matthias Loebe, MD, PhD

CONTENTS

CONTRIBUTORS

Michael A. Acker, MD
William Maul Measey Professor of Surgery Chief
Division of Cardiothoracic Surgery
Professor of Surgery University of Pennsylvania Health System
Philadelphia, Pennsylvania
Chapter 27

Alessandro Barbone, MD
Cardiovascular Department
Istituto Clinico Humanitas IRCCS,
Milan, Italy
Chapter 11

Gill B. Bearnson, PhD
WorldHeart Corporation
Salt Lake City, Utah
Chapter 38

Gerald J. Berry, MD
Director
Cardiac and Pulmonary Pathology
Stanford University Medical Center
Stanford, California
Chapter 17

Gabriele B. Bertoni, MD, PhD
Consultant Vascular Surgeon
Tutor of Surgical Anatomy
Istituto Auxologico Italiano
Università degli Studi di Milano
Milan, Italy
Chapter 6

Emma J. Birks, MRCP, PhD
Professor of Medicine
University of Louisville
Louisville, Kentucky
Chapter 8

Holger Buchholz, MD
Clinical Assistant Professor
Division of Cardiac Surgery
Director of Pediatric Artificial Heart Program, Adult Artificial Heart
Program, Pediatric Heart Failure Program
Univeristy of Alberta, Stollery Children's Hospital, and Mazankowsi
Heart Institute
Alberta, Canada
Chapter 30

John Burdis
Chief Technical Officer
CircuLite, Inc
Saddle Brook, New Jersey
Chapter 35

Daniel Burkhoff, MD, PhD
Chief Medical Officer
CircuLite, Inc.
Saddle Brook, New Jersey
Chapter 35

Sheri S. Crow, MD
Critical Care Medicine
Mayo Clinic
Rochester, Minnesota
Chapter 15

Kurt Dasse, PhD
President and Chief Executive Officer
Levitronix LLC
Waltham, Massachusetts
Chapter 25

Walter P. Dembitsky, MD
Medical Director of Mechanical Circulatory Support
Medical Director of Cardiac Surgery
Sharp Memorial Hospital
San Diego, California
Chapter 14

George Dimeling, MD
Resident
Stanford University Medical Center, CTS Department
Stanford, California
Chapter 10

Arielle Drummond, PhD
Research Engineer
CircuLite, Inc
Saddle Brook, New Jersey
Chapter 35

Gail Farnan, BSN, MBA
Vice President
Marketing
CircuLite, Inc.
Saddle Brook, New Jersey
Chapter 35

Robert Farnan
Director
Endovascular and Cannuia Engineering
CircuLite, Inc.
Saddle Brook, New Jersey
Chapter 35

David J. Farrar, PhD
Vice President
Research and Scientific Affairs
Thoratec Corporation
Pleasanton, California
Chapter 27, Chapter 32

Matthew D. Forrester, MD
Resident
Department of Cardiothoracic Surgery
Stanford University School of Medicine
Stanford, California
Chapter 5, Chapter 22

Monica R. Freeman, MSW, LICSW
Social Worker
Department of Nursing
Mayo Clinic
Rochester, Minnesota
Chapter 21

Peter Göttel, MD
Chief Executive Officer
BerlinHeals
Berlin, Germany
Chapter 31

Thomas Gould
Vice President
Clinical Affairs
Terumo Heart Inc.
Ann Arbor, Michigan
Chapter 37

Robert Halfmann, MD
Director
Global Marketing
Clinical Science and Reimbursement
Berlin Heart GmbH
Berlin, Germany
Chapter 31

Katherine B. Harrington, MD
Resident
Cardiothoracic Surgery
Stanford University
Stanford, California
Chapter 5, Chapter 22

David R. Hathaway, MD
Chief Medical Officer
HeartWare International, Inc.
Framingham, Massachusetts
Chapter 36

Roland Hetzer, MD, PhD
Department of Cardiothoracic and Vascular Surgery
Deutsches Herzzentrum Berlin
Berlin, Germany
Chapter 19

Dora Y. Ho, MD, PhD
Clinical Assistant Professor
Division of Infectious Diseases and Geographic Medicine, Department of Medicine
Stanford University School of Medicine
Stanford, California
Chapter 13

William L. Holman, MD
University of Alabama
Birmingham VA Medical Center
Birmingham, Alabama
Chapter 5

Gordon B. Jacobs, MS
World Heart Corporation
Salt Lake City, Utah
Chapter 38

Robert K. Jarvik, MD
President and Chief Executive Officer
Jarvik Heart, Inc.
New York, New York
Chapter 34

Jal S. Jassawalla, MS, MBA
World Heart Corporation
Salt Lake City, Utah
Chapter 38

Daniel D. Joyce, BFA
Research Assistant
Cardiac Surgery
University of Minnesota
Minneapolis, Minnesota
Chapter 15

David L. Joyce, MD
Study Coordinator
Department of Cardiothoracic Surgery
Stanford University Medical Center
Stanford, California
Chapter 14

Lyle D. Joyce MD, PhD
Professor of Surgery
Division of Cardiovascular Surgery
Mayo Clinic
Rochester, Minnesota
Chapter 7

Biswajit Kar, MD
Assistant Professor of Medicine
Baylor College of Medicine
Director of Cardiac Catheterization Laboratory
Michael E. DeBakey VA Medical Center
Division of Heart Failure and Assist Devices
The Texas Heart Institute at St. Luke's Episcopal Hospital
Houston, Texas
Chapter 4

Pratap S. Khanwilkar, PhD, MBA
Vice President
Rotary Systems and Business Development
World Heart Corporation
Salt Lake City, Utah
Chapter 38

Ali Kilic, Msc
Senir Product Manager
Berlin Heart GmbH
Berlin, Germany
Chapter 30

Tomoya Kitano, MME
Evaheart Medical USA, Inc.
Pittsburgh, Pennsylvania
Chapter 39

Ronald W. Kipp, EE
President
RK Engineering
Willow Street, Pennsylvania
Chapter 2

Jay Kraemer
Vice President
Worldwide Sales and Marketing
MicroMed Cardiovascular, Inc.
Houston, Texas
Chapter 33

Carol Krieger
Vice President
Scientific Affairs
CircuLite, Inc.
Saddle Brook, New Jersey
Chapter 35

Bob Kroslowitz, BS, CCP
Vice President
Clinical Affairs
Berlin Heart Inc
The Woodlands, Texas
Chapter 30, Chapter 31

Thomas P. Laberge, MS, MD
Co-Clinical Director of Anesthesiology
Amplatz Children's Hospital
Assistant Adjunct Professor
University of Minnesota
Minneapolis, Minnesota
Chapter 9

Marco Lanfranconi, MD
Department of Cardiac Surgery
"A. de Gasperis" Niguarda Cà Granda Hospital
Milan, Italy
Chapter 11

Steven Langford, BSEE
Vice President
Clinical Support
Syncardia Systems, Inc.
Tucson, Arizona Area
Chapter 28

James Lee, MS
Director of Engineering
World Heart Corporation
Salt Lake City, Utah
Chapter 38

James W. Long, MD, PhD
INTEGRIS Baptist Medical Center
Oklahoma City, Oklahoma
Chapter 38

Michael K. Loushin, MD
Associate Professor
Anesthesiology
University of Minnesota
Minneapolis, Minnesota
Chapter 9

Bryan E. Lynch, ME, MBA
Partner
First Continental Advisors Inc.
Houston, Texas
Chapter 2

Mark Macedo, RN, BSN
Director
Clinical Affairs
Levitronix LLC
Waltham, Massachusetts
Chapter 25

Hari R. Mallidi, MD
Assistant Professor
Department of Cardiothoracic Surgery
Stanford University School of Medicine
Stanford, California
Chapter 22

John Marks, PhD
Director
Clinical Research
Levitronix LLC
Waltham, Massachusetts
Chapter 25

Filippo Milazzo, MD, PhD
Department of Cardiac Surgery
"A. de Gasperis" Niguarda Cà Granda Hospital
Milan, Italy
Chapter 11

Phillip J. Miller, MS
Vice President
Research and Development
World Heart Corporation
Salt Lake City, Utah
Chapter 38

Seema Mital, MD
Associate Professor
Division of Pediatric Cardiology, Hospital for Sick Children
University of Toronto
Toronto, Canada
Chapter 16

Hiroshi Miyamoto, MD, PhD
Instructor
Department of Gastroenterology and Oncology
University of Tokushima
Tokushima, Japan
Chapter 1

Tadashi Motomra, MD, PhD
Baylor College of Medicine
Michael E. DeBakey Department of Surgery
Houston, Texas
Chapter 1

Johannes Müller, MD, MEng
Chief Operating Officer
Chief Scientific Officer
Berlin Heals
Berlin, Germany
Chapter 31

Karl E. Nelson, RN, MBA
INTEGRIS Baptist Medical Center
Oklahoma City, Oklahoma
Chapter 38

Tomohiro Nishinaka, MD, PhD
Department of Cardiovascular Surgery
Tokyo Women's Medical University
Tokyo, Japan
Chapter 39

Yukhiko Nosé, MD, PhD
Professor, Director
Center for Artificial Organ Development
Michael E. DeBakey Department of Surgery
Baylor College of Medicine
Houston, Texas
Chapter 1

Don B. Olsen, DVM, DSci
President
Utah Artificial Heart Institute
Salt Lake City, Utah
Chapter 2

Phil Oyer, MD
Professor
Department of Cardiothoracic Surgery
Stanford University School of Medicine
Stanford, California
Chapter 10

Steven J. Phillips, MD
Director
Specialized Information Services
Associate Director
National Library of Medicine, National Institutes of Health
U.S. Department of Health and Human Services
Bethesda, Maryland
Chapter 3

Rachel S. Phillips, PhD
Learning Sciences
College of Education
University of Washington
Seattle, Washington
Chapter 3

Evgenij V. Potapov, MD
Specialist in Cardiac Surgery
Department of Cardiothoracic and Vascular Surgery
Deutsches Herzzentrum Berlin
Berlin, Germany
Chapter 19

Daniel H. Raess, MD, FACC, FACS
Senior Medical Director
Abiomed, Inc.
Danvers, Massachusetts
Chapter 23, Chapter 26, Chapter 29

Kumudha Ramasubbu, MD
Section of Cardiology
The Michael E. DeBakey Veterans Affairs Medical Center
Houston, Texas
Chapter 4

Wilfried Roethy, MD
Department of Cardiothoracic Surgery
Medical University of Vienna
Vienna, Austria
Chapter 18

Jennifer Rutledge, MD, FRCPC, FACC
Assistant Professor
Department of Pediatrics
University of Alberta
Alberta, Canada
Chapter 30

Satoshi Saito, MD, PhD
Assistant Professor
Department of Cardiovascular Surgery
Tokyo Women's Medical University
Tokyo, Japan
Chapter 39

Joyce L. Sanchez, MD
Fellow
Infectious Diseases and Geographic Medicine
Stanford University Hospital
Stanford, California
Chapter 13

Hans H. Scheld, MD
Professor
Head of the Department of Thoracic and Cardiovascular Surgery
University Hospital Münster
Münster, Germany
Chapter 12

Heinrich Schima, MD
Center of Medical Physics and Biomedical Engineering
Medical University of Vienna
Vienna, Austria
Chapter 18

Christof Schmid, MD
Head and Director
Department of Cardiothoracic Surgery
University Medical Center Regensburg
Regensburg, Germany
Chapter 12

Robert E. Southard, MD
Assistant Professor of Surgery
Department of Surgery
Washington University in St. Louis
St. Louis, Missouri
Chapter 17

Robert G. Svitek, PhD
Director of Engineering
CardiacAssist, Inc.
Pittsburgh, Pennsylvania
Chapter 24

Marc T. Swartz
Clinical Specialist
HeartWare International, Inc.
Framingham, Massachusetts
Chapter 36

Michael F. Sweeney, MD
Associate Professor
Anesthesiology and Pediatrics
Univeristy of Minnesota Medical School
Attending Anesthesiologist
Fairview University Hospital
Minneapolis, Minnesota
Chapter 9

Hiroyuki Tsukui, MD, PhD
Department of Cardiovascular Surgery
Tokyo Women's Medical University
Tokyo, Japan
Chapter 39

Christina VanderPluym, MD, FRCPC
Division of Cardiology
Pediatric Ventricular Assist Device Program
University of Alberta and Stollery Children's Hospital
Alberta, Canada
Chapter 30

Ettore Vitali, MD
Cardiovascular Department
Istituto Clinico Humanitas IRCCS
Milan, Italy
Chapter 11

David M. Weber, PhD
Chief Operating Officer
Abiomed Inc
Danvers, Massachusetts
Chapter 23

Stephen Westaby BSc, PhD, MS, FRCS, FETCS, FESC , FICA, FACC
Professor of Biomedical Science
Consultant Cardiac Surgeon
Department of Cardiothoracic Surgery
John Radcliffe Hospital
Oxford, England
Chapter 6

Georg M. Wieselthaler, MD
Department of Cardiothoracic Surgery
University Hospital of Vienna
Vienna, Austria
Chapter 18

Ernst Wolner, MD
Department of Cardiothoracic Surgery
University Hospital of Vienna
Vienna, Austria
Chapter 18

Magdi H. Yacoub, FRS
Heart Science Centre
Harefield Hospital
Harefield, England
Chapter 8

Kenji Yamazaki, MD, PhD
Department of Cardiovascular Surgery
Tokyo Women's Medical University
Tokyo, Japan
Chapter 39

Keith A. Youker, PhD
Scientist
Department of Cardiology
The Methodist Hospital Research Institute
Houston, Texas
Chapter 20

PREFACE

Mechanical Circulatory Support: Principles and Applications represents a comprehensive summary of an emerging growth area in cardiovascular medicine. With 5 million Americans suffering from congestive heart failure and substantial limitations on the efficacy of medical therapy, the need for an effective surgical solution has been the singular objective of cardiac surgery for over 50 years. With newer device technology, careful patient selection, and improved postoperative management, mechanical circulatory support has become a viable treatment strategy for thousands of patients. As the field continues to evolve, so do the complexities surrounding the clinical use of these devices. This textbook addresses the common scenarios that are faced by the health care team during the pre-, intra-, and postoperative period after assist device implantation. It also describes the device-specific attributes of the various technologies that are currently in use clinically. By combining a thorough representation of the available published data with the world experience of a group of authors that comprise the leading experts in the field of mechanical circulatory support, this book attempts to compile and summarize the existing knowledge in a way that is accessible to the reader.

This textbook is divided into two sections. The first section addresses the common clinical considerations that occur when managing patients who require assist device therapy. Included here is a historical perspective on the scientific achievement and regulatory process that has contributed to the success of this specialty as well as a detailed perspective on patient selection and perioperative considerations. The second section provides a detailed summary of each of the available assist devices that are at various stages of development worldwide. Included

here is a summary chapter that simplifies the logic behind device selection in an industry that continues to produce an increasing array of short- and long-term therapies.

In producing a textbook of this caliber, we are greatly indebted to the numerous individuals who made this work possible. Since those who are charged with the care of these very sick patients are typically among the most overworked health care professionals, we are truly thankful for the amount of time and energy that each of our contributing authors put in to getting this project completed on schedule. We would also like to thank the editorial and production staff at McGraw Hill for the opportunity to collaborate on this work. In particular, we are indebted to Jim Shanahan, Christie Naglieri, and Laura Libretti.

It goes without saying that this book would never have come to fruition without the mentorship and example of Dr George P. Noon, to whom it is dedicated. Each of the editors owes a particular debt to Dr Noon, who has become an icon in the field of mechanical circulatory support and motivated each of us to persevere in a field that can be as painstaking as it can be rewarding. His leadership, creativity, and exemplary work ethic have inspired a generation of surgeons and will continue to be a force in driving the evolution of this field.

Finally, and most importantly, we are thankful to our families who have supported and encouraged us throughout the production of this textbook.

David L. Joyce, MD
Lyle D. Joyce, MD, PhD
Matthias Loebe, MD, PhD

SECTION I

Clinical Considerations

CHAPTER 1

HISTORY OF MECHANICAL CIRCULATORY SUPPORT

Yukhiko Nosé, Tadashi Motomra, and Hiroshi Miyamoto

Mechanical circulatory support got its start in 1934, when a medical student by the name of Michael Ellis DeBakey developed the concept of a roller pump to facilitate blood transfusions (Fig. 1–1). Two decades later, John Gibbon would first use a cardiopulmonary bypass (CPB) machine based on this same pumping mechanism to repair an atrial septal defect in an 18-year-old woman in 1953, ushering in the era of open-heart surgery. Almost from the dawn of cardiac surgery, the need for a device to provide prolonged circulatory support was recognized, leading several investigators across the world to pursue the dream of an artificial heart. In the evolution that followed, investigators have pursued multiple different strategies to provide mechanical circulatory support, encompassing both intra- and extracorporeal devices, short- and long-term devices, biventricular, left ventricular, and right ventricular support devices, as well as pulsatile and rotary flow (both centrifugal and axial).

PULSATILE VENTRICULAR ASSIST DEVICES

Beginning in the early 1960s, DeBakey and colleagues began developing the concept of an intracorporeal left ventricular assist device (LVAD).[1,2] The early design consisted of double-lumen silastic tubes with outer tubing that acted as housing with only one inlet which was connected to an external air source. The inner silastic tube, which contained the blood chamber, was collapsed by compressed air entering the housing. Starr-Edwards ball valves at either end (inlet and outlet of the housing) established unidirectional flow. This device was first used clinically at the Baylor College of Medicine (BCM) in 1963, implanted in a patient who suffered cardiac arrest 1 day after an aortic valve replacement. DeBakey, together with E. Stanley Crawford, implanted this assist device by anastomosing the inlet tube to the left atrium and the outlet tube to the descending thoracic aorta. During the next few days, left ventricular failure improved, but the patient died on the fourth postoperative day, probably from brain damage that occurred during the cardiac arrest. Realizing that the primary indication for mechanical support at the time came from postcardiotomy cardiac failure, DeBakey began developing a paracorporeal LVAD as a temporary

support device. In 1966, a pneumatic paracorporeal pulsatile LVAD was implanted with successful weaning from cardiopulmonary bypass (Fig. 1–2A,B).[3]

Another of the early methods for achieving circulatory assistance involved developing an auxiliary artificial ventricle.[4,5] This idea was proposed by Kantrowitz and associates in 1963. This auxiliary ventricle consisted of a collapsible bulb, ellipsoidal in shape, in a rigid case whose inner surface followed the same contour. A woven Dacron arterial graft at either end of the major axis connected the inner bulb to the ascending and descending aorta, permitting unrestricted flow through the device. Rhythmic application of compressed air between the inner bulb and outer case caused the bulb to collapse, propelling the blood both proximally and distally. This pumping augmented the coronary arterial blood flow and reduced the left ventricular workload (Fig. 1–3A,B).[6] Kantrowitz implanted this auxiliary ventricle in a patient in 1967. In a first for implantable devices, the patient was able to be discharged home and survived for approximately 80 days. This device was the first attempt at serial blood flow, which permitted intermittent activation, with stopping of the pump during periods of improved hemodynamic conditions.

Multiple variations on the pulsatile LVAD concept were brought to clinical use during the 1980s and 1990s. The Novacor® LVAS (Left Ventricular Assist System) employed an electromechanically driven dual pusher-plate blood pump in what was one of the early implantable LVADs for bridging a patient to transplant. In 1984, this device (developed by P. Portner) was implanted successfully by Phil Oyer at Stanford University in patient Robert St. Laurent, representing the first successful bridge-to-transplantation (BTT).

However, it was the pneumatically powered Thoratec® HeartMate XVE device that gained approval as the first intracorporeal LVAD for destination therapy (DT) in the aftermath of the landmark REMATCH (Randomized Evaluation of Mechanical Assistance for the Treatment of Congestive Heart Failure) trial comparing device therapy to Optimal Medical Management. Variations on this device were first approved as bridge-to-transplant (BTT) in 1994 and 1998. Nevertheless, the large size and limited durability of these pulsatile LVADs prompted a search for alternative engineering designs that would enhance the feasibility of long-term device implantation.

CONTINUOUS FLOW VENTRICULAR ASSIST DEVICES

Rotary blood pumps emerged as an answer to these challenges, taking the form of both axial and centrifugal flow (Table 1–1). The major advantages of these devices over pulsatile are that they are smaller in size, valve free, eliminate the need for a compliance chamber or external vent tube, have lower power

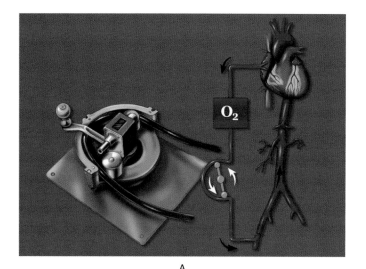

A

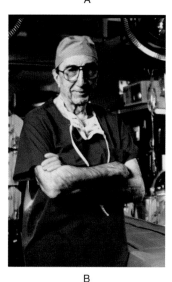

B

FIGURE 1–1. Design of the roller pump proposed by M.E. DeBakey when he was a medical student. (Courtesy of the Baylor College of Medicine Archives.)

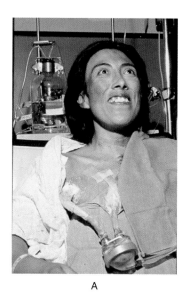

A

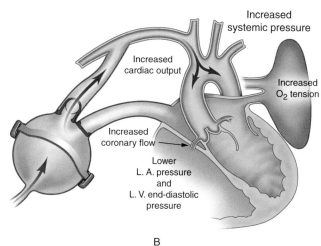

B

FIGURE 1–2. A. Left ventricular bypass pump shown in a patient who had difficulty weaning from cardiopulmonary bypass. This is the first clinically successful paracorporeal LVAD implantation in 1967. (Courtesy of the Baylor College of Medicine Archives.) **B.** Relation between the pump and natural heart. The inlet cannula was connected to the left atrial appendage, and the outlet cannula was connected to the right subclavian artery. (Reproduced with permission from International Center for Medical Technologies [ICMT]).

consumption, and cost less. An axial-flow blood pump operates on the principle of an Archimedes screw and can be produced in a manner that significantly reduces the overall size relative to a pulsatile blood pump. The impeller of the axial-flow pump typically rotates around 10,000 rpm (revolutions per minute). Each rotation of the impeller creates a straightforward moving force on the blood, a feature that permits device miniaturization. The clinical application of an axial pump depends on its basic structure, that is, blood access through direct cannula insertion or via percutaneous insertion. Some of the different types of axial blood pumps that are clinically available are represented in Table 1–2. The first clinical use of a long-term "second-generation" axial flow LVAD occurred in 1998 with the introduction of the MicroMed DeBakey VAD by Noon, Hetzer, and DeBakey. The HeartMate II device has subsequently been FDA (Food and Drug Administration) approved both as DT and BTT.

Centrifugal pumps propel the blood utilizing a spinning top inside the chamber. These types of pumps operate at rpms of approximately one-fifth to one-third of an axial-flow pump. Typically, 2000 to 3000 rpm is needed to generate clinically needed blood flow of approximately 5 ± 1 L/min against 100 ± 20 mm Hg. Because the impeller of a centrifugal pump spins at a much lower speed, its bearing life is expected to be longer than that of an axial pump. A centrifugal pump generates its flow by indirect hemodynamic effect. The vortex bloodstream generated by a rotating impeller provides pressure difference between the outer housing portion (high pressure) and the impeller center portion (low pressure). Consequently, blood circulates from low-pressure region (blood inlet port) to high-pressure region (blood outlet port). The concept of centrifugal pumps was introduced in 1968 by Rafferty. A year later, Perry Blackshear's group in Minnesota developed the first clinically applicable centrifugal pump in 1969. This early-stage centrifugal pump consisted of

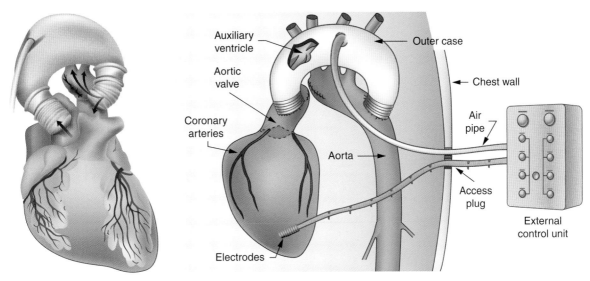

FIGURE 1–3. A. (Left) Kantrowitz' U-shaped auxiliary ventricle. This valve less pumping chamber implanted between the ascending and descending aorta produced effective counterpulsating effects. It augmented coronary arterial blood flow and reduced the left ventricular workload. (Reproduced with permission from International Center for Medical Technologies [ICMT]). **B.** (Right) This device was actuated by an extracorporeal pneumatic actuator. However, this device did not need to be actuated all the time. The patient could connect or remove this pneumatic actuator at will whenever circulatory assistance is needed. (Reproduced with permission from International Center for Medical Technologies [ICMT].)

a shaft that directly connected to an actuator (Fig. 1–4A,B).[7] During subsequent decades, a design that incorporated a magnetic coupling impeller drive was established. The majority of the currently available centrifugal pumps for CPB utilize this impeller driving method, which eliminates direct shaft connection between the impeller and actuator unit and is beneficial for simplifying the total system. The first clinical application of "third-generation" centrifugal flow device technology occurred in 2005 with the successful implantation of a VentrAssist device by Bart Griffith at the University of Maryland.

THE TOTAL ARTIFICIAL HEART

In most cases of end-stage heart failure, left ventricular support alone is sufficient for mechanical unloading and improvement in end-organ perfusion. However, in instances of biventricular failure, right-sided support is needed. Although the current indications for total artificial heart (TAH) implantation are somewhat limited, these devices played an important role in driving the field of mechanical circulatory support.

The first individual to attempt implantation of a mechanical heart was a Soviet investigator named V.P. Demikhov (Table 1–3). In 1937, he described three such experiments in animals, implanting a device that was driven by a rotating shaft powered from outside and inserted through a tube in the chest wall. Demikhov went on to describe five more experiments in 1958 but abandoned these efforts without publishing his work. However, the individual recognized as the original pioneer in the development of a TAH was Willem J. Kolff (Fig. 1–5), who began his work at the Cleveland Clinic Foundation (CCF) and is perhaps best-known for the development of renal hemodialysis. Kolff himself credited Peter F. Salisbury of Cedars Lebanon Hospital, Los Angeles, California, with originally proposing the concept of a TAH in 1955. In that year, Kolff and Salisbury, together with a dozen other scientists and investigators, formed the American Society for Artificial Internal Organs (ASAIO). Kolff and Tetsuzo Akutsu performed the first animal experiments at the CCF, implanting a hydraulically activated TAH into a dog with survival of 90 minutes (Fig. 1–6). Kolff and associates then collaborated with Thompson Ramo Wooldridge (TRW) Corporation in developing a solenoid-driven artificial heart. This was the first electromechanical and totally implantable TAH, except for the power supply (Fig. 1–7A-C).[8] Unfortunately, the technologies available 50 years ago required substantial power of more than 30 W, and overheating of the device represented a substantial limitation. The "ventricle," made of a plastic and polyurethane, lay in oil inside a rigid case. To drive the pump five solenoids pushed disks inward,

TABLE 1–1. Comparison Between Rotary and Pulsatile Pumps

Type	rpm of Impeller	Size of Pump (Priming Volume , in CC's)
Axial-flow pump	10,000 ± 2,000	10 ± 5
Centrifugal pump	2,500 ± 500	25 ± 10
Pulsatile pump	< 150[a]	66 (52[b])

[a] Beat/min.

[b] Effective stroke volume.

rpm, revolution per minute.

TABLE 1–2. Axial Flow Pumps

Classification	Size (weight and volume)	Application	Implant Position	Pump Flow and rpm
Intracardiac micro axial pump				
Hemopump	6 g/5 mL	Post-cardiotomy and during coronary surgery	Intravascular (arterial or right-PA access), transvalvular	3-3.5 L/min (20,000 rpm)
Impella	5 g/2 mL	Minimum invasive surgery	Fully implantable intra-ventricular	4.5 L/min (32,500 rpm)
Implantable axial-type VAD				
INCOR device	200 g, <100 cm³	VAD/BTT/DT	VAD/BTT/DT	5L/min (5,000-10,000 rpm)
MicroMed DeBakey VAD	95 g/15 mL	VAD/BTT	Fully implantable abdominal	5 L/min (10,000-12,000 rpm) Max: over 10 L/min
HeartMate II	165 g/62 mL	VAD/BTT/DT	Fully implantable abdominal	6 L/min (6000-13,000 rpm)
Jarvik 2000	90 g/25 mL	VAD/BTT	Intraventricular	6 L/min (10,000-16,000 rpm)

compressing the oil and thereby squeezing the "ventricle" so that it discharged its fluid into an "artery." While the Cleveland group had been focusing their efforts on the orthotopic TAH, the Houston group (headed by DeBakey) was developing a biventricular bypass artificial heart. Pneumatically driven silastic sac-type pumps were implanted in a right ventricular and left ventricular bypass fashion (Fig. 1–8A,B).[9] Another difference between the TAH of the BCM and the CCF was that the former utilized a texturized blood-contacting surface for their pump, while the latter was pursuing a smooth blood-contacting surface for their pump.

In 1964, the National Heart, Lung and Blood Institute (NHLBI) of the National Institutes of Health (NIH) began to sponsor the development of mechanical devices for short- and long-term circulatory support. This national artificial heart program was initiated by former president Lyndon Johnson upon the suggestion of DeBakey. The initial program was developed by William Hall (head of DeBakey's research at the BCM) and Yukihiko Nosé (head of Kolff's research at the CCF). The

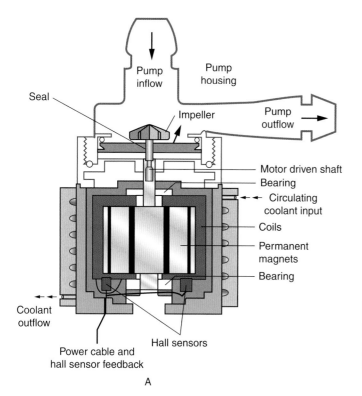

A

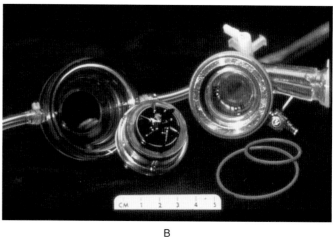

B

FIGURE 1–4. **A.** Blackshear-Medtronic centrifugal pump (cross-sectional drawing). The small impeller inside a pump head was rotated by a DC brushless micromotor with a direct shaft-driven configuration. (Reproduced with permission from International Center for Medical Technologies [ICMT].) **B.** Blackshear-Medtronic centrifugal pump (impeller and housings). (Reproduced with permission from International Center for Medical Technologies [ICMT].)

TABLE 1-3. Historical Timeline of the Key Events in the Development of Mechanical Circulatory Support

1934—M.E. DeBakey (New Orleans) describes dual-roller pump for transfusion of blood. This device subsequently becomes the most widely used type of blood pump for clinical applications of cardiopulmonary bypass and hemodialysis.

1937—V. Demikhov employed an extracorporeal assist device for 5.5 hours to substitute for the cardiac function of a dog.

1953—J. Gibbon, Jr (Philadelphia) performs the first successful clinical use of the heart-lung machine for cardiac surgery (closure of atrial septal defect).

1955—First meeting of the American Society for Artificial Internal Organs is held at the Hotel Chelsea in Atlantic City, New Jersey with 67 founding members.

1957—W.J. Kolff, T. Akutsu, and their research team (Cleveland) successfully implant a hydraulic, polyvinyl chloride total artificial heart (TAH) into a dog, keeping the animal alive for 90 minutes.

1963—D. Liotta and C.W. Hall (Houston) fabricate a tubular left ventricular assist device (LVAD), which is implanted by S. Crawford and M.E. DeBakey, but the patient does not survive. The Smithsonian's National Museum of American History, Artificial Organ Collection has this LVAD, donated by Dr Hall.

1964—Established by the National Heart and Lung Institute, the US Artificial Heart program, led initially by F. Hasting and later C. Dennis and J. Watson, aims to encourage and support further research and development of cardiac replacement devices (L. Harmison, P. Frommer, and F. Altieri all serve important periods of time as acting chief for the Total Artificial Heart program).

1966—A. Kantrowitz (New York) successfully implants into a patient an aortic U-shaped auxiliary ventricle intended as destination therapy for congestive heart failure.

1966—M.E. DeBakey (Houston) performs the first successful clinical implantation of a ventricular assist device (a pneumatically driven paracorporeal diaphragm pump) in a 37-year-old woman who cannot be weaned from cardiopulmonary bypass following aortic and mitral valve replacement. She is supported for 10 days and discharged in less than a month. The original pump implanted in this patient was made by D. Liotta with the help of engineers from Rice University. Later, this pump is refined, and it is called the BCM-Rice pump. A prototype pump is available at the International Center for Medical Technologies in Houston, Texas.

1967—A. Kantrowitz demonstrates clinical effectiveness of the intra-aortic balloon pump in cardiogenic shock patients, with its potential for treatment in acute heart failure.

1969—D.A. Cooley, in the first clinical application of the TAH, implants a pneumatically powered heart designed by D. Liotta (from the laboratory of M.E. DeBakey) as a bridge-to-transplantation (BTT) into a 47-year-old man who survives 64 hours on the TAH and 32 hours following the transplant.

1971—A. Kantrowitz implants the dynamic aortic patch (now called the Kantrowitz CardioVad) in a patient with terminal heart failure. This 63-year-old man is the first patient to be discharged to home with a cardiac assist device intended as destination therapy for congestive heart failure.

1972—J.D. Hill, T.G. O'Brien, and others (San Francisco) report the first successful clinical case using extracorporeal membrane oxygenation (ECMO) for respiratory failure.

1976—The US Food and Drug Administration (FDA), established in 1931, begins regulating medical devices with passage of the 1976 Medical Device Amendments to the Food, Drug & Cosmetic Act, which seeks to provide "reasonable assurance of safety and effectiveness" for all medical devices.

1981—D.A. Cooley implants the Akutsu heart as BTT, complicated by mortality following transplant.

1982—W. DeVries and L.D. Joyce (Salt Lake City) implants the pneumatic Jarvik-7 version of the TAH, developed by W. Kolff and coworkers at the University of Utah as a permanent cardiac replacement into patient Barney Clark who survives 112 days with the device.

1984—First Thoratec PVAD implanted as BTT by J.D. Hill.

1984—In the first successful clinical application of an electrically powered, implantable system, the Novacor LVAS developed by P. Portner is implanted by P. Oywer in patient Robert St. Laurent, representing the first successful BTT.

1985—First implantation of a Jarvik 7-70 in a woman (pediatric implant of the same device in 1986) by L.D. Joyce.

1988—The axial-flow blood pump is described by Richard Wampler at ASAIO.

1994—FDA approval of the pneumatically driven HeartMate LVAD (Thermo Cardiosystems, Inc) for BTT (the first pump with textured blood-contacting surfaces).

1996—REMATCH (Randomized Evaluation of Mechanical Assistance for the Treatment of Congestive Heart failure, E. Rose principal investigator) trial initiated with HeartMate VE (Thoratec Corp). Results published in 2002 showed mortality reduction of 50% at 1 year as compared to patients receiving optimal medical therapy.

(continued)

TABLE 1–3. Historical Timeline of the Key Events in the Development of Mechanical Circulatory Support (continued)

1998–Simultaneous FDA approval of HeartMate VE (Thermo Cardiosystems) and Novacor LVAS (Baxter Healthcare Corp.), electrically powered, wearable assist systems for BTT, utilized in more than 4000 procedures to date.

1998–First clinical implant of miniaturized axial flow ventricular assist device (MicroMed DeBakey VAD) by R. Hetzer, G. Noon, and M. DeBakey.

1999–First clinical application of a fully implantable circulatory support system. LionHeart LVAS implanted into 67-year-old man recipient by R. Koerfer and W. Pae.

2001–The AbioCor totally implantable, electrically powered TAH is implanted into patient Robert Tools by L. Gray and R. Dowling (clinical trial is ongoing.).

2002–FDA approval of the HeartMate VE LVAD for permanent use (Thoratec Corp.).

2005–B. Griffith implants the first third-generation centrifugal flow device (VentrAssist) at the University of Maryland.

2009–The HeartMate II DT pivotal clinical trial (a prospective, randomized evaluation of the HeartMate II left ventricular assist system [LVAS] randomized against the HeartMate® XVE LVAS [control group] on a 2-1 basis) establishes the superiority of second-generation assist device technology.

2011–O.H. Frazier implants dual HeartMate II axial flow pumps as a TAH after excising ventricles.

Modified and used with permission from http://echo.gmu.edu/bionics/exhibits.htm. (Copyright American Society for Artificial Internal Organs [ASAIO].)

development of this program clearly impacted on the rapid improvements that occurred in device technology during the late 1960s. By 1972 totally implantable LVAD programs were initiated, with a reduction in device failure and thromboembolic events and an increase in animal survival. In 1971, US president Richard Nixon and the Russian general secretary agreed that both countries should join together for a peaceful joint high-technology project which would be beneficial to all mankind. They selected the artificial heart program as the project. Thus, the US-USSR Joint Artificial Heart Program was initiated and the first such joint program was held in Houston, Texas, in 1972. Assembly locations for key individuals involved in the artificial heart development program to exchange information on the progress of artificial heart technology were alternated between Moscow and Houston (Fig. 1–9).

Encouraged by the expanded support of the NHLBI, clinically applicable TAHs were attempted for development at four institutions in the United States.[9] In 1969, Denton Cooley (at the Texas Heart Institute) performed the first human TAH implantation, which was used as a bridge to cardiac transplantation. The patient was 47-year-old man with end-stage ischemic cardiomyopathy and left ventricular aneurysm and underwent surgery. The surgery was complicated by failure to wean from a cardiopulmonary bypass. He underwent heart transplant after

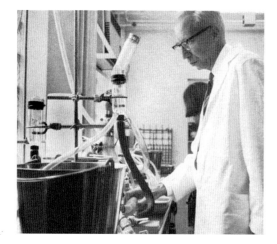

FIGURE 1–5. WJ Kolff squeezing a silastic artificial heart in a mock circuit. (Reproduced with permission from [ICMT] International Center for Medical Technologies.)

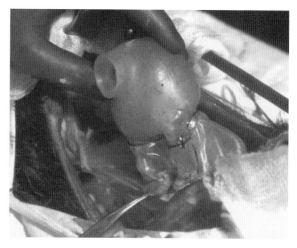

FIGURE 1–6. The first animal implantation of a total artificial heart by W.J. Kolff and T. Akutsu in 1957. (Reproduced with permission from International Center for Medical Technologies [ICMT].)

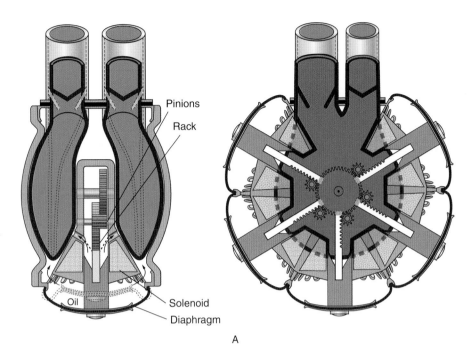

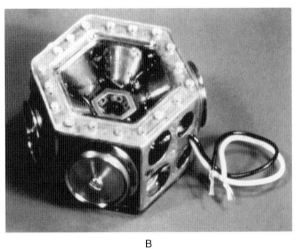

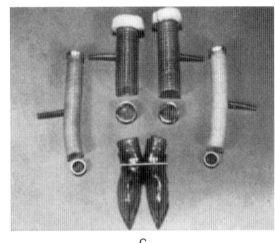

B   C

FIGURE 1–7. **A.** Cross-sectional view of the Kolff solenoid driven TAH. Current in the solenoid pushes diaphragm inward. Pressure transferred by hydraulic fluid forces ventricle sacs to contract and expel blood through tubes at the top. Five solenoids pistons. (Reproduced with permission from International Center for Medical Technologies [ICMT].) **B.** Driving mechanism of the pump which Harry Norton of TRW fabricated. (Reproduced with permission from International Center for Medical Technologies [ICMT].) **C.** The polymer pump components. These parts are made of polyurethane. Two ventricles are located in the same housing. Connecting vessels are corrugated. The valves are of the tricuspid, semilunar type. (Reproduced with permission from International Center for Medical Technologies [ICMT].)

64 hours of support from a pneumatic TAH, manufactured by D. Liotta (Fig. 1–10). Unfortunately, the patient subsequently died of sepsis.

The first permanent implantation of a TAH occurred in 1982 by William DeVries (Fig. 1–11). The Jarvik-7 TAH (Fig. 1–12) was fabricated by Kolff Medical (later Symbion)[10] and was implanted as a permanent device into five patients who were rejected for cardiac transplant between 1982 and 1985. One of these patients survived for 620 days. However, a high incidence of complications, including infection, stroke, and hemorrhage,

combined with a low quality of life for recipients occurred, and the clinical experiment was terminated for permanent use. Since the FDA suspended the production and sale of the Jarvik-7 TAH, CardioWest, Inc, acquired the device in 1992, and the first implant was performed in 1993 as a BTT. The CardioWest TAH is a pneumatically driven, biventricular, pulsatile pump that is implanted in the orthotopic position (Fig. 1–13).[11,12] TAH for permanent therapy has continued to evolve (Fig. 1–14), most recently in 2001 with the implantation of the AbioCor Implantable Replacement Heart by Gray and Dowling in patient

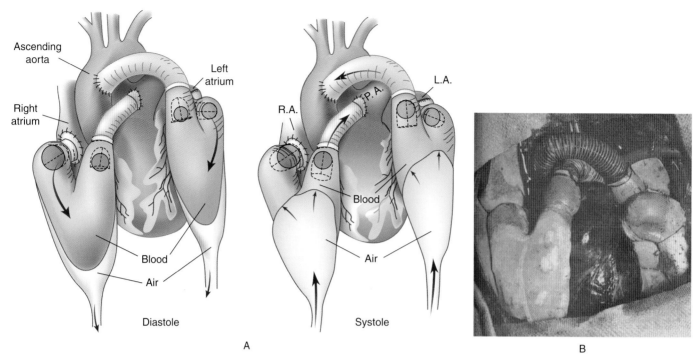

FIGURE 1–8. A. Biventricular bypass artificial heart developed by Houston group headed by Michael E. DeBakey. The right pump was implanted between the right atrium and the pulmonary artery. The left pump was implanted between the left atrium and the ascending aorta. Two pumps are shown in diastole (left) and systole (right). (Reproduced with permission from International Center for Medical Technologies [ICMT].) **B.** Two silastic pneumatic sac hearts are implanted in an experimental animal in the right and the left heart bypass fashion. (Reproduced with permission from [ICMT] International Center for Medical Technologies [ICMT].)

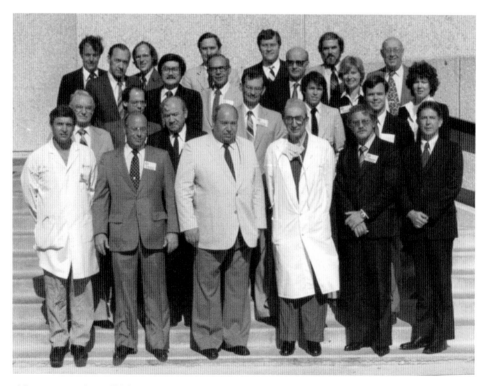

FIGURE 1–9. Members of the US-USSR Joint Artificial Heart Program in 1979. John T. Watson (far right, bottom row). Michael E. DeBakey (third from right, bottom), Valerij I. Shumakov (fourth from right, bottom row), George P. Noon (the far left, bottom row), Robert Jarvik (third from right, second row), William S. Pierce (fourth from right, second row), Donald B. Olsen (third from right, third row), William Hall (fourth from right, third row), Yukihiko Nosé (fifth from right, third row), Peer M. Porter (second from right, top), Frank Altieri (third from right, top). (Reproduced with permission from International Center for Medical Technologies [ICMT].)

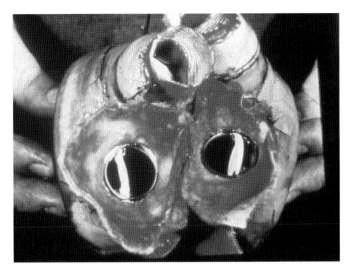

FIGURE 1–10. The first implanted TAH for human. This system was fabricated by D Liotta. (Reproduced with permission from International Center for Medical Technologies [ICMT].)

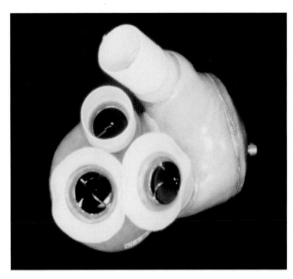

FIGURE 1–12. Jarvik-7 total artificial heart. (Reproduced with permission from International Center for Medical Technologies [ICMT].)

Robert Tools. This device represents the world's first completely self-contained, totally implantable replacement heart.

CONCLUSION

Mechanical circulatory support has made impressive strides as a field since a frustrated Representative John Fogarty exclaimed "We are spending millions of dollars in space and trying to get a man on the moon, and on foreign aid. Here we are losing a million people who are dying every year because of some form of heart disease, and we quibble at trying to get a few million dollars to get going on this project" in 1964. Certainly the

persistence of the early pioneers and the investment of dollars in research funding have paid off with thousands of patients currently having been supported on some type of device. However, the challenges of infection, thromboembolic complications, and

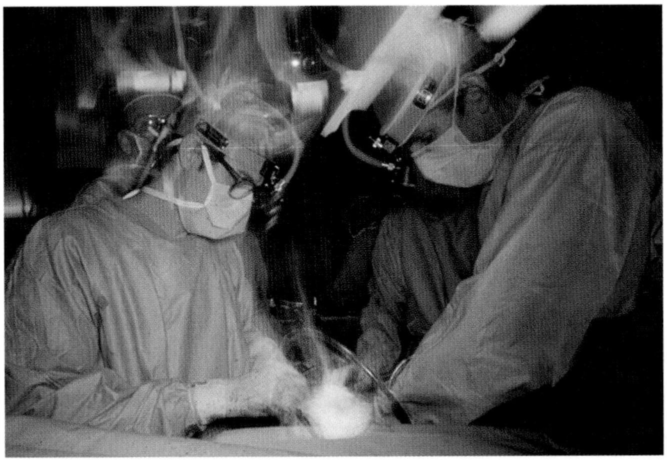

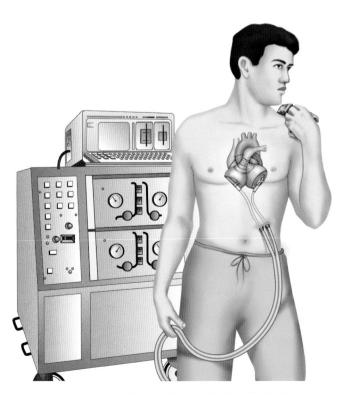

FIGURE 1–13. Schematic drawing of the CardioWest TAH inside a patient and its connection to the pneumatic actuator. (Reproduced with permission from International Center for Medical Technologies [ICMT].)

FIGURE 1–11. W DeVries (right) with L Joyce (left) during the first TAH implantation. (Reproduced with permission from the University of Utah.)

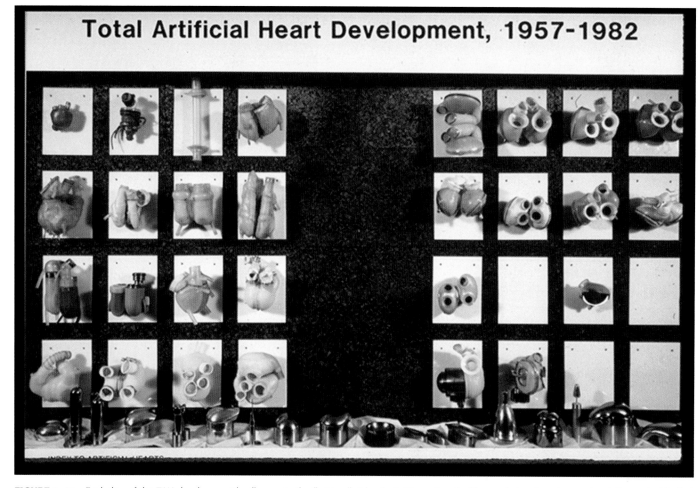

FIGURE 1–14. Evolution of the TAH development leading up to the first Jarvik-7 implant. (Reproduced with permission from International Center for Medical Technologies [ICMT].)

device malfunction remain limitations that the next generation of heart failure specialists will have to confront in bringing this technology to the 5 million Americans who continue to suffer from end-stage heart disease.

REFERENCES

1. Liotta D, Crawford ES, Cooley DA, Debakey ME, De Urquia M, Feldman L. Prolonged partial left ventricular bypass by means of an intrathoracic pump implanted in the left chest. *Trans Am Soc Artif Intern Organs.* 1962;8:90-99.
2. Liotta D, Hall CW, Cooley DA, De Bakey ME. Prolonged ventricular bypass with intrathoracic pumps. *Trans Am Soc Artif Intern Organs.* 1964;10:154-156.
3. DeBakey ME. Left ventricular bypass pump for cardiac assistance. Clinical experience. *Am J Cardiol.* 1971 Jan;27(1):3-11.
4. Kantrowitz A, Kantrowitz A. Experimental augmentation of coronary flow by retardation of the arterial pressure pulse. *Surgery.* 1953;34:678. (Initially presented at the Surgical Forum, American College of Surgeons, New York, Sep 1952. This paper showed the physiological basis for development of intra-aortic balloon counterpulsation in the 1960s.)
5. Kantrowitz A, McKinnon WMP. The experimental use of the diaphragm as an auxiliary myocardium. *Surg Forum.* 1958;9:226.
6. Graedel F, Akutsu T, Chaptal PA, Kantrowitz A. Successful hemodynamic results with a new, U-shaped auxiliary ventricle. *Trans Am Soc Artif Intern Organs.* 1965;11:277-283.
7. Dorman F, Bernstein EF, Blackshear PL, Sovilj R, Scott DR. Progress in the design of a centrifugal cardiac assist pump with trans-cutaneous energy transmission by magnetic coupling. *Trans Am Soc Artif Intern Organs.* 1969;15:441-448.
8. Kolff WJ, Akutsu T, Dreyer B, Norton S. Artificial hearts inside the chest, and use of polyurethane for making hearts, valves and aorta. *Trans Am Soc Artif Intern Organs.* 1959;5:298-303.
9. DeBakey ME, Hall CW, Hellums JD, et al. Orthotopic cardiac prosthesis: preliminary experiments in animals with biventricular artificial heart. *Cardiovasc Res Cent Bull.* 1969 Apr-Jun;7(4):127-142.
10. Mochizuki T, Lawson JH, Olsen DB, et al. A seven-month survival of a calf with an artificial heart designed for human use. *Artif Organs.* 1981 May;5(2):125-131.
11. Jarvik RK, DeVries WC, Semb BK, et al. Surgical positioning of the Jarvik-7 artificial heart. *J Heart Transplant.* 1986 May-Jun;5(3):184-195.
12. Copeland JG, Arabia FA, Tsau PH, et al. Total artificial hearts: bridge to transplantation. *Cardiol Clin.* 2003 Feb;21(1):101-113.

CHAPTER 2

ENGINEERING ELEMENTS OF VAD CONSTRUCTION

Don B. Olsen, Bryan E. Lynch, and Ronald W. Kipp

INTRODUCTION

In order to successfully manufacture an intricate and complex device, such as a left ventricular assist device (LVAD), multiple engineering disciplines (fluidics, magnetics, electromechanical, electronics, and software) must be employed. In addition to each of these individual engineering specialties, which normally work within the isolation of their respective fields, the overall governing design must fit within the bounds and directives of the medical profession. In other words, the form must precisely follow its function.

However, to successfully produce any device, it must be designed so that it can be manufactured. It is the purpose and direction of this remaining task to ensure that the design incorporates the requirements of the medical application, the requirements of the engineering disciplines, and last, but certainly not least, that the total package can be manufactured and assembled into the desired form while being on time and within budget. Precise engineering design and the time and cost to produce that component are usually at loggerheads with each other since the design tolerances are indirectly proportional to their cost; that is, the tighter the tolerance, the greater the cost of the part. Design to manufacture any device, be it either a prototype or production units, must also take into account all of the component and material specifications to ensure that all of the pieces of the puzzle will fit together as a completed functional assembly.

Prudence also dictates that a device as intricate, complicated, and, indeed, as lifesaving as the LVAD requires multiple pieces of engineering software to both design and software test before any product is actually manufactured. In addition to the initial software testing phase of the program, each of the engineering disciplines must be capable of exporting their designs into the next phases of the programs cycles, that is, proof of concept, prototype design(s), prototype build(s), prototype test(s), analysis of the prototype(s) performance data, refinement of the final design, the build final design, the test final design, and produce manufacturing quantities of the LVAD. This chapter reviews the basic principles of manufacturing and describes how these principles are applied toward the construction of an axial-flow LVAD.

BASIC PRINCIPLES OF MANUFACTURING

The manufacturing process required for a ventricular assist device (VAD) could be compared to the construction of a fine piece of jewelry or any complex instrument to be used in small quantities, such as a navigation gyroscope or Hasselblad camera. Even if the demand for VAD technology never exceeds 20,000 or 30,000 devices per year, the need for perfection in manufacturing is a mandatory requirement for this sector. The only way to systematically approach this need for perfection and satisfy the regulatory hurdles of the modern era is to adopt a quality system from the outset of the program. A quality system in its most generic form will ensure that the products manufactured will meet specification and perform as designed every time they are released from production. What happens between receiving raw materials in the backdoor and releasing them from production will depend on how well a quality system matches the manufacturing process, design goals, and financial constraints.

A VAD company's quality system also needs to match the development stage of the device being built. In the prototype stage, a good quality system may be no more than a documentation system used to track and monitor the results of manufacturing as it struggles to constantly modify the product and processes to adapt to the changing needs of the design group. Every VAD developer will proceed in starts and stops as their design is tested, modified, and retested during bench-top and early animal trials. The quality and manufacturing teams must work closely together to accommodate these changes as quickly as possible. It is no mere cliché that *time is money* in this business, so the whole team working together must move quickly and deliberately to modify and improve a product toward the ultimate goal during this stage.

Once a VAD moves into the more advanced stages of human trials, the major design of the implantable device should be complete, but continued experience with the trial will uncover deficiencies both in components and manufacturing processes that must be addressed immediately. A well-established quality system will allow these mid-course corrections to occur with minimal disruption of the manufacturing process. Typically, the gating item for any design modification will come from the regulatory group as it moves its submissions through the governing process.

Many devices have failed simply because necessary changes could not be implemented and tested quickly enough to satisfy a schedule dictated by the corporate burn rate. It is also true that many companies fail because they fail to settle their design quickly enough. It is up to a strong management team to determine when the development is acceptable for certain components, when development must continue for others, and when a design must be revisited for modification. Every device will likely be in some state of design flux during its life cycle, underscoring a flexible, team-oriented quality and manufacturing process.

The design of the device must satisfy the broad physiologic needs of the patient; it must also be *manufacturable*. In fact, the manufacturability of a VAD could prove to be one of the single most difficult aspects of the project. Like any new manufacturing project, building the first one or two or even a dozen *perfect* devices may not be difficult because these first few devices benefit from an unusual and likely unsustainable amount of time and attention. It is not until the typical manufacturing pressures of material cost, labor costs, time, design changes and improvements, and manufacturing improvements come to bear that the true challenge of manufacturing a VAD starts to become apparent.

The basics of building elements of a VAD are not unlike building large quantities of any product; the engineering has to be excellent before the manufacturing will be excellent. The components must be designed so they will fit together without *adjustment*. The tolerance stack-ups must be managed so that the skill required to assemble a device will be minimized. Processes must be developed, documented, and made easily repeatable.

A VAD requires developing a manufacturing plan that will include a complete description of how to manufacture the device, step by step, including requirements for the facility, machines, and tools required. The manufacturing plan will grow to become a series of detailed work instructions that are tracked by work-order travelers for each subassembly that constitutes the device. These work instructions represent some of the most important documents in the company because they contain all the information defining how the product is actually built. They should contain all the production knowledge, including the *tribal knowledge* that invariably becomes a part of any device.

The fabrication technology available to build a VAD today is spectacular. Like any precision device, precision machines and computer-aided design (CAD) work together to ensure an accurate, replicable process. The computational fluid dynamics (CFD) available today will typically dictate the shape of all blood-contacting surfaces. These surfaces will be critical to gently adding energy to the blood through pumping so that it can flow throughout the body. The reliable and reproducible translation from a CFD model in the computer to a solid three-dimensional (3D) metal impeller or diffuser component is imperative in developing and manufacturing a VAD. Once the design phase has produced a viable impeller design, the shape of the impeller is typically defined by a set of parametric equations that describe the shape of a blade or fin. These parametric equations are used by 3D CAD software to generate surfaces so a solid component definition results. This solid component, in this case an impeller, would be impossible to make without a numerically controlled multiaxis mill to take the codes generated by the CAD software and guide a cutting tool along a path that will remove metal from a rod, leaving only the complex shapes of the blades for complete computer-aided manufacturing (CAM). In most cases, the completed component will have such a complex shape that measurements to validate the dimensions are impossible to obtain. There are light and laser methods available to validate a machined part, but after validation, a reproducible system matched with a few key dimensions will ensure consistency in fabricating that part.

MANUFACTURING THE MAGNETICALLY SUSPENDED IMPELLER AXIAL LEFT VENTRICULAR ASSIST DEVICE

■ BACKGROUND

Fluidic Components

The axial-flow LVAD consists of three major fluidic components or regions within the device: the inducer, the impeller, and the diffuser (Fig. 2–1). The purpose of the inducer is to induce a laminar flow of blood into the impeller region of the LVAD. The rotating impeller region, under the control of built-in software within the physiologic controller, will automatically adjust the pressure and blood flow rate required by the LVAD recipient. The diffuser region of the LVAD receives the blood from exit tips of the rotating impeller blades and creates a laminar flow output from the pump. The shapes for these three critical components are very intricate, and by definition they also have to be very precise. In addition to the critical dimensions and tolerances for each of these fluidic components, these components must be manufactured to ensure adequate hemostasis, given that these surfaces come into contact with the bloodstream. These bloodstream-contacting surfaces need to be highly polished to ensure that clots do not form, and that hemolysis is not induced on the LVAD surfaces. All of the above-mentioned design parameters force the LVAD's fluidic components into the realm of precision and high tolerance manufacturing, and given the shape and form of these parts, several unique manufacturing and *proof of concept* methods are employed.

Magnetic Suspension and Electromechanical Components

The suspension system for the LVADs impeller employs a combination of permanent and temporary electromagnets to radially and axially levitate the impeller; therefore, the impeller floats within a magnetic field. The magnetic portions of the LVAD consist of rotor components that are embedded within the impeller structure, and the stator components that are

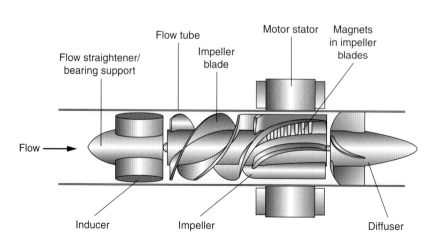

FIGURE 2–1. Diagram of the MicroMed DeBakey VAD, illustrating the three major fluidic components of an axial-flow device. (Reproduced with permission from DeBakey ME.[1] Copyright © Elsevier.)

placed within the housing. The shielding of the stator magnetic components from the blood pathway is accomplished by placing a titanium barrier, or can, in between the stator and rotor components. The stator barrier can take the form of a very thin-walled (0.012 in radial) can, or it can be integrated into the form of one of the fluidic components. In this regard, the region that we refer to as the inducer is in reality the inducer/active magnetic bearing (AMB) region, where the structure of the fluidic inducer houses the AMB stator components.

The magnetically levitated impeller provides two very important characteristics for the LVAD. (1) Rotational losses due to bearing friction are, by definition, eliminated. (2) The design of radial and axial magnetic bearings provides for a clean and unimpeded single blood flow pathway, and therefore, the possibility of trapping and damaging blood cells within these structures is completely eliminated. The components for the magnetic suspension system require high-precision manufacturing of the rare-earth permanent magnet bearings (PMBs) and the active electromechanical components of the AMB suspension system. Also included within the precision manufacturing scope are the electromechanical and magnetic components of the motor stator and the permanent magnet and active magnetic rotor assemblies that are embedded within the impeller.

Electronics and Control Software

The electronics portion of the LVAD is divided into three separate component parts that synergistically work together to control the functionality of the LVAD. The position of the impeller (radial and axial) is monitored by two Hall effect (HE) sensor arrays that are mounted at each end within the housing. The positional information obtained by these HE arrays is used by the external AMB controller to adjust the coil currents within the AMB to radially move and align the impeller into its desired position. The axial (thrust) position of the impeller is governed by the passive PMB stator and rotor magnet assemblies, and since this magnetic bearing is not externally controllable; that is, it is passive, the axial position of the impeller is provided to the physiologic controller as dynamic information. The delivered pressure and volume of blood is governed by the motor speed. The physiologic controller software will adjust this parameter via the motor controller hardware, which is external to the LVAD.

Engineering and Design Software

One of the last, but not least, of the engineering disciplines that must be brought to task, to successfully engineer, manufacture, and produce a working LVAD, is the software. The LVAD software can be divided into two classifications: (1) operational software that is burned into the microprocessor(s) for the physiologic, AMB, and motor controllers (which is outside the hardware scope of this writing); and (2) engineering and design software are key tools that must be utilized for any project of this magnitude and complexity.

The design and engineering for the LVAD, as pertains to item 2 can be broken down into four major groups: fluidics, magnetics, electromechanical, and electronics, wherein each of these engineering specialties has their own software programs that must produce reasonable and reliable results. The one overlying parameter that is paramount to any complex 3D design, such as the LVAD, is that these individual programs must be capable of exporting or integrating their designs to the next phase of the engineering design. Exporting could be, in its simplest terms, a 2D-part drawing. However, the intricate design and complex structures of the fluidic components within the LVAD require a precision and machining flexibility that only extremely close tolerance CAM machines can produce. An example of the CFD used to mathematically predict fluid flow through the HeartMate II device is shown in Fig. 2–2.

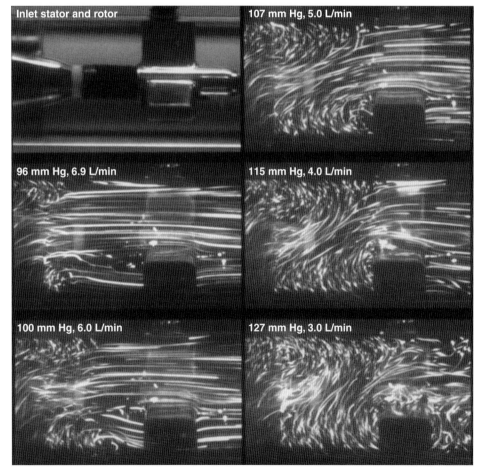

FIGURE 2–2. Flow visualization study of HeartMate II; area of inlet stator and rotor are seen with various pressure-flow conditions. Note variation in flow pattern. The microvortices predicted by CFD were not apparent. (Reproduced with permission from Griffith BP.[2] Copyright © Elsevier.)

Unfortunately, the fluidic design and analytical software, which is referred to as computer-aided engineering (CAE), does not typically produce an output that can be directly imported into CAM machines. In this case, as well as in other CAE programs that are cited herein, another engineering tool has to be brought to bear. As previously mentioned, this software tool is called CAD. There are many different and well-known variations of CAD programs that run from a simplistic drafting and drawing aid such as 2D AutoCAD, to the very powerful and robust 3D CAD programs. An example of such a robust 3D CAD program is called SolidWorks. SolidWorks cannot only handle importation of complex 3D solid shapes; it can also produce 3D CAM files that can be exported into the machines that will eventually manufacture the parts. Additionally, SolidWorks can produce 3D assemblies that show exactly how a complex device can and will be assembled, *without actually ever assembling one piece of physical hardware*. The other engineering software programs, magnetics, electromechanical, and electronics, all have the same design problem in that they require an overall CAD program to seamlessly integrate their component parts and assemblies into one unified structure. The parts for the LVAD were engineered by other programs; software *built and assembled*, and then exported as drawing and/or CAM files using SolidWorks.

The final piece of the engineering software that was utilized on this program is called finite element analysis (FEA). The basic premise behind this powerful engineering tool is that the whole is equal to the sum of the parts. Therefore, the way to characterize and understand a complex engineering problem is to break down the problem into small, defined, *elemental* pieces, which are then *reassembled* into interacting elements whose characteristics are governed and determined by the elements' material and the environmental conditions surrounding those elements. Assuming that all of the other modeling parameters (material characteristics, geometry, environmental conditions) are established, then the element size, or how detailed the model is resolved, will determine the resolution of the FEA results. If the element size were infinitely small, the model would be infinitely resolved. However, an infinitely small element infers an infinite number of elements, and therefore a *finite*, or specified number, of elements is used to obtain reasonably accurate results.

The definition of accuracy, or resolution refinement, depends on the need and requirements of the results. A first-run analysis may only be used to determine the validity of the model, and whether or not the results *ballpark* the engineered predictions. Subsequent FEA runs would then be taken to much higher levels of validity, where the accuracy would be determined by the number of elements or *nodes* that are solved, and the computer time allowed for the run. A second or third pass for a small FEA model could involve 30,000 or greater nodes and hours of computer time. Today, the power of the personal computer has allowed these calculations to be done on the desktop. However, not that long ago FEA was delegated only to the realm of supercomputers, where minutes of computer time equated to tens of thousands of dollars. Well-known FEA programs typically solve material questions about physical properties that are sometimes intuitively apparent to a skilled engineer.

However, magnetic material properties and their interaction is one of those engineering quirks where intuition and empirical data are more than likely to run amok. A program that helps magnetic engineers understand these counterintuitive issues is magnetic finite element analysis (MFEA). MFEA was used very extensively to check the static and dynamic performance of all of the magnetic components, as well as to determine the interaction between the magnetic and nonmagnetic components of the LVAD.

■ PROOF OF CONCEPT MODELS

Fluidic Components

In order to prove the design concepts that were incorporated into the LVAD, two basic engineering structures were first built and tested. The first proof-of-concept design was the fluidic portions of the LVAD (inducer, impeller, diffuser), and this was accomplished by building a solid model of these component parts. This simplistic fluidic model did not contain any of the other LVAD operational parts; that is, the magnetic bearings and internal motor components were excluded. In order to rotate the impeller within the housing, an external drive was physically attached to the rear portion of the impeller, and as such, the moniker that was attached to this structure was the *Pump on a Stick* (Fig. 2–3).

As mentioned previously, the fluidic portions of the LVAD are precise, extremely complex, and very challenging to successfully manufacture. However, from a proof-of-concept viewpoint, we only needed a method of testing and proving the performance of these pumping components. The method we chose to accomplish this task is referred to as *rapid prototyping*, which, as the name implies, allows the model to be produced relatively quickly and inexpensively before actually building and assembling the real component structures.

Rapid prototyping incorporates two state-of-the-art technologies: CAD design software and CAM machines that produce

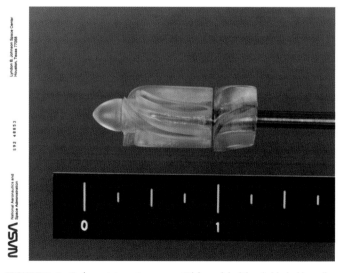

FIGURE 2–3. Early prototype *Pump on a Stick* model of the six-bladed impeller and diffuser for the MicroMed DeBakey VAD. (Courtesy of micromedcv.com.)

the desired parts. Rapid prototype manufacturing machines are devices that build parts one axial layer at a time; that is, these machines can be thought of as ink-jet printers that *stack* layer upon layer of material to realize the desired 3D form. In actuality, these devices use a precisely guided laser and a bath of heat-activated epoxy to produce their parts.

There are two rapid prototyping issues that need to be presented. The first deals with the structure of these parts, and the second deals with the material characteristics: (1) Building a part layer by layer produces a step or striated part. These steps give the part *rough* inconsistent surfaces that could be damaging to the blood cells. (2) Pumping a liquid of similar density would prove the LVAD fluidic concepts, while avoiding actual blood products. Selection of both the pumping fluid and the rapid prototyping materials was accomplished in conjunction with these respective industries.

Magnetic and Electromechanical

The second proof-of-concept model that was manufactured and tested was the magnetic and electromechanical portions of the pump. This rig was referred to as the magnetic bearing test rig. However, the name is a little misleading, since it also incorporates the motor rotor and stator portions of the LVAD. The technology that was used to manufacture these parts brings to bear several different state-of-the-art technologies: (1) the PMB and the motor rotor subassemblies, which both require *exotic* rare earth magnets to be manufactured to very tight mechanical and magnetic material tolerances; and (2) the electromechanical AMB and the motor stator components, which also require very tight mechanical tolerances and high-quality magnetic materials.

Magnetic Components

Specifications and drawings for the magnetic components and assemblies were supplied directly to magnetic manufactures. The manufacturing techniques for these parts are beyond the scope of this writing since they involve many internal company proprietary processes. However, the basic processes that are used to create permanent magnetic devices entail the forming of powdered magnetic materials, such as nickel, iron, and boron (NiFeB), into the proper form (shape), and then firing the powder to form a ceramic. Postprocessing of the ceramic then entails grinding the rough shape into its specified dimensions and then magnetizing this material to its desired parameters. Magnetic assemblies are then created by bonding the magnetic parts into a composite. The PMB and the motor rotor for the LVAD are created using this, or a similar, technique.

Electromechanical Components

Laminated Silicone Iron Blocks The six-pole motor stator and the AMB stator and rotor components are manufactured using the following technique. Thin (0.005 in) sheet metal of high-quality magnetic material (silicone iron [SiFe]) provides the material platform for these parts. The SiFe material is first cut into a convenient form (strips) that will allow enough surface area for the parts being produced. These strips are then heated in a time-controlled oven to a temperature, which will magnetically anneal them. This magnetic annealing process does two things simultaneously: (1) it induces the desired magnetic properties into the material; and (2) it physically stress-relieves the strips. After the annealing process, the strips are then stacked and bonded together into a laminate block that will be further processed in the next step which is called wire electric discharge machining (EDM).

EDM Techniques The process of EDM involves the burning away of an electrically conductive material through the use of a precision-guided electrode. There are two forms of EDM. One uses a solid electrode whose form is the negative or the inversion of the desired part, and this type of EDM is referred to as the plunge, classic, or just plain EDM technique. The electrode materials that are generally used for this plunge EDM process consist of either a solid high-quality carbon composites or solid copper. The burning or erosion of the unwanted material takes place within a nonconductive liquid coolant bath, such as deionized water, which prevents the part's material from warping and becoming *work* stressed.

The forms and shapes that can be created with a properly designed and executed plunge EDM technique are as varied and complex as anything that can be imagined; that is, a state-of-the-art EDM machine can operate in X, Y, and Z planes, and also include rotation about the Z axis. However, there is a drawback to this machine, in that the plunging electrodes will deteriorate during use, and they have to be periodically replaced. Obviously, the more material that is burned away during this EDM process requires more of the electrode to also be eroded and the more time that will be spent on the machine. Multiple electrodes (rough, medium, and finish surface) are generally used during this process, and, given the shape and complexities of any given part, there could easily be multiple electrodes being used to form separate portions of the part structure.

A subset of the plunge EDM technique is called wire EDM, and, as the name implies, a wire is used for the electrode. The wire EDM process uses a very long (10,000 ft), one pass and then discarded wire to cut 2D (X and Y) shapes from a solid piece of material. The other restraint placed on a wire EDM part is that only the straight line (Z axis) shapes can be created.

As mentioned in the opening paragraph of this section, laminated SiFe blocks are the basis for the AMB and motor stator components. The laminated SiFe stacks or blocks are placed into a wire EDM machine to have their proper forms extracted. These forms are prescribed by the engineering and CAD software, and they are supplied to the wire machine as CAM software and engineering drawings.

■ PROTOTYPE LVAD COMPONENTS

The prototype LVAD components are a hybrid composition of rapid prototyped fluidic components, the magnetic and electromechanical parts, and an assortment of classically machined parts (Fig. 2–4). The purposes of this device are to prove by testing the operational capabilities of the combined technologies and to discover any operational anomalies. This device is for laboratory testing only. The major difference between the rapid

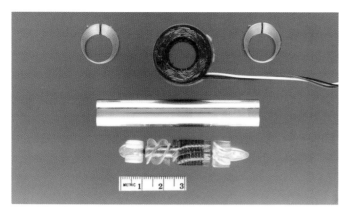

FIGURE 2–4. MicroMed DeBakey VAD prototype with magnets embedded in the impeller blades and a three-bladed inducer in front of the impeller. The flow tube, clamps, and circular motor stator are also displayed. (Courtesy of micromedcv.com.)

prototype (plastic) parts that were constructed for the prototype *Pump on a Stick* and the parts manufactured for this phase of the program is that the former parts were solid and monolithic, whereas the new parts that were created represented hollowed-out entities or inserts. The hollows within the parts were then filled with the magnetic, electromagnetic components, or the insert, such as the diffuser, became a part of the housing structure, and wherever possible the final (titanium) assembly component parts were used. This is the interim phase of the manufacturing program, where all of the component parts will be assembled and tested as a system for fluidic, electrical, electronic, and software performance and interaction.

■ FINISHED LVAD COMPONENTS

The major difference between the prototype and finished component is the replacement of the plastic fluidic pieces with their titanium counterparts. A brief synopsis of the most relevant techniques is discussed below as a primer into how to build the critical titanium components (impeller and diffuser) within the LVAD. The inducer, which is also a critical fluidic component, can be realized by using a straightforward machining approach.

Machining the Impeller and Diffuser

One of the obvious techniques to manufacture the impeller and diffuser components is to have them machined by a 3D precision CAM-driven milling machine. However, there are three major machining problems that can't be overcome using this technology. (1) The tight twist of impeller blades at its front will not allow even the smallest of cutting tools to be inserted into this space. (2) The internal blades of the diffuser are even more problematic than the impeller to machine since they consist of internal blades that consist of a helical twist. (3) Even if these parts could be machined (which they could not be), they would have to be hand-polished to a finish of 10 μm or better.

Investment Casting or the Lost-Wax Method

The second approach uses old technology with a new technology twist. Investment casting, or the lost-wax method, involves using

a precise (*positive*) representation in wax of the object that you want to cast as the starting point. A mold base is created by surrounding this positive wax object with a liquid-like material that eventually solidifies into a hardened outer object that will create a *negative* of the starting object. The final step is to then pour into this mold a hot liquid metal that will melt, evaporate, and replace the wax, and if everything is done correctly, the results will yield a metal object that is the exact duplicate (*positive*) of the starting object. This technique has come down to us over the ages as an artists' tool for replicating sculptures, and it does have merit in many technical applications. However, there are several shortcomings to this technique that cannot be overlooked. (1) A precise wax representation of the object must be created for each and every object to be cast. (2) Thin-walled intricate structures are problematic. (3) Surface finishes can be nonuniform. (4) The mold bases are destroyed in order to remove the cast object. Despite all of these shortcomings, this approach to creating the impeller and diffuser castings has merit.

Investment Casting

The wax impellers and diffusers that started the lost wax process are created on a unique rapid prototyping machine that is very similar in concept to the rapid prototyping machine that created the plastic parts discussed previously. The difference between the two rapid prototyping methods is that instead of using a laser to solidify a bath of heat-activated epoxy, the rapid prototyping wax machine puts down layer upon layer of wax, in a fashion similar to an ink-jet printer that creates solid objects of the desired shape. Like the plastic parts, this creates a stepped wax solid which in turn will then create a stepped metallic surface. Indeed, when inspecting the surfaces of the cast parts made with this process, a stepped pattern is readily visible. However, the random surface discontinuities within these parts cannot be attributed to the steps within the wax structure alone.

One way to avoid the stepped wax pattern is to make a precision and polishe mold that will create the wax objects in a clean, step-free manner. The problem with this technique is that the "investment" portion of this name has correctly identified one of its issues, in that the cost for precision molds of this caliber requires a lot of machine and hand polishing time. Obviously for a prototype application, the rapid prototype response represents the correct application of this technology. However, in the long run investment casting may prove its worth both in dollars and time.

Motor and Stator AMB Coils

The motor and AMB stator coils provide the driving force to respectively rotate and radially position the impeller. The coils are wound on precision mandrels that provide the correct form for assembly and insertion into the component parts of the LVAD. Great care is taken to ensure that coil precision and uniformity of form were maintained.

Internal and External Electronics

The internal electronics for the LVAD consist of two HE arrays that provide radial location information about the impeller.

The two HE arrays are axially offset from each other so that they provide axial location information about the impeller. The HE arrays consist of four HE devices geometrically arranged in a 90-degree pattern about the centerline of the LVAD, and they are located on a precision printed circuit board (PCB). The PCB is mounted into a precision nylon holder that aligns and electrically isolates the HE devices. The wiring to and from the HE arrays is passed through the LVAD housing and connected to the external electronics. The external electronics consist of multiple hardware devices that provide sensing derivation from the raw HE data, driving voltages and currents for the motor and AMB stators as well as the physical location for the microprocessors that run the physiologic, motor, and AMB software.

CONCLUSION

Manufacturing an implantable, life-supporting product like a VAD is a process that requires a complete understanding of manufacturing, planning, regulatory guidance, machining, fabrication, hiring, teamwork, and financing. Every VAD on the market today started as a series of unique prototypes, built by dedicated individuals with the dream of saving lives and in the process satisfying a market for heart assist devices. Whether positive displacement, centrifugal or axial flow, these devices must be biocompatible, reliable, and producible. The transition from prototype to production can be as challenging as the implementation of animal trials and early human trials.

REFERENCES

1. DeBakey ME. A miniature implantable axial flow ventricular assist device. *Ann Thorac Surg* 1999;68:637-640.
2. Griffith BP. HeartMate II left ventricular assist system: from concept to first clinical use. *Ann Thorac Surg* 2001;71:S116-S120.

CHAPTER 3

REGULATORY ISSUES IN CARDIAC ASSIST DEVICE APPLICATION

Steven J. Phillips and Rachel S. Phillips

INTRODUCTION

From the beginning of civilization people have been concerned about the quality and safety of food, medicine, and devices. In 1202, King John of England proclaimed the first English food law, the Assize of Bread, which prohibited adulteration of bread with ingredients such as ground peas or beans. Regulation of food in the United States dates from early colonial times.

Until the 20th century, drugs and devices were regulated primarily by state and local governments. Drugs and devices "could be bought and sold like any other consumer good."[1] Federal controls over the drug supply began with the inspection of imported drugs in 1848. Table 3–1 describes some of the milestones in the history of food and drug regulation in the United States. The Food and Drug Administration (FDA) began regulating the use of artificial organs in 1976.

Artificial organs have been used to treat chronic illnesses for nearly half a century. The use of the artificial kidney, artificial heart, cardiac pacemaker, artificial hips and knees, cochlear implants, and intraocular lenses offer treatments for a variety of debilitating illnesses. In the field of heart failure, ventricular assist devices (VADs) offer options for the treatment of cardiovascular illnesses that account for the leading cause of death in the United States.

New technology has allowed the development of smaller, lighter, and more dependable devices. This includes new pumping technologies, new power sources, and the combination of mechanical and biological therapies which join the latest in tissue and cellular engineering technologies with the most recent advances in pumping systems. Along with these scientific advances are parallel changes in the regulatory laws.

THE FOOD AND DRUG ADMINSTRATION

The Food and Drug Administration (FDA) is responsible for protecting the public health by ensuring the safety, efficacy, and security of human and veterinary drugs, biological products, medical devices, our nation's food supply, cosmetics, and products that emit radiation. The FDA is also responsible for enhancing public health through education and help to speed innovations that make medicines and devices more effective, more affordable, and safer.

The FDA is a scientific, regulatory, and public health agency that oversees items accounting for 25 cents of every dollar spent by consumers. The FDA was established in 1930 and is a part of the US Department of Health and Human Services (HHS). The agency grew from a single chemist in the US Department of Agriculture in 1862 to a staff of approximately 9000 employees and a budget of $1.3 billion in 2001.

Approximately one-third of the agency's employees are stationed outside of the Washington, DC area in over 150 field offices and laboratories, including 5 regional offices and 20 district offices. Agency scientists evaluate applications for a wide variety of products, including new human and animal drugs and biologics, complex medical devices, food and color additives, and infant formulas. In addition, the FDA annually monitors the manufacturing, importing, transporting, storing, and selling of an estimated $1 trillion worth of products at a cost to taxpayers of about $3 per person. Investigators and inspectors visit more than 16,000 facilities a year and coordinate with state governments in an attempt to increase the number of facilities checked every year.

Table 3–2 lists the FDA divisions.

HISTORY OF DEVICE REGULATION

Until 1938, the Post Office Department and the Federal Trade Commission oversaw cosmetics and medical devices. With the passage of the Federal Food, Drug, and Cosmetic (FD&C) Act in 1938, cosmetics and devices came under FDA authority. While premarket approval (PMA) did not apply to devices as they did for drugs, in every other sense, the 1938 FD&C Act equated devices to drugs for regulatory purposes. This unfortunate analogy of devices as drugs persisted until the FDA Modernization Act (FDAMA) of 1997 acknowledged the distinction between devices and drugs.

Quack products were the subjects of most of the FDAs device regulatory actions until the 1960s. As the FDA had to deal with both increasing medical device quackery and a proliferation of medical technology in the post–World War II years, Congress considered a device law when it passed the 1962 drug amendments. Although the 1962 legislation failed to develop, the secretary of the Department of Health, Education, and Welfare (HEW) commissioned a study group on medical devices, which recommended in 1970 that medical devices be classified according to their comparative risk. Medical devices were then regulated accordingly. The 1976 Medical Device Amendments, a result of a therapeutic disaster in which thousands of women were injured by the Dalkon Shield intrauterine device, provided three classes of medical devices, each requiring a different level of regulatory scrutiny.

◼ FOOD AND DRUG MODERNIZATION ACT OF 1997

The Food and Drug Modernization Act (FDAMA) of 1997 reauthorized the Prescription Drug User Fee Act of 1992 and mandated the most wide-ranging reforms in agency practices since 1938. FDAMA distinguished drugs from devices. FDAMA

TABLE 3–1. Milestones in FDA History

1820: *US Pharmacopeia* established.

1848: *Drug Importation Act* requires US Customs Service inspection to stop entry of adulterated drugs.

1862: *President Lincoln* appoints a chemist, Charles M. Wetherill, to serve in the new Department of Agriculture, the predecessor of the FDA.

1938: *The Federal Food, Drug, and Cosmetic (FD&C) Act* is passed by the Congress.

1940: The *FDA transferred* from the Department of Agriculture to the Federal Security Agency, with Walter G. Campbell appointed as the first commissioner of Food and Drugs.

1968: *Reorganization* of federal health programs places FDA in the Public Health Service.

1976: *Medical Device Amendments* passed to ensure safety and effectiveness of medical devices, including diagnostic products. The amendments require manufacturers to register with FDA and follow quality control procedures. Some products must have premarket approval by FDA; others must meet performance standards before marketing.

1990: The *Safe Medical Devices Act* is passed requiring postmarket surveillance and the reporting of incidents death, serious illness, or serious injury related to a medical device. The act authorizes FDA to order device product recalls and other actions.

1997: The *FDA Modernization Act (FDAMA)* reauthorizes the Prescription Drug User Fee Act of 1992 and mandates the most wide-ranging reforms in agency practices since 1938. Provisions include measures to accelerate review of devices, regulate advertising of unapproved uses of approved drugs and devices, and regulate health claims for foods.

2002: The *Medical Device User Fee and Modernization Act (MDUFMA)* of 2002 amended FDAMA of 1997. MDUFA established user fees for premarket reviews and allowed inspections to be conducted by accredited third parties.

recognized the dynamic process of device development and mandated timely market access for so-called breakthrough devices, including their incremental improvements. FDAMA has been helpful in device development in that it requires the FDA to meet with a device sponsor early in the approval cycle to identify from the start the scientific evidence needed to prove effectiveness.

Other significant portions of the 1997 Modernization Act included the streamlining of the review process for less risky devices and the elimination of low-risk devices from review altogether. FDAMA accelerated the review of devices by exempting certain devices from premarket notification requirements. With FDAMA manufacturers could rely on FDA-recognized performance standards to fulfill 510(k) review requirements.

TABLE 3–2. FDA, an Agency Within the Department of Health and Human Services, Consists of Eight Centers and Offices

Center for Biologics Evaluation and Research (CBER)

Center for Devices and Radiological Health (CDRH)

Center for Drug Evaluation and Research (CDER)

Center for Food Safety and Applied Nutrition (CFSAN)

Center for Veterinary Medicine (CVM)

National Center for Toxicological Research (NCTR)

Office of the Commissioner (OC)

Office of Regulatory Affairs (ORA)

FDAMA authorized third-party reviews, which allowed the FDA to use expert panels in the drug approval process and, more recently, in the device approval process. FDAMA required the FDA to consider the least burdensome means to prove device effectiveness. This is a giant step from the mindset of the past when the FDA sought absolute assurance of a device's effectiveness. The provisions of FDAMA, and others not discussed here, have brought timeliness, predictability, and efficiency to the medical device approval process.

■ THE MEDICAL DEVICE USER FEE AND MODERNIZATION ACT OF 2002

On October 26, 2002 the Medical Device User Fee and Modernization Act (MDUFMA) of 2002 became law. MDUFMA authorized the FDA to charge a fee for medical device Premarket Notification 510(k) reviews. In 2003 the user fee for 510(k) review was $2187.00.

Incidents in which a device may have caused or contributed to a death or serious injury must be reported to FDA under the Medical Device Reporting program. In addition, certain malfunctions must also be reported. The MDR regulation is a mechanism for FDA and manufacturers to identify and monitor significant adverse events, involving medical devices. The goals of the regulation are to detect and correct problems in a timely manner. Further information on the Medical Device Reporting process can be found at http://www.fda.gov/cdrh/devadvice/351.html.

The Center for Devices and Radiological Health (CDRH) created a website, www.fda.gov/cdrh/mdufma/index.html, dedicated to MDUFMA. Included in this website are links to reference materials and background information on MDUFMA, including a full text of the law, summary of the law, and the legislative history of MDUFMA. In addition, there is a frequently asked questions (FAQ) document, which should help one address questions regarding the new law. As the FDA proceeds with implementation of MDUFMA, the CDRH expects to update the website regularly.

DEFINITION OF A MEDICAL DEVICE

The Medical Device Amendments of 1976 categorized medical devices based on risk. It required devices to meet certain performance standards and mandated recordkeeping and adverse event reporting.

According to the definition in the FD&C Act, section 201(h) a "device" is

An instrument, apparatus, implement, machine, contrivance, implant, in vitro reagent, or other similar or related article, including any component, part or accessory, which is intended for use in the diagnosis of disease or other conditions, or in the cure, mitigation, treatment, or prevention of disease, in man or other animals, or intended to affect the structure or any function of the body and which does not achieve its primary intended purposes through chemical action and which is not dependent upon being metabolized for the achievement of its primary intended purpose.[2]

As this complex definition suggests, many different types of products are regulated as medical devices. Medical devices include over 100,000 products in more than 1700 categories. The products regulated by FDA as medical devices range from simple everyday articles, such as thermometers, tongue depressors, and heating pads, to more complex devices, such as pacemakers, intrauterine devices, diagnostic imaging devices, kidney dialysis machines, respirators, and artificial hearts.

THE CENTER FOR DEVICES AND RADIOLOGICAL HEALTH

The FDA Center for Devices and Radiological Health (CDRH) has responsibility for regulating medical devices and promoting and protecting public health by helping to ensure that medical devices are safe and effective. CDRH carries out its mission by evaluating new devices before they are marketed, ensuring quality control in manufacturing through inspection and compliance activities, monitoring adverse events in already marketed products, and taking action, when necessary, to prevent injury or death. A device manufacturer must comply with all applicable requirements of the FD&C Act, including, but not limited to, establishing registration and device listing, premarket review, use of good manufacturing practices, and the reporting of adverse events.

The range and complexity of problems, which can arise from their use and are as diverse as medical devices. These problems include mechanical failure, faulty design, poor manufacturing quality, adverse effects from materials implanted in the body, improper maintenance/specifications, user error, compromised sterility/shelf life, and electromagnetic interference among devices.

Medical devices are classified into classes I, II, and III. Regulatory control increases as you go up in class level. The device classification regulation defines the regulatory requirements for a general device type. Most class I devices are exempt from Premarket Notification 510(k), most class II devices require Premarket Notification 510(k), and a majority of class III devices require Premarket Approval (PMA).[3]

If a device requires the submission of a Premarket Notification 510(k), it cannot be commercially distributed until the FDA acknowledges that the device is substantially equivalent to an approved device. A 510(k) must demonstrate that the device is equivalent to one in legal commercial distribution in the United States.

■ CLASS I DEVICES

The FDA has exempted almost all class I devices from the premarket notification requirement. If a device falls into a generic category of an exempted class I device, a premarket notification application and FDA clearance is not required before marketing the device in the United States. However, the manufacturer of that device is required to register its establishment.

■ CLASS II DEVICES

The FDA has published a list of class II devices, subject to certain limitations, that are exempt from the premarket notification requirements under the FDAMA of 1997. The FDA believes that these exemptions will relieve manufacturers from the need to submit premarket notification submissions for these devices and will also enable the FDA to redirect resources that would be spent on reviewing such submissions to more significant public health issues. The FDA is taking this action in order to meet a requirement of the Modernization Act. Class II devices are *not* exempt from good manufacturing practice requirements.

If a device manufacturer plans to send a 510(k) application[4] to FDA for a class I or II device, the manufacturer may have a 510(k) review by an accredited third party or accredited person. The 510(k) review by an accredited person is exempt from any FDA fee; however, the third party may charge a fee for its review.

The FDA has accredited 12 organizations to conduct a primary review of 670 types of devices. By law, the FDA must issue a final determination within 30 days after receiving a recommendation from an accredited person.[5]

■ CLASS III DEVICES

PMA is the FDA process of scientific and regulatory review to evaluate the safety and effectiveness of medical devices. Products requiring PMAs are class III devices. Class III devices are those that support or sustain human life, are of substantial importance in preventing impairment of human health, or present a potential or unreasonable risk of illness or injury. Because of the level of risk associated with class III devices, the FDA has determined that general and special controls alone are insufficient to ensure the safety and effectiveness of class III devices. Therefore, these devices require a PMA application under section 515 of the FD&C Act in order to obtain market clearance.

PMA is the most stringent device marketing application required by FDA. PMA approval is based on a determination by the FDA that the PMA contains sufficient valid scientific evidence to ensure that the device is safe and effective for its intended use(s). An approved PMA is, in effect, a private license granting the applicant (or owner) permission to market the device. The PMA owner, however, can authorize use of its data by another party.[6]

FDA regulations provide 180 days to review the PMA and make a determination. Typically, the review time is longer than 180 days. Before approving or denying a PMA, the appropriate FDA advisory committee must review the PMA at a public meeting and provide the FDA with the committee's recommendation on whether the FDA should approve the submission. After the FDA notifies the applicant that the PMA has been approved or denied, a notice is published on the Internet both announcing the data on which the decision is based and providing interested persons an opportunity to petition FDA within 30 days for reconsideration of the decision.

■ INVESTIGATIONAL DEVICE EXEMPTION

An investigational device exemption (IDE) allows an experimental device to be used in a clinical study in order to collect safety and effectiveness data required to support a PMA application or a Premarket Notification 510(k) submission to FDA. Clinical studies are most often conducted to support a PMA. Investigational use also includes clinical evaluation of certain modifications or new intended uses of already legally marketed devices.

Clinical trials using unapproved medical devices on human subjects are performed under an IDE. Clinical studies with devices of significant risk must be approved by FDA and by an institutional review board (IRB) before the study can begin. Studies with devices of no significant risk must be approved by the hospital IRB only before the study can begin.

An approved IDE permits a device to be shipped lawfully for the purpose of conducting investigations of the device without complying with other requirements of FD&C that apply to devices in commercial distribution. Manufactures need not submit a PMA or Premarket Notification 510(k), register their establishment, or list the device while the device is under investigation. Sponsors of IDEs are also exempt from the Quality System (QS) Regulation except for the requirements for design control.[7]

DISCUSSION

Medical technology has advanced at an incredible pace during the last 50 years. The medical miracles of tomorrow depend on the clinical and regulatory environment of today. The provisions that recognize the unique dynamics of device development as compared to pharmaceuticals represent some of the most revolutionary language in the new laws. The distinction between devices and drugs is significant. The two cannot be compared and, for the benefit of the patient, must be held to different standards. Over time, a drug remains the same. On the other hand, devices do develop incrementally. A device should begin a clinical trial as a safe and effective prototype. This prototype should be improved during the trial process so it can evolve to a superior finished product. This is not true for a drug. An aspirin or any other drug reach is in its completed form. The aspirin one took this morning is the same chemical formula as the one swallowed 10 years ago. A drug, once formulated, remains the same. Change its chemical formula, and you have a different drug. The 1997 FDAMA recognized the dynamic process of device development, thus allowing unregulated incremental improvements in a prototype device allowing it to evolve into a "state-of-the-art" finished product.

The FDAMA also recognized the need for timely market access of so-called "breakthrough" devices with their incremental improvements. The FDAMA law has been helpful in that it requires the FDA to meet with a device sponsor early in the approval cycle to identify from the beginning, the scientific evidence needed to prove effectiveness. This has reduced needless and time-consuming requests by the FDA for data later in the process. The FDAMA also requires the FDA to consider whether premarket data requirements can be reduced if postmarket tools are employed. This is another potentially significant time saver.

The Modernization Act also streamlined the review process for less risky devices, known as "510(k) s." Those with the least risk—all "class I" and some "class II" devices—have been exempted from the review process, thus freeing valuable agency resources to concentrate on higher-risk and breakthrough devices. Manufacturers may now rely on FDA-recognized performance standards as a means of fulfilling 510(k) review requirements. In another effort to preserve agency resources, the FDA's third-party review authority has been expanded to include a wider range of medical devices.

For both breakthrough devices and the less risky 510(k) products, the FDAMA requires the agency to consider the "least burdensome" means to prove device effectiveness.[8] This is a giant step from the mindset of the past when the FDA sought an absolute science or, in other words, absolute assurance of a device's effectiveness. But science rarely, if ever, is perfect. That is why the Congress, in the 1976 device law, directed the FDA to seek reasonable assurance of safety and effectiveness when approving devices. Physicians depend on good scientific data but must use common sense and adapt science to the needs of the patient and the device innovation process. Toward that end, it is enormously helpful that manufacturers can now distribute certain information from peer-reviewed journals describing unapproved uses for devices or drugs.

All of the provisions of FDAMA, many of which are not addressed here, bring timeliness, predictability, and efficiency to the medical device approval process. In the recent past, delays in product approvals and an unpredictable and inefficient US regulatory processes forced many companies to move clinical trials and manufacturing strategies overseas. Cutting-edge technologies, scores of jobs, significant venture capital, and our revenue base in this country have fallen victim to the move outside of the United States. This is a sad testimony to a vibrant biomedical industry that has been one of the few US industries to consistently post a positive trade deficit.

The 1997 FDAMA and subsequent legislation based on the FDAMA have ignited a resurgence of innovative spirit within the US medical device community. The hope is that this reform will permit US investigators to regain the creative momentum that excites our young researchers and gives vibrancy to our teaching institutions. The successful implementation of the FDAMA can make unnecessary product delays, repetitive clinical research, and an exodus of scientific leadership something of the past.

REFERENCES

1. US Regulatory Affairs History, Fundamentals of Regulatory Affairs, chapter 1.
2. http://www.fda.gov/cdrh/devadvice/313.html
3. http://www.fda.gov/cdrh/devadvice/314.html
4. http://www.fda.gov/cdrh/devadvice/314.html21 CFR Parts 862-892
5. http://www.fda.gov/cdrh/thirdparty
6. http://www.fda.gov/cdrh/devadvice/pma/
7. http://www.fda.gov/cdrh/devadvice/ide/index.shtml
8. http://www.fda.gov/cdrh/devadvice/pma/. 21 CFR Part 814

CHAPTER 4
LVAD PATIENT SELECTION CRITERIA

Kumudha Ramasubbu and Biswajit Kar

A major factor determining the success of left ventricular assist device (LVAD) implantation lies in appropriate patient selection. LVAD therapy is indicated in patients with end-stage, refractory heart failure (HF). The art of selecting the correct patient involves three main factors: (1) identifying the patient with severe enough HF to confer mortality benefit from LVAD therapy; (2) ensuring that the disease process is not so far progressed that LVAD implantation fails to result in a morbidity and mortality benefit but rather in increased complications; and (3) ensuring that there are no contraindications to LVAD implantation. To date, published data on patient selection criteria are scarce. This chapter thus mainly focuses on evidence gathered from available data and personal experience.

The two main indications for LVAD placement in patients with chronic end-stage HF are bridge-to-transplantation (BTT) and destination therapy (DT). Before a patient is deemed a candidate for BTT, the patient should undergo rigorous assessment of all organ systems to ensure that there are no contraindications for cardiac transplant (Table 4–1). Transplant candidates who should be considered for LVAD placement as BTT are those too ill to wait for a heart and undergo transplant (acute decompensation, postcardiotomy cardiogenic shock) and those who are expected to have extended waiting times on the transplant list (large patient, blood type O, high panel reactive antibody [PRA]). LVAD for DT is indicated in patients who have contraindications for cardiac transplant such as advanced age or significant comorbidities. The inclusion criteria used in the REMATCH trial (Randomized Evaluation of Mechanical Assistance for the Treatment of Congestive Heart Failure) have been generally accepted to identify appropriate candidates for DT (Tables 4–2 and 4–3).[1,2]

IDENTIFYING PATIENTS WITH END-STAGE HEART FAILURE

Perhaps the most difficult decision involves the timing of LVAD surgery. LVAD implantation earlier in the disease process may lead to improved LVAD outcomes but may not result in mortality benefit compared to medical management. LVAD placement

too late in the disease process (for example in severe shock states) may result in high risk of early mortality.[3] Deng et al evaluated 39 patients who had a LVAD placed as BTT. Survival to transplant was 77% in the elective group followed by 56% in the urgent group and 33% in the emergent group who received LVADs for acute cardiogenic shock.[4] These data underline the need for early identification of high-risk HF patients as potential candidates for elective LVAD implantation.

What are indicators of high risk? HF patients are considered to be end-stage or refractory if they remain symptomatic or display hemodynamic derangement despite maximal tolerated medical therapy. The inability to tolerate neurohormonal antagonists such as angiotensin-converting enzyme inhibitors, angiotensin receptor blockers, and β-blockers also identifies patients with advanced heart failure.[2,5] A further identifier of high risk is the refractoriness to oral medications and requirement of continuous inotropic therapy.[6] Furthermore, patients who develop signs of renal dysfunction have been shown to have a high mortality risk and may thus benefit from LVAD placement.[7,8]

Patients evaluated for BTT and DT require hemodynamic and functional assessment to ensure that the HF stage is advanced enough to benefit from LVAD placement. The hemodynamic criteria identify patients with low cardiac output and evidence of volume retention despite maximum possible medical support. This group also includes patients who require chronic administration of inotropes or support with an intra-aortic balloon pump (IABP) to maintain hemodynamic parameters within normal range. The currently accepted hemodynamic criteria include a pulmonary capillary wedge pressure of greater than 20 mm Hg, systolic blood pressure less than 80 mm Hg, and cardiac index less than 2.0 L/min/m^2. However using hemodynamic criteria alone may be misleading. On the one hand, a group of patients have been identified with low cardiac output without severe HF symptoms or evidence of end-organ damage, who appear to have a relatively good prognosis. On the other hand, there are patients with relatively preserved hemodynamic parameters with severe HF symptoms and evidence of progressive end-organ dysfunction who have poor long-term prognosis.[9] Therefore the hemodynamic criteria need to be viewed in conjunction with other clinical criteria discussed below.

Clinical criteria for LVAD implantation include the presence of New York Heart Association (NYHA) functional classes III and IV HF symptoms, that is, symptoms with minimal exertion or at rest.[2,10] Objectively, cardiopulmonary exercise testing is used to identify patients with severe functional impairment due to HF. The initial study by Lund et al concluded that patients with a peak oxygen consumption (MVO$_2$) of less than 14 mL/kg/min would confer most benefit from cardiac transplant. Patients in this group had a 1-year survival of 70% compared to 94% in the transplant group. Similarly, in the REMATCH trial, patients were included for potential LVAD placement if they had a peak MVO$_2$ of 12 mL/kg/min or less, or were dependent on inotropes

TABLE 4–1. Listing Criteria for Heart Transplantation: International Society for Heart and Lung Transplantation Guidelines for the Care of Cardiac Transplant Candidates–2006

Cardiopulmonary exercise testing	$MVO_2 \leq 14$ mL/kg/min in patients intolerant of a β-blocker
	$MVO_2 \leq 12$ mL/kg/min in presence of a β-blocker
	$\leq 50\%$ of predicted peak MVO_2 in young patients (< 50 years) and women
Invasive hemodynamic criteria	Relative contraindication: PVR > 5 Wood units or the PVR index (PVRI) >6 or the transpulmonary gradient > 16-20 mm Hg
	If the PVR can be reduced to < 2.5 Wood units with a vasodilator but the systolic blood pressure falls to < 85 mm Hg, the patient remains at high risk of right heart failure (RHF) and mortality
Age	≤ 70 years of age
Neoplasm	Tumor recurrence is low based on tumor type, response to therapy, and negative metastatic workup
	No arbitrary time period for observation given
Weight	BMI < 30 kg/m^2 or percent idea body weight (PIBW) $< 140\%$
Diabetes	Relative contraindication: diabetes with end-organ damage other than nonproliferative retinopathy or poor glycemic control (HbA1C > 7.5) despite optimal effort
Renal function	Relative contraindication: irreversible renal dysfunction (Glomerular filtration rate <40 mL/min)
	Exclude intrinsic renal disease with renal ultrasonography, estimation of proteinuria, and evaluation for renal arterial disease
Cerebrovascular disease	Contraindication to transplantation: severe symptomatic cerebrovascular disease not amenable to revascularization
Peripheral vascular disease	Relative contraindication: presence limits rehabilitation and revascularization is not a viable option
Psychosocial	Relative contraindication: active tobacco smoking
	Contraindication: active substance abusers (including alcohol)
	Contraindication: patients who have demonstrated inability to comply with drug therapy on multiple occasions
Neurocognitive	Relative contraindication: mental retardation or dementia

(Reproduced with permission from Mehra et al.[46] Copyright © Elsevier.)

TABLE 4–2. Inclusion Criteria for Destination LVAD Therapy in the REMATCH Trial

New York Heart Association (NYHA) class	Class IV despite optimal medical therapy
	Classes III-IV for at least 28 days and have received at least 14 d of support with an IABP or with dependence on intravenous inotropic agents, with two failed weaning attempts
Left ventricular ejection fraction	$\leq 25\%$
Peak oxygen consumption	≤ 14 mL/kg/min
Clinical criteria	Continued need for intravenous inotropic therapy due to symptomatic hypotension, decreasing renal function, or worsening pulmonary congestion
Cardiac transplantation contraindicated	Age > 65 y
	Insulin-dependent diabetes mellitus with end-organ damage
	Chronic renal failure with a serum creatinine > 2.5 mg/dL for at least 90 d before randomization
	Major comorbidity (physical or psychiatric) that would make the patient ineligible for cardiac transplantation

(Reproduced with permission from Rose et al.[1] Copyright © Elsevier; Rose et al.[2] Copyright © Massachusetts Medical Society. All rights reserved.)

TABLE 4–3. Exclusion Criteria for LVAD Destination Therapy in the REMATCH Trial

Cause of heart failure	Due to or associated with uncorrected thyroid disease, obstructive cardiomyopathy, pericardial disease, amyloidosis, or active myocarditis
Technical obstacles	Posing a high surgical risk in the judgment of the certified surgeon
Hepatic dysfunction	*INR > 1.3 or PT > 15 s within 24 h before randomization*
	Evidence of intrinsic hepatic disease: liver enzyme values (aspartate aminotransferase, alanine aminotransferase, or total bilirubin) > five times the upper limit of normal within 4 d before randomization
	Biopsy-proved liver cirrhosis
Body size	Body surface area < 1.5 m^2
Weight	Body mass index > 40 kg/m^2
Pulmonary dysfunction	Severe chronic obstructive pulmonary disease; forced expiratory volume < 1.5 L/min
Women	*If premenopausal, positive serum pregnancy test*
Pulmonary hypertension	*Fixed pulmonary hypertension with pulmonary vascular resistance > 8 Wood units, unresponsive to pharmacologic intervention, documented within 90 d before randomization*
Surgical history	*History of cardiac transplantation, left ventricular reduction procedure, or cardiomyoplasty*
	Presence of implanted mechanical aortic valve that will not be converted to bioprosthesis at time of LVAD implantation
	Patient under consideration for conventional revascularization procedure, therapeutic valvular repair, left ventricular reduction procedure (ie, Batista procedure), or cardiomyoplasty
	Abdominal operation planned
Neurologic disease	Occurrence of stroke within 90 d before randomization
	History of cerebrovascular disease with major (> 80%) extracranial or carotid stenosis documented by Doppler study
Cognitive impairment	Confirmation by neurologist of impairment of cognitive function, presence of Alzheimer disease or any other form of irreversible dementia, or both
Peripheral vascular disease	Evidence of untreated abdominal aortic aneurysm > 5 cm as measured by abdominal ultrasound within 30 d before randomization
	Major peripheral vascular disease accompanied by pain on rest or leg ulceration
Infection	Suspected or active systemic infection 48 h before randomization
Hematology	Platelet count < 50 × 10^3/mm^3 within 24 h before randomization
Renal dysfunction	Serum creatinine > 3.5 mg/dL
	Long-term dialysis
Other medical therapy	*Receiving calcium channel blocker (except amlodipine besylate) or type I (eg, quinidine, procainamide hydrochloride, disopyramide phosphate) or type III antiarrhythmic agent (eg, encainide hydrochloride, flecainide acetate, propafenone hydrochloride, moricizine hydrochloride) within 28 d before randomization*
Psychiatric disease	Recent history of psychiatric disease (including drug or alcohol abuse) that is likely to impair compliance with study protocol
Expected survival	*Presence of condition other than heart failure that would limit survival to < 3 y*
Other	*Receiving therapy with investigational intervention or participating in another clinical study*

In italics are exclusion criteria that were used in REMATCH but may not apply in regular clinical practice.

(Reproduced with permission from Rose et al.[1] Copyright © Elsevier.)

or IABP. Of note the 1-year survival in the control group was only 25% compared to 52% in the LVAD group.[2]

PREDICTORS OF POOR OUTCOME AFTER LVAD IMPLANTATION

To date, several publications have retrospectively evaluated preoperative predictors of poor outcome after LVAD implantation (Table 4–4). Leading causes of increased morbidity and mortality are evidence of end-organ dysfunction (renal failure, hepatic dysfunction, multiorgan failure), ventilator dependence, and right HF. It is important to be aware of these predictors in order to identify patients who are too high risk to undergo LVAD placement. Moreover, in patients with these risk factors (RF),

an attempt can be made to improve and stabilize deranged risk factors before proceeding to LVAD implantation.

Preoperative renal insufficiency has been consistently related to high morbidity and mortality in LVAD patients. Elevated creatinine,[11] decreased creatinine clearance,[12] elevated BUN,[13] and decreased preoperative urine output[3] have been associated with worse postoperative outcomes. Patients with end-stage renal disease or requiring dialysis have been considered to be very high risk due to increased risk of complications, especially infectious complications. For these reasons, in the REMATCH destination therapy trial patients with a creatinine of greater than 3.5 mg/dL were excluded.[2] The dilemma lies in determining if the renal dysfunction is due to poor cardiac output and is thus reversible once sufficient renal blood flow is restored or is a result of intrinsic kidney disease and is thus irreversible.

TABLE 4–4. Retrospective Studies That Identified Predictors of Poor Outcome After LVAD Implantation

Reference	Number of Patients	Indication for LVAD	Type of LVAD	Predictors of Poor Outcome
Pennington et al[47]	44	BTT	32 Thoratec, 11 Novacor, and 2 Jarvik	WBC, platelet count
Frazier et al[14]	280	BTT	HMXVE	Age, prior open-heart surgery, baseline creatinine, and baseline total bilirubin
Oz et al[48]	56		HM IP and VE	Oliguria (UOP < 3 0 mL/h), ventilator dependence, elevated CVP > 16 mm Hg, elevated PT > 16 s, reoperation status and WBC > 15,000/mm³
McCarthy et al[49]	100	BTT	HMXVE	Need for RVAD support, reoperation for bleeding, dialysis, device failure
				Multivariate RF for death: postoperative dialysis, device failure, RVAD requirement
				RF for death after LVAD implantation but before discharge from ICU: mechanical ventilation, UOP < 30 mL/h (borderline RF), Oz scale score > 5
				Preoperative ECMO and baseline creatinine
Deng et al[39]	464	Not mentioned	Novacor	Age at implant > 65, preimplant AMI, preexisting RHF, acute postcardiotomy shock, preimplant sepsis with concomitant respiratory failure
Deng et al[50]	655	80% BTT and 12% DT	Various	Concurrent RVAD placement, age, female, lower platelet count, higher WBC, blood type A, diabetes, preimplant ventilator, higher creatinine
				DT multivariate analysis: age
Rao et al[37]	130	BTT	HMXVE	New univariate predictors: previous LVAD or RVAD, postcardiotomy shock, AMI, ICMP
				Multivariate predictors: ventilation, previous LVAD

AMI, acute myocardial infarction; BTT, bridge-to-transplantation; CVP, central venous pressure; DT, destination therapy; ECMO, extracorporeal membrane oxygenation; HM IP, heartmate intraperitoneal; ICMP, ischemic cardiomyopathy; ICU, intensive care unit; LVAD, left ventricular assist device; PT, prothrombin time; RF, risk factor; RHF, right heart failure; RVAD, right ventricular assist device; UOP, urinary output; VE, vented electric; WBC, white blood count.

(Reproduced with permission from Lund et al.[38] Copyright © Elsevier.)

Preexisting right heart failure (RHF) or the need for a right ventricular assist device (RVAD) postoperatively is associated with increased mortality as well as a significant increase in postoperative complications (reoperation for bleeding and renal failure). The incidence of RHF after LVAD implantation has been reported to be 10% to 20%[14,15] and is the cause of death in up to 20% of LVAD patients.[16] The etiology of RHF in this setting is multifactorial and involves changes in septal motion/ventricular interdependence, depressed right ventricular (RV) contractility, and increased RV afterload/pulmonary vascular resistance. Risk factors for RHF after LVAD placement have been identified as preoperative mechanical support, female gender, younger age, smaller stature, and nonischemic etiology of HF.[17,18] Hemodynamic parameters associated with RHF are low RV stroke work index, low mean pulmonary artery pressure, low diastolic pulmonary artery pressure, higher right atrial pressure, and dilated RV with increased RV preload and afterload.[17-19] Interestingly, elevated systolic pulmonary artery pressure, elevated pulmonary vascular resistance (PVR), and elevated transpulmonary gradient did not predict RHF. This may suggest that these patients have decreased RV contractility preventing them from mounting higher pulmonary artery pressures. Mortality is very high in patients who develop RV failure after LVAD placement.[18, 20,21] Thus, in patients with significant preoperative RV dysfunction, measures to improve RV function must be instituted such as the use of inotropes and vasodilators. Other options include the preemptive insertion of an RVAD during LVAD implantation or deeming the patient to be too high risk for LVAD placement.

Hepatic dysfunction has also been consistently associated with poor outcome after LVAD placement. Elevated total bilirubin level and elevated liver enzymes (greater than three times upper limits of normal) have been demonstrated as independent risk factors for adverse outcomes.[10,11,13] Moreover, a prolonged prothrombin time (PT) or elevated international normalized ratio (INR) has been associated with increased morbidity and mortality.[3] Pathophysiologically, hepatic congestion from elevated right heart pressures can lead to impairment in hepatic synthetic function, resulting in reduced production of coagulation factors and abnormal INR. This can result in increased perioperative bleeding requiring transfusions which can worsen RV function, poor LVAD filling, and ultimately lead to renal dysfunction and multiorgan failure.[22] Methods of preventing this downward spiral include optimizing volume status, using medications to support RV function, cautious repletion of blood and clotting factors, and the preemptive placement of an IABP or RVAD.

Preoperative ventilator requirement has consistently been associated with worse postoperative outcome, which may be a reflection of the patient's overall poor status rather than isolated poor pulmonary status. With respect to obstructive and restrictive pulmonary diseases, there are no specific recommendations for risk stratification. However, further investigation is recommended for patients with pulmonary function test results less than 50% of predicted and some authors suggest that severe obstructive and restrictive pulmonary disease may even be a contraindication to LVAD placement.[23,16] Similarly, there is

no consensus on risk stratification of patients with elevated preoperative PVR. Some authors attempt to decrease PVR of less than 3 Wood units before committing patients to LVAD implantation,[24] while others believe that elevated PVR does not preclude LVAD placement since elevated PVR may decline over time with LVAD support.[16] In any case, in patients with elevated PVR extreme prudence must be exercised in evaluating for RV dysfunction and timely treatment of RV dysfunction.

In addition to these more robust risk factors, there are other indicators of higher risk such as age, gender, body size, history of previous open-heart surgery, and presence of peripheral vascular disease (PVD) and neuropsychiatric illness which can aid in patient selection. The impact of age on survival after LVAD placement has been controversial. However, the largest analysis to date of the International Society of Heart and Lung Transplantation (ISHLT) LVAD database of 655 patients observed advanced age as a significant risk factor for post-LVAD mortality. In the BTT group, 50% of patients older than 50 years underwent cardiac transplant at 1 year, but nearly 40% died with the LVAD. In patients younger than 30 years, nearly 75% received cardiac transplant and only 13% died with LVAD at 1 year. In the DT group of 78 patients, age remained a major risk factor for mortality by multivariate analysis (survival at 1 year: < 65 years old, 41%; > 65 years old, 26%).[25]

The data on gender-dependent outcome of LVAD patients is scarce since the majority of patients enrolled in the pulsatile LVAD studies have been men partly because of the body surface area (BSA) restriction of greater than 1.5. Morgan et al evaluated the impact of gender on post-LVAD outcome and noted a significantly lower survival in women after LVAD implantation (78.5% vs 62.2%) as well as a lower rate of successful BTT compared to men (72.8% vs 57.8%).[26] The authors proposed that differences in disease process and timeliness of HF management might account for the worse outcome in female patients. Of note, several reports analyzing RV function in LVAD patients noticed that a greater percentage of women appear to develop RHF with subsequent worse outcome.[15,17] The reason for this is not clear.

Weight at both extremes appears to increase risk of poor outcome after LVAD placement. A body mass index (BMI) of greater than 40 kg/m^2 has been associated with a higher incidence of wound infections. On the other end of the spectrum, a low BMI (< 22 kg/m^2), which is often associated with cachexia, appears to have a worse effect on outcome than obesity.[27,28] The pathogenesis of cardiac cachexia appears to be multifactorial, including poor oral intake due to poor appetite, early satiety (due to hepatomegaly), increased work of breathing, and elevated cytokines.[29] In cardiovascular surgery patients, malnutrition has been associated with poor wound healing and increased risk of infection.[27,28] Similarly, in LVAD patients low albumin (< 3.3), a reflection of malnutrition, has been reported as a RF for mortality.[23] Thus, there is a great strive toward improving patients' nutritional status before proceeding to LVAD implantation.

Redosternotomy for LVAD implantation has been associated with worse outcomes.[3] The presence of dense adhesions in these patients requires lengthy dissection, resulting in increased bleeding as well as increasing time on cardiopulmonary bypass. This in turn can lead to coagulopathy further aggravating perioperative bleeding. Attempts to reduce these operative risks include staged reoperation and nonthoracic, extraperitoneal insertion of the LVAD through a left upper quadrant incision.[30,31] Thus, patients with history of previous sternotomies need to be identified and the possibility of a staged operation or a nonthoracic LVAD insertion should be considered.

Patients considered for LVAD therapy should be screened for PVD. Severe PVD may be a contraindication to LVAD implantation. For example, iliac artery occlusion would preclude femoral artery cannulation for cardiopulmonary bypass which is frequently required in these patients. Other areas that are important for patient selection include neurologic and psychosocial evaluation as well as gender- and age-appropriate cancer screening. Ideally, patients should have intact neurocognitive function, no significant psychiatric illness, demonstrate compliance, and be free of chemical dependency. A sound and able social network is also necessary for a stable home environment and providing assistance in case of emergencies.

SPECIFIC PATIENT SELECTION CRITERIA FOR CONTINUOUS-FLOW DEVICES

In addition to the general LVAD patient selection criteria largely derived from pulsatile LVAD data, there are several factors that have to be considered specifically for continuous-flow devices. Because of the higher thrombogenic potential of continuous-flow LVADs, anticoagulation is necessary in all patients. Thus patients selected for a continuous-flow LVAD must be candidates for anticoagulation. Along the same line, a preexisting hypercoagulable state may exacerbate thrombotic complications and may thus be a contraindication for implantation of continuous-flow LVADs.[32,33]

In contrast to a BSA limit of greater than 1.5 m² in pulsatile LVADs, continuous-flow LVADs are approved even for smaller individuals with a BSA less than 1.5 cm² because of the small size of the device itself. This has significantly broadened the group of patients who can benefit from LVAD therapy (specifically women and children). Of note, several of the axial-flow LVADs have been approved for pediatric use.[34]

The long-term effects of continuous-flow physiology are essentially unknown and may result in a unique set of problems defining patient selection. Several case series of patients with continuous-flow devices have noted a relatively high incidence of hemolysis caused by destruction of red blood cells by the pump and thrombus formation within the pump.[33] Thus patients with hemolytic disorders due to intrinsic erythrocyte abnormalities or extrinsic etiologies may not be good candidates for continuous-flow devices. Furthermore, an association

between continuous-flow devices and intestinal arterio-venous malformations has been suggested. Therefore, continuous-flow devices may not be the first choice in patients with preexisting arteriovenous malformations.[35]

The effect of continuous-flow physiology on stenotic atherosclerotic lesions is unknown. In the pulsatile state, stenoses of greater than 70% are accepted as flow limiting. However, this may not be the case in the setting of continuous-flow hemodynamics. Kar et al, on the basis of clinical observation and computerized flow simulation, suggest that lesions of milder severity could pose significant problems in the setting of continuous flow.[36] Thus aggressive evaluation for PVD and revascularization may be necessary prior to implantation of a continuous-flow device. The majority of these unique observations in patients with continuous-flow devices has been anecdotal and will have to be substantiated in larger patient numbers before specific recommendations regarding patient selection devices can be made.

COMPOSITE RISK SCORES FOR LVAD PATIENT SELECTION

Rather than using individual criteria to predict risk, the convergence of multiple risk factors probably gives a more accurate prediction of risk. Based on this premise, composite risk scores have been developed to help reliably predict risk and guide patient selection for LVAD implantation. Oz et al evaluated 56 patients undergoing LVAD placement, identified five high-risk indicators, and allotted them different weights to develop a risk factor–selection scale (RFSS). The risk factors and their weighting are displayed in Table 4–5. Survivors (n = 42) had an average RFSS of 2.45 ± 1.73 compared with 5.43 ± 2.85 in nonsurvivors (n = 14) ($P < .0001$). The authors classified patients with RFSS 5 or greater as high risk and reported that most of these patients died after LVAD implantation ($P < .001$).[3]

More recently, Rao et al revised the risk score by Oz et al using a more current cohort of 130 LVAD patients at a single center. They noted that most of the previous risk factors continued

TABLE 4–5. Risk factors and Their Respective Weighting Used to Calculate the Initial and Revised Risk Factor Summation Score

Previous Risk Factor Summation Score		Revised Risk Factor Summation Score	
Variable	Weighting	Variable	Weighting
Preoperative urine output<30 mL/h	3	Ventilated	4
CVP >16 mm Hg	2	Postcardiotomy shock	2
Ventilated	2	Previous LVAD	2
PT > 16 s	2	CVP > 16 mm Hg	1
Redo surgery	1	PT > 16 s	1

(Reproduced with permission from Rao et al.[37] Copyright © Elsevier.)

to be valid except for renal insufficiency defined by poor preoperative urine output and remote sternotomy. The authors proposed that a change in patient management in response to the older risk score (aggressive treatment of volume overload and continuous veno-venous hemofiltration [CVVH]) might have attenuated the poor outcome associated with low preoperative urine output. However, postoperative renal failure was a strong predictor of outcome. Moreover, new univariate predictors were identified: history of previous LVAD or RVAD and postcardiotomy shock. Multivariate predictors of mortality were mechanical ventilation and previous LVAD of which mechanical ventilation was found to be the strongest multivariable predictor of death. The revised risk score (see Table 4–5) was noted to have an improved discrimination and slightly higher accuracy. The risk of mortality was 46% in patients with a score greater than 5 versus 12% with a score less than 5. This publication points out that the risk factors must be reanalyzed periodically as the learning curve of LVAD implantation and intensive care management improves.[37]

Aaronson et al developed the Heart Failure Survival Score (HFSS) using 7 noninvasive parameters to guide in the patient selection for cardiac transplantation (Table 4–6). Using the HFSS, patients were divided into three groups of low, medium, and high risk. One-year event-free survival was 88-93% in the low-risk, 60% to 72% in the medium-risk, and 35% to 43% in the high-risk group.[9] In a subsequent evaluation, the HFSS was determined serially in patients listed and waiting for cardiac transplantation. Patients who remained at low risk at two serial evaluations demonstrated the best prognosis (87% freedom from death and 81% freedom from LVAD or urgent transplant at 1 year) followed by patients whose risk improved from medium/high to low (overall 1-year event-free survival rate of 72%). The worst prognosis was noted in two groups of patients: (1) low-risk patients who deteriorated to medium or high risk (1-year event-free survival rates of 61% [by HFSS] and 45% [by Vo_2]) and (2) patients who remained at medium or high risk (1-year event-free survival rates were 58% [by HFSS] and 68% [by peak Vo_2]). In the current setting of scarcity of available hearts for transplantation, the HFSS can be used to identify end-stage heart failure patients with a high mortality risk who could be maintained with an LVAD until a heart becomes available. Furthermore, the HFSS can be determined serially in patients awaiting cardiac transplantation, and identify patients with poor prognosis who may benefit from LVAD implantation.[38]

Deng et al analyzed 366 LVAD patients from the Novacor European Registry and identified five preimplant risk factors as independent predictors of postimplant mortality: respiratory failure with septicemia (OR 11.2), RHF (OR 3.2), age over 65 years (OR 3.01), acute postcardiotomy (OR 1.8), and acute infarction (OR 1.7). Patients without any of these risk factors had a 1-year survival after LVAD implantation of 60%. Patients who had at least one risk factor had a 1-year survival of 24%.[39] In a further analysis, Gracin et al calculated the APACHE (Acute Physiology and Chronic Health Evaluation) score in patients undergoing LVAD implantation. Patients with APACHE score in the moderate range (11-20) demonstrated a greater survival benefit (40%) than severely ill patients with a score greater than 20 (20% benefit) or those who were not very ill with a score less than 10 (0% benefit).[40]

The Seattle Heart Failure Score (SHFS) was developed at the University of Washington as a strategy for predicting 1-, 2-, and 3- year survival in patients with various types of heart failure therapy.[41] This model utilizes a set of clinical parameters, including age, gender, heart failure etiology, BMI, EF, blood pressure, serum sodium, cholesterol, hemoglobin, and percent lymphocytes to derive anticipated 1- to 3-year survival. In addition, the user may manipulate various forms of therapy for heart failure in order to study the impact on survival. Using the REMATCH patient population, this risk stratification model has been validated for LVAD therapy as well as medical therapy (Fig. 4–1).[42]

Lietz et al developed a cumulative risk score to predict 90-day in-hospital mortality by evaluating 222 patients undergoing pulsatile LVAD implantation for destination therapy. Nine risk factors were identified by multivariable analysis and were given a weighted risk score (Table 4–7A). The cumulative risk score stratified patients into four operative risk categories (low, medium, high, and very high) with

TABLE 4–6. Heart Failure Survival Score (HFSS) Variables Used for Risk Stratification

Variable	Adjusted Hazard Ratio (95% CI)	Wald χ^2	p value
Ischemic cardiomyopathy	2.00 (1.35, 2.97)	11.71	.0006
Resting heart rate (beats/min)	1.02 (1.01, 1.04)	11.45	.0007
LVEF (%)	0.96 (0.93, 0.98)	10.65	.0011
Mean blood pressure (mm Hg)	0.98 (0.96, 0.99)	8.94	.0028
IVCD	1.84 (1.22, 2.76)	8.55	.0035
Peak Vo_2 (mL kg^{-1} min^{-1})	0.95 (0.91, 0.99)	6.76	.0093
Serum sodium (mmol/L)	0.95 (0.92, 1.00)	4.76	.0292

HFSS = ([0.0216 × heart rate at rest] + [–0.0255 × mean arterial blood pressure] + [–0.0464 × left ventricular ejection fraction] + [–0.0470 × serum sodium] + [–0.0546 × peak Vo_2] + [0.6083 × presence (1) or absence (0) of intraventricular conduction defect (QRS interval ≥ 120 ms due to left or right bundle branch block, nonspecific intraventricular conduction delay, or ventricularly paced rhythm)] + [0.6931 × presence (1) or absence (0) of ischemic cardiomyopathy]).

The seven products are summed and the absolute value is taken as the HFSS.

HFSS ≥ 8.10: low risk.

HFSS 7.20-8.09: medium risk.

HFSS ≤ 7.19: high risk.

(Reproduced with permission from Lund et al.[38] Copyright © Elsevier.)

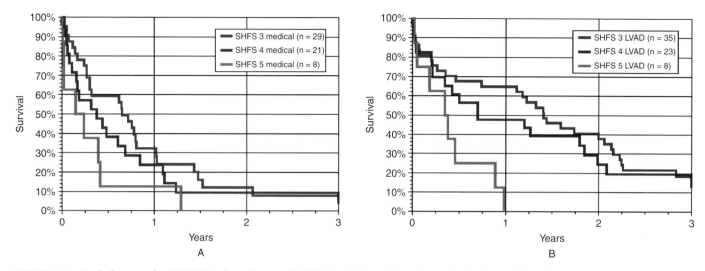

FIGURE 4–1. Survival among the REMATCH cohort when stratified by Seattle Heart Failure Score (SHFS) for medical and LVAD therapy. (Reproduced with permission from Rose et al.[71] Copyright © Elsevier.)

90-day survival rates ranging from 94% in low-risk patients to 18% in very-high-risk patients (Table 4–7B).[43]

Klotz et al developed a risk calculator for death in ICU after LVAD implantation based on a multivariate regression analysis of 13 variables that were found to be significant risk factors among a population of 241 LVAD patients (Fig. 4–2).[44] These risk factors included age (> 50 years), clinically/procedurally relevant data (ischemic cardiomyopathy, redo surgery, extracorporeal membrane oxygenation [ECMO], IABP, previous cardiac surgery, ventilation, emergency implant, inotropic support, renal replacement therapy, preoperative resuscitation, transfusion),

and laboratory values (blood urea nitrogen > 40 mg/dL, creatinine > 1.5 mg/dL, lactate > 3 mg/dL, platelets < 100, white blood cell count > 13, C-reactive protein > 8 mg/dL, hemoglobin < 12 g/dL, hematocrit < 35%, lactate dehydrogenase > 500 U/L, creatine kinase > 200 U/L, troponin > 20 ng/mL). Using a weighted risk score derived from these variables, a maximum score of 50 points represented a patient with the highest possible risk. Patients with a score of less than 15 were considered low risk for ICU mortality (15.8%), those with scores of 16 to 30 were considered moderate risk (48.2%), and those with greater than 30 points were considered high risk (65.2%).[44]

The bulk of data for patient selection prior to LVAD placement stems from patients with pulsatile devices. One study evaluated the predictive accuracy of various cumulative scores (developed in patients with pulsatile devices) in patients undergoing implantation of continuous-flow devices. Schaffer et al retrospectively calculated five cumulative scores in 86 patients who had undergone implantation of continuous-flow devices and assessed their accuracy in predicting 30-day, 90-day, and 1-year mortality.[45] The study demonstrated that the SHFS fared best in stratifying patients into low- and high-risk categories and in predicting postimplantation mortality, whereas both the SHFS and APACHE scores best predicted 1-year mortality.

TABLE 4–7A. Multivariable Analysis of Risk Factors for 90-Day In-Hospital Mortality After LVAD as DT (n = 222)

Patient Characteristics	Odds Ratio (CI)	P	Weighted Risk Score
Platelet count ≤ 148 × 10³/μL	7.7 (3.0-19.4)	<.001	7
Serum albumin ≤ 3.3 g/dL	5.7 (1.7-13.1)	<.001	5
International normalization ratio >1.1	5.4 (1.4-21.8)	.01	4
Vasodilator therapy	5.2 (1.9-14.0)	.008	4
Mean pulmonary artery pressures ≤25 mm Hg	4.1 (1.5-11.2)	.009	3
Aspartate aminotransferase >45 U/mL	2.6 (1.0-6.9)	.002	2
Hematocrit ≤34 %	3.0 (1.1-7.6)	.02	2
Blood urea nitrogen >51 U/dL	2.9 (1.1- 8.0)	.03	2
No intravenous inotropes	2.9 (1.1-7.7)	.03	2

Reproduced with permission from Lietz et al.[43]

TABLE 4–7B. Operative Risk Categories With Corresponding Cumulative Risk Score for 90-Day In-Hospital Mortality After LVAD Implantation as DT and Survival to Hospital Discharge and 1-Year Survival Depicted by the Operative Risk Categories[a]

Operative Risk Categories	Risk Score	No.	In-Hospital Mortality Within 90 Days				Survival, %		
			Observed, n	Predicted, n	% Probability (CI)		To Discharge, %	90 d	1 y
Low	0-8	65	2	1.6	2 (1.1-5.4)		87.5	93.7	81.2
Medium	9-16	111	12	13.7	12 (8.0-18.5)		70.5	86.5	62.4
High	17-19	28	10	7.9	44 (32.8-55.9)		26	38.9	27.8
Very high	>19	18	22	22.8	81 (66.0-90.9)		13.7	17.9	10.7

[a]Analysis limited to 208 patients available measure of pulmonay artery pressure and serum albumin level.

(Reproduced with permission from Lietz et al.[43])

SUMMARY

Patient selection for LVAD therapy requires comprehensive evaluation of the severity of HF in order to identify patients who have advanced enough HF to benefit from LVAD implantation but are not too far progressed. Certain risk factors have been noted to predict higher risk of morbidity and mortality in patients after LVAD placement. Moreover, several composite risk scores have also been developed to aid in identifying patients who may benefit from LVAD placement and in predicting prognosis after LVAD implantation. These observations have helped in recognizing these risk factors and targeting them in an attempt to improve LVAD outcomes. A constant reevaluation of the risk factors will be necessary as LVAD technology changes, the use of LVADs in end-stage HF patients becomes more widespread, and as management of LVAD patients continues to improve.

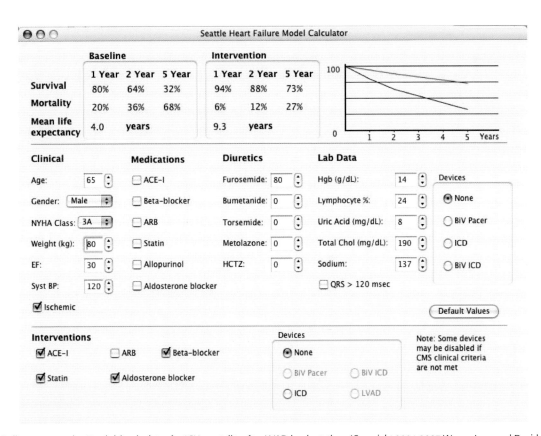

FIGURE 4–2. Online preoperative Excel risk calculator for ICU mortality after LVAD implantation. (Copyright 2004-2007 Wayne Levy and David Linker. University of Washington, Seattle, Washington.)

Historically, patient selection criteria have been derived from experience with pulsatile LVADs. However, as the experience with continuous-flow devices is growing, unique risks associated with these devices are emerging. Future research will more accurately identify specific patient selection criteria pertaining to continuous-flow devices.

REFERENCES

1. Rose EA, Moskowitz AJ, Packer M, et al. The REMATCH trial: rationale, design, and end points. Randomized Evaluation of Mechanical Assistance for the Treatment of Congestive Heart Failure. *Ann Thorac Surg.* 1999;67(3):723-730.

2. Rose EA, Gelijns AC, Moskowitz AJ, et al. Long-term mechanical left ventricular assistance for end-stage heart failure. *N Engl J Med.* 2001;345(20): 1435-1443.

3. Oz MC, Goldstein DJ, Pepino P, et al. Screening scale predicts patients successfully receiving long-term implantable left ventricular assist devices. *Circulation.* 1995;92(9 Suppl):II169-II173.

4. Deng MC, Weyand M, Hammel D, et al. Selection and management of ventricular assist device patients: the Muenster experience. *J Heart Lung Transplant.* 2000;19(8 Suppl):S77-S82.

5. Butler J, Young JB, Abraham WT, et al. Beta-blocker use and outcomes among hospitalized heart failure patients. *J Am Coll Cardiol.* 2006; 47(12):2462-2469.

6. Stevenson LW, Miller LW, Svigne-Nickens P, et al. Left ventricular assist device as destination for patients undergoing intravenous inotropic therapy: a subset analysis from REMATCH (Randomized Evaluation of Mechanical Assistance in Treatment of Chronic Heart Failure). *Circulation.* 2004;110(8):975-981.

7. Heywood JT. The cardiorenal syndrome: lessons from the ADHERE database and treatment options. *Heart Fail Rev.* 2004;9(3):195-201.

8. Butler J, Forman DE, Abraham WT, et al. Relationship between heart failure treatment and development of worsening renal function among hospitalized patients. *Am Heart J.* 2004;147(2):331-338.

9. Aaronson KD, Schwartz JS, Chen TM, Wong KL, Goin JE, Mancini DM. Development and prospective validation of a clinical index to predict survival in ambulatory patients referred for cardiac transplant evaluation. *Circulation.* 1997;95(12):2660-2667.

10. Stevenson LW. Patient selection for mechanical bridging to transplantation. *Ann Thorac Surg.* 1996;61(1):380-387.

11. Reedy JE, Swartz MT, Termuhlen DF, et al. Bridge to heart transplantation: importance of patient selection. *J Heart Transplant.* 1990;9(5):473-480.

12. Miller LW. Patient selection for the use of ventricular assist devices as a bridge to transplantation. *Ann Thorac Surg.* 2003; 75(6 Suppl):S66-S71.

13. Farrar DJ. Preoperative predictors of survival in patients with Thoratec ventricular assist devices as a bridge to heart transplantation. Thoratec Ventricular Assist Device Principal Investigators. *J Heart Lung Transplant.* 1994;13(1 Pt 1):93-100.

14. Frazier OH, Rose EA, Oz MC, et al. Multicenter clinical evaluation of the HeartMate vented electric left ventricular assist system in patients awaiting heart transplantation. *J Thorac Cardiovasc Surg.* 2001;122(6):1186-1195.

15. Dang NC, Topkara VK, Mercando M, et al. Right heart failure after left ventricular assist device implantation in patients with chronic congestive heart failure. *J Heart Lung Transplant.* 2006;25(1):1-6.

16. Oz MC, Rose EA, Levin HR. Selection criteria for placement of left ventricular assist devices. *Am Heart J.* 1995;129(1):173-177.

17. Ochiai Y, McCarthy PM, Smedira NG, et al. Predictors of severe right ventricular failure after implantable left ventricular assist device insertion: analysis of 245 patients. *Circulation.* 2002;106(12 Suppl 1):I198-I202.

18. Fukamachi K, McCarthy PM, Smedira NG, Vargo RL, Starling RC, Young JB. Preoperative risk factors for right ventricular failure after implantable left ventricular assist device insertion. *Ann Thorac Surg.* 1999;68(6):2181-2184.

19. Nakatani S, Thomas JD, Savage RM, Vargo RL, Smedira NG, McCarthy PM. Prediction of right ventricular dysfunction after left ventricular assist device implantation. *Circulation.* 1996;94(9 Suppl):II216-II221.

20. Morgan JA, John R, Lee BJ, Oz MC, Naka Y. Is severe right ventricular failure in left ventricular assist device recipients a risk factor for unsuccessful bridging to transplant and post-transplant mortality. *Ann Thorac Surg.* 2004;77(3):859-863.

21. Kavarana MN, Pessin-Minsley MS, Urtecho J, et al. Right ventricular dysfunction and organ failure in left ventricular assist device recipients: a continuing problem. *Ann Thorac Surg.* 2002;73(3):745-750.

22. Goldstein DJ, Seldomridge JA, Chen JM, et al. Use of aprotinin in LVAD recipients reduces blood loss, blood use, and perioperative mortality. *Ann Thorac Surg.* 1995;59(5):1063-1067.

23. Miller LW, Lietz K. Candidate selection for long-term left ventricular assist device therapy for refractory heart failure. *J Heart Lung Transplant.* 2006;25(7):756-764.

24. Aaronson KD, Patel H, Pagani FD. Patient selection for left ventricular assist device therapy. *Ann Thorac Surg.* 2003;75(6 Suppl):S29-S35.

25. Deng MC, Edwards LB, Hertz MI, et al. Mechanical circulatory support device database of the International Society for Heart and Lung Transplantation: third annual report—2005. *J Heart Lung Transplant.* 2005;24(9):1182-1187.

26. Morgan JA, Weinberg AD, Hollingsworth KW, Flannery MR, Oz MC, Naka Y. Effect of gender on bridging to transplantation and posttransplantation survival in patients with left ventricular assist devices. *J Thorac Cardiovasc Surg.* 2004;127(4):1193-1195.

27. Engelman DT, Adams DH, Byrne JG, et al. Impact of body mass index and albumin on morbidity and mortality after cardiac surgery. *J Thorac Cardiovasc Surg.* 1999;118(5):866-873.

28. Reeves BC, Ascione R, Chamberlain MH, Angelini GD. Effect of body mass index on early outcomes in patients undergoing coronary artery bypass surgery. *J Am Coll Cardiol.* 2003;42(4):668-676.

29. Sharma R, Anker SD. Cytokines, apoptosis and cachexia: the potential for TNF antagonism. *Int J Cardiol.* 2002;85(1):161-171.

30. Cohn W, Gregoric ID, Frazier OH. Staged reoperation: a novel strategy for high-risk patients. *Ann Thorac Surg.* 2007;83(4):1558-1559.

31. Frazier OH, Gregoric ID, Cohn WE. Initial experience with non-thoracic, extraperitoneal, off-pump insertion of the Jarvik 2000 Heart in patients with previous median sternotomy. *J Heart Lung Transplant.* 2006;25(5):499-503.

32. Frazier OH, Myers TJ, Westaby S, Gregoric ID. Clinical experience with an implantable, intracardiac, continuous flow circulatory support device: physiologic implications and their relationship to patient selection. *Ann Thorac Surg.* 2004;77(1):133-142.

33. Wilhelm MJ, Hammel D, Schmid C, et al. Long-term support of 9 patients with the DeBakey VAD for more than 200 days. *J Thorac Cardiovasc Surg.* 2005;130(4):1122-1129.

34. Fraser CD, Jr, Carberry KE, Owens WR, et al. Preliminary experience with the MicroMed DeBakey pediatric ventricular assist device. *Semin Thorac Cardiovasc Surg Pediatr Card Surg Annu.* 2006;109-114.

35. Letsou GV, Shah N, Gregoric ID, Myers TJ, Delgado R, Frazier OH. Gastrointestinal bleeding from arteriovenous malformations in patients supported by the Jarvik 2000 axial-flow left ventricular assist device. *J Heart Lung Transplant.* 2005;24(1):105-109.

36. Kar B, Delgado RM, III, Radovancevic B, et al. Vascular thrombosis during support with continuous flow ventricular assist devices: correlation with computerized flow simulations. *Congest Heart Fail.* 2005;11(4):182-187.

37. Rao V, Oz MC, Flannery MA, Catanese KA, Argenziano M, Naka Y. Revised screening scale to predict survival after insertion of a left ventricular assist device. *J Thorac Cardiovasc Surg.* 2003;125(4):855-862.

38. Lund LH, Aaronson KD, Mancini DM. Validation of peak exercise oxygen consumption and the Heart Failure Survival Score for serial risk stratification in advanced heart failure. *Am J Cardiol.* 2005;95(6):734-741.

39. Deng MC, Loebe M, El-Banayosy A, et al. Mechanical circulatory support for advanced heart failure: effect of patient selection on outcome. *Circulation.* 2001;103(2):231-237.

40. Gracin N, Johnson MR, Spokas D, et al. The use of APACHE II scores to select candidates for left ventricular assist device placement. Acute Physiology and Chronic Health Evaluation. *J Heart Lung Transplant.* 1998;17(10):1017-1023.

41. Levy WC, Mozaffarian D, Linker DT, et al. The Seattle Heart Failure Model: prediction of survival in heart failure. *Circulation.* 2006;113(11):1424-1433.

42. Levy WC, Mozaffarian D, Linker DT, Farrar DJ, Miller LW. Can the Seattle heart failure model be used to risk-stratify heart failure patients for potential left ventricular assist device therapy? *J Heart Lung Transplant.* 2009;28(3):231-236.

43. Lietz K, Long JW, Kfoury AG, et al. Outcomes of left ventricular assist device implantation as destination therapy in the post-REMATCH era: implications for patient selection. *Circulation.* 2007;116(5):497-505.

44. Klotz S, Vahlhaus C, Riehl C, Reitz C, Sindermann JR, Scheld HH. Pre-operative prediction of post-VAD implant mortality using easily accessible clinical parameters. *J Heart Lung Transplant.* 2010;29(1):45-52.

45. Schaffer JM, Allen JG, Weiss ES, et al. Evaluation of risk indices in continuous-flow left ventricular assist device patients. *Ann Thorac Surg.* 2009;88(6):1889-1896.

46. Mehra MR, Kobashigawa J, Starling R, et al. Listing criteria for heart transplantation: International Society for Heart and Lung Transplantation guidelines for the care of cardiac transplant candidates—2006. *J Heart Lung Transplant.* 2006;25(9):1024-1042.

47. Pennington DG, McBride LR, Peigh PS, Miller LW, Swartz MT. Eight years' experience with bridging to cardiac transplantation. *J Thorac Cardiovasc Surg.* 1994;107(2):472-480.

48. Oz MC, Goldstein DJ, Pepino P, et al. Screening scale predicts patients successfully receiving long-term implantable left ventricular assist devices. *Circulation.* 1995;92(9 Suppl):II169-II173.

49. McCarthy PM, Smedira NO, Vargo RL, et al. One hundred patients with the HeartMate left ventricular assist device: evolving concepts and technology. *J Thorac Cardiovasc Surg.* 1998;115(4):904-912.

50. Deng MC, Edwards LB, Hertz MI, et al. Mechanical circulatory support device database of the International Society for Heart and Lung Transplantation: third annual report—2005. *J Heart Lung Transplant.* 2005;24(9):1182-1187.

CHAPTER 5

INTERAGENCY REGISTRY FOR MECHANICALLY ASSISTED CIRCULATORY SUPPORT: CURRENT STATUS AND FUTURE DIRECTIONS

Katherine B. Harrington, Matthew D. Forrester, and William L. Holman

INTRODUCTION

The Interagency Registry for Mechanically Assisted Circulatory Support (INTERMACS) database is a national registry for patients who receive the US Food and Drug Administration (FDA) approved mechanical circulatory support devices (MCSD) as destination therapy (DT), bridge-to-transplantation (BTT), bridge-to-candidacy (BTC), or bridge-to-recovery (BTR). The registry is a collaboration that is funded by the National Heart, Lung, and Blood Institute (NHLBI), regulated by the FDA, reimbursed by the Center for Medicaid and Medicare Services (CMS), and helmed by the advanced heart failure and mechanical circulatory support professional community. MCSDs in trials pending FDA approval are not included in INTERMACS, although an increasing number of new device trials are designed with variables (patient demographics, adverse events, and outcome) that can be compared with INTERMACS data.

There have been several precursors to the INTERMACS database. From 1986 to 1995, a voluntary registry for the clinical use of mechanical ventricular assist devices and the total artificial heart was run by the International Society for Heart and Lung Transplantation (ISHLT) and the American Society for Artificial Internal Organs.[1,2] This yielded six reports encompassing more than 2000 patients.[3] In 2001, the Scientific Council on Mechanical Circulatory Support of the International Society for Heart and Lung Transplantation (ISHLT) established a Mechanical Circulatory Support Device database, which published three annual reports in which data on 655 device implants from 60 centers around the world were presented.[4-6]

Following the pivotal Randomized Evaluation of Mechanical Assistance for the Treatment of Congestive Heart Failure (REMATCH) trial, which showed implantation of left ventricular assist devices (LVADs) as destination therapy was a viable option for heart failure treatment,[7] there was recognition that patients receiving an MCSD would need long-term follow-up. In addition

to the benefits over maximal medical management, the REMATCH trial also highlighted the considerable mortality and adverse event rate associated with MCSD, notably infection, coagulopathies, and device malfunction. Thus, with the emergence of MCSD as legitimate long-term therapy, the patients' often complete dependence on the devices, and the room for improvement in considerable mortality and morbidity, a comprehensive, mandatory, and adequately funded clinical registry was deemed imperative.

In 2003, when CMS extended coverage for MCSD as destination therapy, they called for all patients receiving an MCSD as destination therapy to be entered in a nationally audited registry. On June 1, 2005 the University of Alabama at Birmingham received the competitive contract as the data collection and clinical coordination center, with the United Network of Organ Sharing (UNOS) as the clinical research organization charged with maintaining the database. The database began prospectively enrolling patients on June 23, 2006, and to date data on well over 1000 devices have been published.[8] On March 27, 2009 CMS mandated that all US hospitals approved for MCSD as destination therapy enroll their patients in the INTERMACS database. At this point, 107 centers are participating and over 3000 patients have been entered.[9]

DESIGN AND STRUCTURE

The goals of the registry are to "investigate, facilitate, and improve the application of mechanical circulatory support as a long-term therapy to improve the duration and quality of life for patients with advanced heart failure."[10] As a registry, the hope is to facilitate the adoption of evidence into clinical practice more quickly than a randomized clinical trial, as well as provide a means for postmarket surveillance and provide data on the comparative effectiveness and patient selection for MCSD.

Upon enrollment, patient profile data, implant and device data, and scheduled follow-up information are collected. Adverse events are reported at the time of occurrence for infection, device failure, neurologic event, and death. Additional adverse events including bleeding, arrhythmia, myocardial infarction, right heart failure, hepatic dysfunction, respiratory failure, renal dysfunction, hemolysis, and venous thrombosis are indentified and collected at specific follow-up intervals (Table 5–1). All data and hospitals go through an auditing process, and there is a formal peer review process for adverse event adjudication. Shared access to the overall data is available to all participants, and quarterly reports are sent to all sites, as well as to the collaborating federal partners and industry collaborators. Individual institutions also receive site specific reports of their own data for hospital performance committees or joint commission compliance quality reporting. In addition, participation in the INTERMACS database fulfills the FDA requirement for reporting device-related events.

Another important function of INTERMACS is as a comparison group for new MCSDs in FDA Investigational Device Exemption (IDE) trials. This role is emerging but will likely become increasingly useful as more devices receive approval. Plans are also under way for INTERMACS to participate in

TABLE 5-1. Major Adverse Events Collected in INTERMACS Registry

Arterial non-CNS thromboembolism
Bleeding
Cardiac arrhythmia
Device malfunction
Hemolysis
Hepatic dysfunction
Hypertension
Major infection
Myocardial infarction
Neurological dysfunction
Pericardial collection
Psychiatric episode
Renal dysfunction
Respiratory failure
Right heart failure
Venous thrombosis
Wound dehiscence

(Reproduced with permission from Kirklin et al.[10] Copyright © Elsevier.)

postmarket approval (PMA) studies of FDA-approved devices. PMA research reflects real-world experience with MCSDs that is typically not addressed in prospective IDE trials because patient numbers are lower, follow-up tends to be shorter, and entry criteria are more restrictive.

PATIENT STRATIFICATION AND SELECTION

Whereas medical treatment of heart failure is commonly tested and approved in patients with moderate heart failure and then extended to more severe patients, the efficacy of MCSD therapy to provide clinically meaningful survival and improved quality of life even for the sickest patients has already been established.[7] However, MCSD implantation exposes the patient to significant risk. Most of the mortality accrues in the early postoperative period, and multiple studies have shown it is related closely to degree of organ dysfunction and urgency of implant.[2] There is hope that moving the window of intervention toward less emergent, less severe cases will improve overall mortality. However, MCSD implantation exposes the patient to significant morbidity as well, which also accrues over time. Thus, one of the main goals of the INTERMACS database is to identify predictors of good outcomes and risk factors for adverse events, and then to use these data to refine patient selection to maximize outcome.

A crucial predictor for the success of MCSD implantation is patient selection. The spectrum of eligible patients with "severe" heart failure is quite broad, encompassing patients living at home with mild fluid overload and functional limitations to

critically ill hospitalized patients on intravenous inotropic support and temporary circulatory support. Seven patient profiles with three modifiers have been designed for the INTERMACS registry.[11] These levels further stratify patients who are candidates for MCSD by defining subsets within New York Heart Association (NYHA) classes III and IV (Table 5–2). Levels one through five are all degrees of NYHA class IV. The levels are defined over time on optimal medical therapy. This includes angiotensin-converting enzyme inhibitors, β-blockers, diuretics, digoxin, biventricular pacing for eligible patients, and revascularization or surgical repair of mechanical complications following myocardial infarction. The levels attempt to define the important clinical milestones which trigger escalation of therapy, and movement between the levels is defined by failure of various levels of optimal medical therapy.

■ INTERMACS PROFILE 1

This is the most dramatic profile, these patients are in critical cardiogenic shock, are unstable, and have life-threatening hypoperfusion. They are frequently on rapidly escalating doses of inotropic medications and are not stabilized even with temporary circulatory support (TCS) devices (eg, intra-aortic balloon pump [IABP]). Critical hypoperfusion is confirmed by acidosis, rising lactate levels, oliguria, and possibly rising liver function tests indicative of "shock liver."

■ INTERMACS PROFILE 2

These patients are "dependent" on inotropic therapy with stable hemodynamics but declining nutritional status, renal function, and fluid retention. This level can also define patients with declining status who are unable to tolerate inotropic therapy due to tachyarrhythmias or clinical ischemia. These patients may also have TCS in place, with temporary hemodynamic stabilization but continual decline of nutritional, fluid, and renal status.

■ INTERMACS PROFILE 3

Patients in level 3 are "stable" on midlevel doses of inotropic support (eg, ≤ 5 μg/kg/min of dopamine or dobutamine or < 0.5 μg/kg/min of milrinone) but exhibit failure to wean from these inotropes. Failure to wean must be well documented after multiple attempts at weaning are aborted due to hypotension, worsening symptoms, or progressive organ dysfunction. It is important to distinguish this subset of patients who are truly stable on midlevel inotropic support from those who are undergoing a subtle decline in nutrition, fluid balance, and renal dysfunction, and thus considered level 2. Patients in level 3 can either be hospitalized or represent stable patients on home intravenous inotropic therapy. These patients can have multiple repeat hospitalizations to stabilize episodes of fluid retention or renal dysfunction. Patients who require temporary circulatory devices would by definition be hospitalized.

■ INTERMACS PROFILE 4

Level 4 represents patients who are at home on oral therapy with resting symptoms. These patients also have orthopnea and

TABLE 5–2. INTERMACS Level of Limitation

INTERMACS Profile	Brief Description	Profile Description	Time Frame to Intervention
1. Critical cardiogenic shock	"Crash and burn"	Persistent hypotension despite escalating inotropic support and eventually IABP, critical organ hypoperfusion	Definite intervention needed with hours
2. Progressive decline	"Sliding on inotropes"	Intravenous inotropic support with acceptable hemodynamics, but continuing decline in fluid status, renal function, or nutrition	Definite intervention needed with days
3. Stable but inotrope dependent	"Dependent stability"	Stability reached with mild to moderate inotropic doses, but failure to wean	Definite intervention needed over weeks to months
4. Recurrent advanced heart failure	"Frequent flyer"	Able to wean inotropes but frequent relapses	Definite intervention needed over weeks to months
5. Exertion intolerant	"Housebound"	Severely limited activity tolerance. Comfortable at rest. Mild volume overload	Variable urgency
6. Exertion limited	"Walking wounded"	Less severe activity tolerance but fatigues easily. No volume overload	Variable urgency
7. Advanced NYHA III	"Placeholder"	Without recent unstable fluid balance	Transplantation or circulatory support may not be currently indicated

ABP, intra-aortic balloon pump; NYHA, New York Heart Association.

(Reproduced with permission from Stevenson et al.[11] Copyright © Elsevier.)

dyspnea during basic activities of daily living (ADLs). Some, but not all, of these patients require frequent hospitalizations. They may have physically restricting lower extremity edema or ascites with concomitant abdominal bloating, nausea, anorexia, and precarious nutritional status. These patients may gradually deteriorate such that they are unable to be stabilized at a recurrent hospitalization and thus require a "higher" profile label.

INTERMACS PROFILE 5

Patients in this subset have no symptoms at rest but with fluid overload and often underlying renal dysfunction. They have a severely limited activity tolerance and difficulty performing ADLs. They are exertion intolerant and are largely housebound.

INTERMACS PROFILE 6

Level 6 represents patients who also have no symptoms at rest and also no signs of fluid overload. They have slightly improved exercise tolerance compared to level 5 and are able to perform ADLs with minimal discomfort and likely are able to walk outside the house.

INTERMACS PROFILE 7

These patients have low ejection fraction and history of previous decompensation but are currently clinically stable and comfortable

with a reasonable amount of activity. There are plans to expand this group further based on exercise tolerance or an objective scoring system.

■ MODIFIERS

In the original INTERMACS profile classification scheme there was one modifier for frequent arrhythmias. Following the first interval analysis of the data, it was deemed necessary to add two more: temporary circulation support and the need for frequent rehospitalization.

The arrhythmia modifier is used for recurrent ventricular tachyarrhythmias which can be a major contributor to clinical risk in a certain subset of advanced heart failure patients. This includes sustained ventricular tachycardia or ventricular fibrillation and can be a modifier for all seven levels. Currently, this will most likely lead to an implantable cardioverter-defibrillator and be represented by recurrent shocks, usually more than twice weekly. Malignant arrhythmias were thought to be a contraindication to use of MCSD, but more recent data suggest these patients do well, and indeed the arrhythmias often resolve after stabilization. In the first annual report, 20% of all patients were limited by ventricular arrythmias.[10]

The TCS modifier describes patients on devices designed only for temporary support in the hospital and thus can only modify levels 1, 2, and 3 when hospitalized. This modifier includes patients on IABP, extracorporeal membrane oxygenation (ECMO), TandemHeart, Impella, Levitronix, and BVS5000 or AB5000.

The frequent hospitalization, or "frequent flier" (FF) modifier, is only applied to outpatients and thus only applicable to level 3 patients at home, levels 4 through 6, and, by definition, rarely level 7. These are patients requiring frequent emergency room visits or hospitalizations for treatment of fluid overload such as intravenous diuresis, ultrafiltration, paracentesis, or thoracentesis or temporary intravenous vasoactive therapy. "Frequent" is defined as at least two visits/admissions in the past 3 months or three in the past 6 months.[11]

PREDICTING OUTCOMES

Patient selection is a critical factor in MCSD outcomes. The objective is to select patients who are appropriate surgical candidates but are most likely to benefit from current device therapies. Over the years, many efforts have been made to risk-stratify preoperative MCSD candidates. Several novel scoring systems have been developed along with efforts to use preexisting scoring systems.

Several independently derived scoring systems have been developed and vetted to predict outcomes in critically ill patients and then applied to VAD populations, such as the Acute Physiology and Chronic Health Evaluation II (APACHE II) score, Seattle Heart Failure Model (SHFM) score, Heart Failure Survival Score (HFSS), the Model for End-Stage Liver Disease (MELD) score, and the Sequential Organ Failure Assessment (SOFA) score. Other scoring systems have been generated from cohorts of VAD patients to risk-stratify patients after device implantation, such as the Columbia University VAD score, Lietz-Miller risk score, and the INTERMACS profiles, as well as several individual center risk scores.

The APACHE II score was developed using a multi-institutional cohort of 5815 patients and sought to measure the severity of disease in intensive care unit patients. It consists of 13 variables: temperature, mean arterial pressure, heart rate, respiratory rate, partial pressure of arterial oxygen, arterial pH, serum sodium, serum potassium, serum creatinine, hematocrit, white blood cell count, Glasgow coma score, and age. A significant increase in hospital deaths was shown in congestive heart failure patients whose APACHE II score exceeded 20.[12] This score was applied to a cohort of 31 patients who received the VE HeartMate I LVAD as BTT versus 50 patient treated with optimal medical management. Gracin and colleagues found that patients with APACHE II scores between 10 and 20 treated with LVADs received a mortality benefit over medical therapy.[13]

The SHFM was derived from a cohort of 1125 NYHA IIIb or IV patients. Twenty-one preoperative variables weighted by hazard ratio were used to calculate a risk score: age, gender, NYHA class, weight, ejection fraction, systolic blood pressure, presence of ischemic cardiomyopathy, daily furosemide equivalent dose, inotrope use, statin use, allopurinol use, angiotensin-converting enzyme inhibitor use, angiotensin receptor blocker use, β-blocker use, potassium-sparing

diuretic use, implantable cardioverter-defibrillator use, hemoglobin, serum lymphocyte percentage, serum uric acid, serum cholesterol, and serum sodium. Two modifiers are added for LVAD patients: IABP use and mechanical ventilation. Once the score is calculated, it can be inserted into a formula to calculate predicted survival:

$$S(t) = e^{\wedge}[-0.045 * t * e^{\wedge}(\text{SHFM score})]$$

The MELD score has been used to calculate adverse event rates for cirrhotics undergoing major surgery and is thought to be a good measure of multisystem dysfunction. A single-center report evaluated the prognostic valve of MELD score on LVAD candidates. They showed that higher MELD scores were associated with decreased survival at 6 months, increased transfusion requirements, increased rate of renal replacement therapy, and longer intensive care unit and total hospital stay.[14] These data were validated with comparison against a similar cohort from the INTERMACS database.

The SOFA score has been established as a valid score for multisystem organ failure. It has been shown to be a good predictor of early (within the first week) postoperative mortality after VAD. A SOFA score of ≥ 11 had a specificity of 96.7% and a sensitivity of 92.9% for predicting early mortality.[15]

Columbia University VAD score was derived from a cohort of 130 patients with the VE HeartMate I device implanted as BTT.[16] Points are assigned for five preoperative factors that were shown to predict preoperative mortality:

- Ventilation—4
- Post cardiotomy shock—2
- Previous LVAD—2
- Central venous pressure greater than 16mm Hg—1
- Prothrombin time greater than 16 seconds—1

Patients were stratified into high (> 5 points) and low (≤ 5 points) risk groups, with the high-risk group having a significantly increased operative mortality (46% vs 12%).

The Lietz-Miller score was derived from a cohort of 222 patients with the XVE HeartMate I device implanted as DT.[17] They assigned points to nine preoperative factors that were associated with 90-day in-hospital mortality:

- Platelets fewer than 148,000/μL—7
- Albumin less than 3.3 g/dL—5
- International normalized ratio (INR) greater than 1.1—4
- Vasodilator therapy—4
- Mean pulmonary artery pressure less than 25 mm Hg—3
- Aspartate aminotransferase greater than 45 U/L—2
- Hematocrit less than 34%—2
- Serum urea nitrogen greater than 51 mg/dL—2
- And lack of intravenous inotropic support—2

Patients were risk-stratified into four groups, low (0-8 points), medium (9-16 points), high (17-19), and very high (> 19) risk. Survival at 1 year was 81.2%, 62.4%, 27.8%, and 10.7%, respectively.

A single-center cohort study comparing the Lietz-Miller, Columbia VAD, APACHE II, SHFM, and INTERMACS scores on a retrospective cohort of all patients receiving continuous flow LVADs showed that the SHFM score was the best predictor of actual mortality.[18] Patients determined to be high risk by INTERMACS (levels 1 and 2), APACHE II, and SHFM had a significantly higher mortality rate. SHFM was able to predict mortality at 30 days, 90 days, and 1 year, whereas APACHE II and INTERMACS were able to predict mortality at 90 days and 1 year. High- and low-risk groups formed using the Columbia VAD score and Lietz-Miller score had no statistically significant difference between their outcomes.

Several studies have investigated the ability of the INTERMACS scale to predict outcomes following MCSD implantation.[2,19] A multi-institutional study using the INTERMACS data set showed the patient risk factors for mortality following MCSD implantation were age (RR = 1.41), ascites (RR = 2.04), increased bilirubin (RR = 1.49), and INTERMACS level 1 (RR = 1.59). Further interval analysis of the INTERMACS data showed the patient profile had a statistically significant impact on survival.[20]

Alba and colleagues looked specifically at the usefulness of the INTERMACS scale levels 1 through 4 to predict patient outcomes after MCSD implantation. Levels 1 and 2 were grouped into group A and levels 3 and 4 were grouped into group B. Mortality at 30 days was significantly higher in group A (38% vs 11%), and Cox regression models showed overall poorer survival (HR = 2.7). The main causes of death were multisystem organ failure in group A and infection in group B. This group also calculated the Columbia University VAD score for each patient and found it had a strong association with INTERMACS level, but that was not accurate in discriminating risk in more stable heart failure patients (INTERMACS ≥ 3) due to the acuity of the variables.

Many of the calculators are complex and may be limited to academic purposes. The INTERMACS scoring system is easily assessed at the bedside. With various scoring and classification systems it is also difficult to compare results between various studies, as their cohorts are heterogeneous. The INTERMACS profiles also seek to standardize the patient populations compared in studies of various devices to more accurately examine outcomes.

CURRENT INTERMACS OUTCOMES

Since creation of the INTERMACS, data have been published from more than 1000 primary LVAD implants and over 1400 patients who received primary and secondary devices.[8] Two annual reports have been published,[8,10] as well as several studies based on the data set.[19-21] The majority (1324) of devices are implanted as primary devices with 1092 LVADs, 3 RVADs, 179 biventricular assist devices (bi-VADs), and 50 total artificial hearts (TAHs). An additional 94 secondary devices were implanted. In both the first and second annual reports, the vast majority of devices were implanted in patients in INTERMACS levels 1 and 2. The most recent data show of the 1092 primary LVADs implanted, 30% were implanted in level 1 patients, 40% in level 2, 15.4% in level 3, 9.7% in level 4, and fewer than 5% in levels higher than 4.[8] There

TABLE 5–3. INTERMACS Level at Time of Implant for Primary LVAD

INTERMACS Level	Number	Percentage (%)
1. Critical cardiogenic shock	328	30.0
2. Progressive decline	437	40.0
3. Stable but inotrope dependent	168	15.4
4. Recurrent advanced heart failure	106	9.7
5. Exertion intolerant	21	1.9
6. Exertion limited	12	1.1
7. Advanced NYHA III	20	1.8
Total	1092	100.0

NYHA, New York Heart Association.

(Reproduced with permission from Kirklin et al.[8] Copyright © Elsevier.)

has been a trend between the first and second annular reports; the proportion of level 1 implants has decreased from 38% to 27% of the total devices (Table 5–3). This may reflect a recognition of the higher mortality risk for patients in INTERMACS level 1 demonstrated in the first annual report.[10] The preimplant device strategy continued to be focused on bridge-to-transplant (BTT) and bridge-to-candidacy (BTC) with only 10% initially chosen as destination therapy (DT).[8] The role of MCSD therapy for patients with NYHA class III heart failure (INTERMACS levels 5-7) has not been fully defined (Table 5–4). INTERMACS data will certainly have an important part in resolving this issue.

There has been a major change in device composition of the database since the HeartMate II axial flow pump received clinical approval by the FDA in April 2008. No axial flow pump was FDA approved for the first several years of the INTERMACS database, but following its approval there has been a dramatic increase in continuous or axial flow pumps (85% of primary LVADs between July 2008 and January 2009) such that at the time of the second annual report continuous flow pumps now represent the majority (51.6%) of primary LVADs in the database.[8] This will certainly have implications for ongoing outcomes data.

The most common adverse events in the INTERMACS database following MSCD implant remain bleeding and infection, followed by cardiac arrhythmia and respiratory failure. Continuous flow devices demonstrated lower rates of device malfunction, infection, hepatic dysfunction, and neurologic events compared to pulsatile flow devices.[8] The durability of rotary pumps is expected to improve over time, thereby increasing the value received for each patient.

Overall actuarial survival of the primary LVAD cohort was 83% at 6 months, 74% at 1 year, and 55% at 2 years. Primary LVAD patients had significantly better mortality than their bi-VAD counterparts.

TABLE 5–4. INTERMACS Level at Time Implant and Device Strategy

INTERMACS Level	BTT	BTC	DT	BTR	RT	Other	Total
1. Critical cardiogenic shock	120	162	21	16	8	1	328
2. Progressive decline	217	173	39	5	2	1	437
3. Stable but inotrope dependent	85	58	23	1	0	1	168
4. Recurrent advanced heart failure	41	50	12	3	0	0	106
5. Exertion intolerant	11	9	1	0	0	0	21
6. Exertion limited	5	5	2	0	0	0	12
7. Advanced NYHA III	17	1	2	0	0	0	20
Total	496	458	100	25	10	3	1092

NYHA, New York Heart Association.

(Reproduced with permission from Kirklin et al.[8] Copyright © Elsevier.)

transition from pulsatile to continuous flow MCSD. Between the first and second annual reports, the percentage of devices implanted in patients in level 1 has decreased dramatically with a shift toward patients in levels 2 through 7. The emerging role of INTERMACS as a comparison group for devices in FDA trials and the use of INTERMACS for PMA studies are increasingly important to the field of MCS. The unique collaboration of regulatory agencies, clinicians, and industry is guiding the most effective use of MCSDs to improve the duration and quality of life for patients, while optimizing the cost and value to society.

BTT patients had better survival than their BTC and DT therapy cohorts at 3 months (91% vs 85% vs 85%), 6 months (90% vs 78% vs 72%), and 12 months (84% vs 72% vs 64%). Survival stratified by INTERMACS level shows an increased risk of early mortality in patients in level 1 at the time of implant. Multivariate analysis showed that older age, greater severity of right ventricular failure (higher right atrial pressure and higher bilirubin), and cardiogenic shock were predictors for early death (Fig. 5–1). Fifty-two percent of BTT patients, 35% of BTC patients, and 10% of DT patients had undergone transplant within 1 year of device implant.[8]

The INTERMACS registry has already proved capable of indentifying predictors of good outcomes and risk factors for adverse outcomes. It also has captured the period of dramatic

REFERENCES

1. Pae WE, Pierce WS. Combined registry for the clinical use of mechanical ventricular assist pumps and the total artificial heart. *J Heart Transplant.* 1986 Jan;5(1):6-7.
2. Holman WL, Kormos RL, Naftel DC, et al. Predictors of death and transplant in patients with a mechanical circulatory support device: a multi-institutional study. *J Heart Lung Transplant.* 2009 Jan;28(1):44-50.
3. Pae WE, Jr, Pierce WS. Combined Registry for the clinical use of mechanical ventricular assist pumps and the total artificial heart: first official report—1986. *J Heart Transplant.* 1987 March;6(2):68-70.
4. Deng MC, Edwards LB, Hertz MI, Rowe AW, Kormos RL. Mechanical Circulatory Support Device database of the International Society for Heart and Lung Transplantation: first annual report—2003. *J Heart Lung Transplant.* 2003 June;22(6):653-662.
5. Deng MC, Edwards LB, Hertz MI, et al. Mechanical circulatory support device database of the International Society for Heart and Lung Transplantation: third annual report—2005. *J Heart Lung Transplant.* 2005 Sep;24(9):1182-1187.
6. Deng MC, Edwards LB, Hertz MI, et al. Mechanical Circulatory Support Device database of the International Society for Heart and Lung Transplantation: second annual report—2004. *J Heart Lung Transplant.* 2004 Sep;23(9):1027-1034.
7. Rose EA, Gelijns AC, Moskowitz AJ, et al. Long-term use of a left ventricular assist device for end-stage heart failure. *N Engl J Med.* 2001 Nov 15;345(20):1435-1443.
8. Kirklin JK, Naftel DC, Kormos RL, et al. Second INTERMACS annual report: more than 1,000 primary left ventricular assist device implants. *J Heart Lung Transplant.* 2010 Jan;29(1):1-10.
9. The INTERMACS website. 9-1-0010. Ref Type: Online Source.
10. Kirklin JK, Naftel DC, Stevenson LW, et al. INTERMACS database for durable devices for circulatory support: first annual report. *J Heart Lung Transplant.* 2008 Oct;27(10):1065-1072.
11. Stevenson LW, Pagani FD, Young JB, et al. INTERMACS profiles of advanced heart failure: the current picture. *J Heart Lung Transplant.* 2009 June;28(6):535-541.
12. Knaus WA, Draper EA, Wagner DP, Zimmerman JE. APACHE II: a severity of disease classification system. *Crit Care Med.* 1985 Oct;13(10):818-829.
13. Gracin N, Johnson MR, Spokas D, et al. The use of APACHE II scores to select candidates for left ventricular assist device placement. Acute Physiology and Chronic Health Evaluation. *J Heart Lung Transplant.* 1998 Oct;17(10):1017-1023.
14. Matthews JC, Pagani FD, Haft JW, Koelling TM, Naftel DC, Aaronson KD. Model for end-stage liver disease score predicts left ventricular assist device

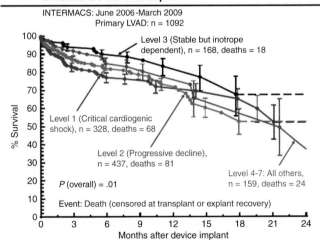

INTERMACS Level at Implant

FIGURE 5–1. Actuarial survival by INTERMACS level in LVAD implant. (Reproduced with permission from Kirklin et al.[8] Copyright © Elsevier.)

operative transfusion requirements, morbidity, and mortality. *Circulation.* 2010 Jan 19;121(2):214-220.

15. Qedra N, Reus T, Ilmaz K, Roman T, Uppe H, Etzer R. Preopeperative Application of modified Sequential Organ Failure Assessment score (SOFA) in prediction of early postoperative mortality after implantation of ventricular assist devices (VAD). *J Heart Lung Transplant.* 2008 Feb;27(2 Suppl I):S61.

16. Rao V, Oz MC, Flannery MA, Catanese KA, Argenziano M, Naka Y. Revised screening scale to predict survival after insertion of a left ventricular assist device. *J Thorac Cardiovasc Surg.* 2003 April;125(4):855-862.

17. Lietz K, Long JW, Kfoury AG, et al. Outcomes of left ventricular assist device implantation as destination therapy in the post-REMATCH era: implications for patient selection. *Circulation.* 2007 July 31;116(5):497-505.

18. Schaffer JM, Allen JG, Weiss ES, et al. Evaluation of risk indices in continuous-flow left ventricular assist device patients. *Ann Thorac Surg.* 2009 Dec;88(6):1889-1896.

19. Alba AC, Rao V, Ivanov J, Ross HJ, Delgado DH. Usefulness of the INTERMACS scale to predict outcomes after mechanical assist device implantation. *J Heart Lung Transplant.* 2009 Aug;28(8):827-833.

20. Holman WL, Pae WE, Teutenberg JJ, et al. INTERMACS: interval analysis of registry data. *J Am Coll Surg.* 2009 May;208(5):755-761.

21. Holman WL, Kirklin JK, Naftel DC, et al. Infection after implantation of pulsatile mechanical circulatory support devices. *J Thorac Cardiovasc Surg.* 2010 June;139(6):1632-1636.

CHAPTER 6
DESTINATION THERAPY

Stephen Westaby and Gabriele B. Bertoni

Successful intervention in acute coronary syndromes together with the improved management of dysrhythmia provides an increasing pool of heart failure patients spread through a greater age range.[1] Young adults with palliated congenital heart disease, myocarditis, or idiopathic dilated cardiomyopathy enter the lower end of the spectrum. Heart failure beyond the benefits of medical therapy is a frightening and desperately debilitating condition. These patients have very poor quality of life, becoming progressively more dependent on hospital admissions for stabilization and outpatient nursing for palliative care.

The prevalence and incidence of heart failure in Western countries is 1% and 0.15% respectively.[2] In the United States, an estimated 5 million people are affected, 60% of whom have systolic dysfunction and reduced left ventricular ejection faction (LVEF). Two-thirds have ischemic heart disease where myocardial infarction is the trigger for left ventricular structural remodeling. Remodeling is progressive but can be attenuated by treatment with ACE inhibitors and β-blockers which reduce myocardial wall tension.

Advanced heart failure is characterized by the presence of structural myocardial disease and symptoms that limit daily activity (New York Heart Association [NYHA] III and IV, or stage D disease; Fig. 6–1 and Table 6–1) despite attempted maximum medical therapy.[3] This description applies to between 300,000 and 800,000 patients in the United States and approximately 60,000 in the United Kingdom. Twenty percent of stage D patients are younger than 65 years. In the United States, they may be in hospital awaiting cardiac transplant or at home receiving intravenous milrinone infusion for symptomatic relief left ventricular shape and volume are important predictors of survival. In both ischemic and idiopathic dilated cardiomyopathy patients, increased chamber sphericity and the onset of mitral regurgitation are markers of worse prognosis. Mitral regurgitation occurs secondary to altered left ventricular geometry, papillary muscle dysfunction, and eventual annular dilatation. Volume overload causes progressive dilatation and decreased survival. Patients with an LVEF of less than 30% and left ventricular end-systolic volume index (LVESVI) of greater than 150 mL/m^2 have a 5-year survival of only 54%.[4]

For end-stage patients, cardiac transplantation provides the benchmark for increased longevity and symptomatic relief.[5] But, by the very nature of heart failure, the vast majority of patients are either too old or have organ dysfunction or comorbidity which excludes them from this operation. There is an enormous therapeutic gap between at least 60,000 stage D patients younger than 65 years in the United States and around 2200 organ donors (12,000 and < 200 in the United Kingdom, respectively).[6] In the

light of recent medical and surgical advances, the evidence base for transplantation is less secure than it appeared to be 30 years ago. Clear indications include refractory cardiogenic shock, dependence on intravenous inotropic support (both status I) or persistent class IV symptoms with a peak oxygen consumption of less than 10 mL/kg/min. Without treatment, these patients have a projected mortality varying from imminent to more than 50% at 6 months while transplant survival exceeds 80% at 1 year and is almost 50% at 10 years.[5]

Most patients awaiting transplant are ambulatory on oral therapy (status II) and have a less impaired peak oxygen consumption (11-14 mL/kg/min). In this category, the benefits of committal to a transplant waiting list are less certain. In Germany, Deng showed that status II patients who were accepted for transplant but did not receive a donor heart had similar 3- and four-year risk-adjusted survival rates.[7] In 2000, the average waiting time (869 days) for a group O blood type transplant recipient exceeded by far the projected life span of that patient at the time of wait listing. Survival was achieved only by mechanical bridging with a left ventricular assist device (LVAD). In contrast, many status II patients actually improved (symptomatically and prognostically) given the detailed medical management provided by a specialist heart failure service.[8] Others with clearly defined hibernating myocardium or anterior scar can be selected out for revascularization or left ventricular restoration surgery.[9]

Many centers stress the need for reevaluation of waiting list candidates by repeated measurement of peak oxygen uptake. Patients are deemed too well for transplant if they remain stable with a sustained improvement of peak oxygen uptake by more than 2 mL/kg/min (as many as 30% of status II candidates). Shah et al showed that survival at 1 and 3 years for status II patients removed from the transplant waiting list after 6 months of optimized treatment was 100% and 92%, respectively.[8] Patients with idiopathic dilated cardiomyopathy frequently showed spontaneous improvement with much better long-term outlook than for ischemic cardiomyopathy.

The new millennium has brought a paradigm shift in the approach to patients with severe heart disease. The development of nontransplant surgical options is now the clear priority. One reason for this change is the important observation that the adult heart is not necessarily a postmitotic organ and that regeneration of cardiac myocytes may occur given the appropriate signaling processes.[10] Left ventricular unloading with a blood pump can reverse the remodeling process while new cardiomyocytes can be developed from nonmyocyte precursors.[11] The goal of both medical and surgical treatment is to arrest or reverse the progression of the remodeling process. Currently, there are few guidelines and no clear algorithms as to which operation best suits an individual patient who no longer gains symptomatic relief from medical treatment. Coronary surgery may improve the contractility of stunned or hibernating myocardium in 60% to 70% of cases as long as the LVESVI is below 100 mL/m^2.[4] A critical mass of reversibly ischemic myocardium must be present to achieve global improvement in left ventricular function. Heart failure patients without angina or reversible ischemia do not have improved outlook with coronary surgery.

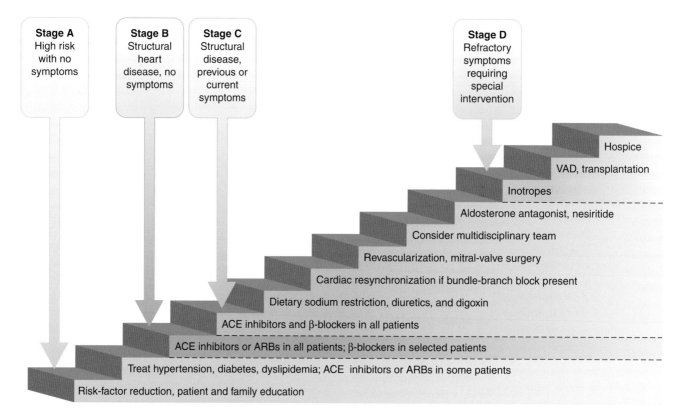

FIGURE 6–1. Stages of Heart Failure and Treatment Options. **Stage A:** High risk for heart failure in the absence of structural heart disease or symptoms of heart failure. **Stage B:** Structural heart disease in the absence of symptoms. **Stage C:** Structural heart disease and current or previous symptoms of heart failure (NYHA class I, II, III, or IV). **Stage D:** Refractory symptoms of heart failure at rest despite maximal medical therapy, are hospitalized, and require specialized interventions or hospice care (NYHA class IV). (Reproduced with permission from Jessup M, Brozena S. Heart failure. *N Engl J Med.* 2003 May 15;348(20):2007-2018. Copyright Massachusetts Medical Society. All rights reserved.)

In ischemic patients with noncontractile anterolateral segments, left ventricular restoration surgery can reduce left ventricular size and improve shape (globular to elliptical). This operation is best performed before the LVESVI rises above 120 mL/m² though

TABLE 6–1. NYHA Classification

NYHA Class	Symptoms
I	No symptoms and no limitation in ordinary physical activity, eg, shortness of breath when walking, climbing stairs, etc
II	Mild symptoms (mild shortness of breath and/or angina) and slight limitation during ordinary activity
III	Marked limitation in activity due to symptoms, even during less-than-ordinary activity, eg, walking short distances (20-100 m) Comfortable only at rest
IV	Severe limitations. Experiences symptoms even while at rest. Mostly bed-bound patients

NYHA, New York Heart Association.

success has been achieved in much larger hearts.[12] On average, the LVEF increases by 20% to 35%. This immediate and substantial change contrasts with the delayed and unpredictable improvement after revascularization for hibernation. Despite these operations and the use of mitral valve repair in idiopathic dilated cardiomyopathy, there are many patients for whom conventional surgery has little to offer. In this case, long-term mechanical circulatory support may offer a realistic opportunity for symptomatic relief and improved survival.[13]

THE ROLE OF MECHANICAL CIRCULATORY SUPPORT

Mechanical blood pumps were developed in the late 1960s with the intention to treat terminally ill patients for whom donor organs were unavailable.[14] DeBakey achieved the first postcardiotomy mechanical bridge-to-recovery with a pulsatile LVAD in 1966. Cooley and Liotta first used a total artificial heart for bridge-to-cardiac transplantation in 1969. After more than $160 million of federal funds had been invested in artificial heart development, DeVries at the University of Utah performed the first definitive total artificial heart operation (Jarvik-7) in December 1982. Only four permanent Jarvik-7 implants were performed (with survival to 2 years) though 160 had been used for bridge-to-transplantation before thromboembolism, infection, and durability issues precluded widespread use as a permanent substitute.[15] With improved technology, complete mechanical cardiac replacement recently resumed with the AbioCor total artificial heart. This has so far provided implant durations of up to 17th months.[15] Despite the use of transcutaneous energy transfer, mechanical reliability and thromboembolism continue to frustrate biventricular replacement so that left ventricular support is the preferable option for most patients. Cardiac excision and replacement is an irretrievable step whereas unloading with an LVAD may promote myocardial improvement, particularly in patients with myocarditis or idiopathic dilated cardiomyopathy.[16]

The pulsatile implantable LVADs recently licensed for permanent, or "destination therapy" (DT) by the US Food and Drug Administration (FDA) resulted from the National Heart, Lung and Blood Institute (NHLBI) development program for long-term circulatory support initiated in the 1970s. Two of these systems, the vented electric HeartMate (Thoratec Corporation, Pleasanton, California) and Novacor (World Heart Corporation, Ottawa, Canada) LVADs were volume displacement blood pumps that provided cardiac output with pulse pressure.[17] They are implanted in series but empty and completely replace the native left ventricle. Unidirectional blood flow is achieved with valved conduits. A thick percutaneous lead transmits the electric power line and external vent (which equalizes air pressure behind the pusher plate) through the abdominal wall. These LVADs are implanted via median sternotomy and upper abdominal incision into a pre- or intraperitoneal pocket beneath the left hemidiaphragm. The inflow cannula crosses the diaphragm and is inserted into the apex of the left ventricle. The outflow conduit conveys blood from the pump's blood sac to the ascending aorta. During normal operation, the pump completely empties the left ventricle and provides pulsatile blood flow at physiological levels of up to 12 L/min.

The original goal of these devices was to provide long-term circulatory support for end-stage cardiomyopathy patients who were not transplant candidates. Their temporary use as a bridge-to-cardiac transplantation provided a clinical laboratory to evaluate safety and effectiveness, device durability, and the patients' quality of life.[18]

For those presenting with chronic low output state and multiple organ failure, recovery of end-organ function occurs gradually at a rate that depends on the duration and severity of preexisting heart failure. Most patients return to NYHA class I and are able to wait at home for a transplant. Hospital discharge improves the patient's psychosocial status, reduces costs, and decreases the incidence of hospital-based infections. Recovery of the hemodynamic, nutritional, metabolic, and cellular abnormalities of heart failure has, in turn, improved the outcome after cardiac transplant.[19] Approximately 75% of patients survive the waiting time to transplant and most are discharged from the hospital. Nevertheless, adverse events occur frequently and for transplant candidates a shorter duration of support is optimal.

These first-generation devices have been subject to three major complications.[20] Pyogenic infection developing in the percutaneous driveline may subsequently involve the bloodstream, pump pocket, or blood sac. Antibiotic treatment often leads to fungal supra infection. Neurological events (either cerebral hemorrhage or embolic infarction) occur with both devices. Catastrophic mechanical failure may originate in the driveline, the controller, the inflow or outflow valves/conduits, or the pusher-plate pumping mechanism.

THE SIGNIFICANCE OF THE REMATCH TRIAL

In 1998, the FDA approved the HeartMate VE LVAD for bridge-to-cardiac transplantation. This portable system allowed the patient to leave hospital with an acceptable quality of life and presented the opportunity for its use in otherwise untreatable, severely symptomatic patients deemed ineligible for transplant. Accordingly, the REMATCH (Randomized Evaluation of Mechanical Assistance for the Treatment of Congestive Heart Failure) trial was conducted in 20 experienced LVAD centers which randomized 120 NYHA class IV patients to either the HeartMate VE LVAD or continued medical therapy.[21] The primary endpoint was death from any cause. Secondary endpoints included the incidence of serious adverse events, the number of days in hospital, the quality of life, symptoms of depression, and NYHA functional status. Adverse events were considered serious if they caused death or permanent disability, were life threatening, or required prolonged hospitalization. At enrolment, 68% of patients were dependent on intravenous inotropes with or without an intra-aortic balloon pump (IABP). The remainder who were well enough to undergo exercise testing had a peak myocardial oxygen consumption (MVO_2) of 9.18 ($\pm$ 1.98) mL/kg/min, a value that is highly predictive of early death. This prediction was borne out by the 75% 1-year mortality for medically treated patients, which exceeds that for AIDS and breast, lung, and colon cancer. Sixty-eight patients with a mean age of 66 ($\pm$ 9.1) years received the LVAD. No patient in either group crossed over and none underwent cardiac transplant.

Median survival was 409 days in the LVAD group and 150 days in the medical therapy patients. Two-year mortality, the primary endpoint, was 38% lower in the LVAD group, but only 23% of these patients survived for 2 years. Nevertheless, use of the LVAD was associated with a 48% relative reduction in the risk of death during the follow-up period and a 27% absolute reduction in mortality at 1 year (Fig. 6–2). This treatment effect is nearly four times that of β-blockers or angiotensin-converting enzyme (ACE) inhibitors and suggests that, for every 1000 patients with advanced heart failure, the use of an LVAD would prevent at least 270 deaths annually. These survival data set the precedent for the use of an "off-the-shelf" device to treat advanced heart failure with a potential application which exceeds transplant by a factor of 50:1.

In contrast to the substantial survival benefits, the anticipated improvement in quality of life was limited by LVAD-related complications. Infection caused 41% of the LVAD deaths in REMATCH and, by 2 years, the probability of LVAD mechanical failure causing death or reoperation was 35%. Of the 68 LVAD patients, 10 required a second major surgical procedure to replace the pump. In addition, there was a 42% incidence of bleeding complications by 6 months and an overall stroke rate of 10%.

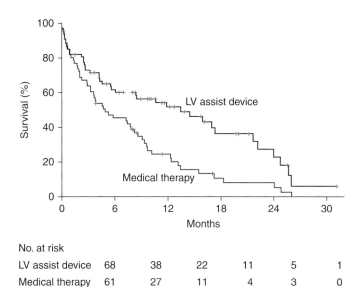

FIGURE 6–2. Kaplan-Meier Analysis of Survival in the REMATCH trial comparing left ventricular (LV) assist devices and optimal medical therapy. (Reproduced with permission from Rose et al.[21] Copyright Massachusetts Medical Society. All rights reserved.)

During the course of REMATCH recruitment, it was clear that early mortality occurred largely through failure to turn around moribund patients with multiorgan failure. With more sensible patient selection, the initial 2-year survival of 21% improved to 43% later in the recruitment phase.

By implanting before the antimortem state and with improved postoperative management, an 85% 1-year and 65% 2-year survival has been described at the University of Utah with the same device. Nevertheless, the inherent limitations of driveline infection and mechanical failure have driven the pursuit of newer pump technology with even better outcomes.

NEW BLOOD PUMPS TECHNOLOGY

Recognizing the limitations of pulsatile blood pumps, the Devices and Technology Branch of the NHLBI (1994) invited submissions for the development of innovative new LVADs. The design criteria sought to provide the ideal fully implantable long-term circulatory support device. From the engineering standpoint, the pumping mechanism had to be relatively simple, mechanically reliable, and durable with an efficient power supply. For the patient, the implantable components should be small, silent, and noninvasive. For the surgeon, the device must be easy to implant with the potential for safe removal in the event of functional improvement in the native heart. The blood contact surfaces must produce minimal blood trauma or immunogenicity. Lastly, cost-effectiveness should be possible through prolonged, safe, and widespread use in the community.

Blood pump bioengineering has evolved rapidly. Currently, there are more than 30 new LVADs undergoing bench, animal, or clinical testing. Axial-flow and centrifugal devices have been developed with blood-washed microceramic bearings, electromagnetic

suspension, and now hydrodynamic suspension to offer greater durability and minimal thrombogenicity. The power packs and controllers are easily portable. The risk of driveline infection has been reduced by finer, more flexible electric cables, transcutaneous energy transmission, or skull-mounted pedestals. Concern that pulse pressure was required to main end-organ function in the human has been dispelled by both laboratory and clinical experience.[22] Pump output from these devices varies between 3 to 8 L/min requiring only 6 to 10 W of power. In some devices, the patient can regulate pump speed according to activity level, and there is an inverse relationship between continuous-flow rate and pulsatility in the circulation.[23]

Currently, there are several second-generation devices in clinical use worldwide for the indication of DT. DT data from the Jarvik-2000 device was recently published in Europe, with 46 patients demonstrating a 0% rate of pump malfunction or infection, five patients with duration of support more than 3 years (with longest event-free survival at 7.5 years), and 19 patients with ongoing support, three patients who were successfully transplanted, and 22 deaths.[24] The HeartMate II device was recently randomized in a 2:1 implantation ratio against the HeartMate XVE in a prospective randomized DT study. Patients with continuous-flow devices demonstrated superior actuarial survival rates at 2 years (58% vs 24%, $P = .008$) with lower adverse events and less frequent device replacement.[25]

PATIENT SELECTION FOR DESTINATION THERAPY

To date, there are no absolute guidelines to help identify which heart failure patients should be referred for DT. Clearly, stages C and D patients who are amenable to conventional surgery by ventricular remodeling, revascularization of hibernating myocardium, or mitral valve repair should be preferentially treated along those lines leaving mechanical circulatory support or cardiac transplant in reserve.[4] However, the majority of patients have no target lesion, have little prospect of improvement in left ventricular function, and are not eligible for transplant. These patients are often left untreated irrespective of their age or severity of symptoms. Given the "off-the-shelf" mechanical alternative, this evaluation process deserves a logical, ethical, and economic consideration of the following types of questions: Is use of a blood pump fundamentally different from that of a pacemaker or implantable defibrillator? Shouldn't those with acute myocarditis or idiopathic dilated cardiomyopathy be allowed a trial for left ventricular recovery before transplant is undertaken? Is it necessary to exclude transplant candidates from clinical trials of long-term circulatory support?

Analysis of mortality in LVAD patients shows that many die from irreversible organ dysfunction or comorbidity in the early postoperative setting. These patients likely would have benefited from device insertion earlier in their disease course. Under the current scheme, patients considered for DT must be considered ineligible for cardiac transplantation and in an advanced state of decompensation. Many already have undergone previous cardiac surgery, multisite pacing, an implantable defibrillator, or are admitted to the hospital with intravenous inotropic support or a balloon pump. However, as data from the REMATCH study suggest, patients who are declined for transplant may also have an unacceptable risk for LVAD surgery. This applies particularly to patients in irreversible cardiogenic shock for more than 12 hours, those with established renal failure or sepsis, and those with cachexia or liver dysfunction.

With increasing experience, it is clear that an implant for DT should be performed on an elective basis, not as a salvage procedure. The patient must be a reasonable candidate for cardiac surgery with acceptable risk. With safer more user-friendly devices and less invasive implantation techniques, LVAD deployment should be considered in patients other than those who are end-stage in their disease. Reasonable selection criteria for ambulatory but severely restricted patients out of hospital would be NYHA class IV symptoms for more than 60 days on maximum tolerated medical treatment, LVEF 25% or less, peak Vo_2 14 mL/kg/min or less, or intravenous inotrope dependence (Table 6–2).

Given that circulatory support and improved end-organ function have improved the results of cardiac transplantation, it is illogical and perhaps unethical to exclude transplant-eligible patients from clinical trials of LVAD therapy. In our own experience, a number of patients accepted for transplant expired on the waiting list because of protocol limitations that prohibited them from receiving a device. Subsequently, the notion of a "bridge to decision" has emerged, whereby nontransplant-eligible candidates can improve on an LVAD before being reassessed for transplant and listed in the event that a donor heart becomes available. Some LVAD patients may inevitably follow the transplant route through progressive right heart failure. Irrespective of transplantation, there are at least 60,000 stage D patients younger than 65 years in the United States and 12,000 in the United Kingdom who may wish to be considered for an LVAD. Preliminary evidence shows LVADs to be cost-effective by reducing hospital dependency and allowing the patient to return to a productive life. Multisite pacing and implantable defibrillators are already widely accepted despite limited symptomatic benefit. Blood pumps are far more effective in

TABLE 6–2. Patient Selection for Destination Therapy

Indications for Destination Therapy

Advanced heart failure symptoms (class IIIB or IV) with one of the following:

(1) On optimal medical management (OMM), including dietary salt restriction, diuretics, digitalis, β-blockers, spironolactone, and ACE inhibitors, but failing to respond

(2) Class III or IV heart failure and dependent on intra-aortic balloon pump (IABP) and/or inotropes

(3) Intolerant of angiotensin-converting enzyme (ACE) inhibitors or β-blockers

Body surface area (BSA) > 1.2 m²

Ineligible for cardiac transplant

Vo_2 max < 14 mL/kg/min or < 50% of predicted Vo_2 max with attainment of anaerobic threshold (AT)

Left ventricular ejection faction (LVEF) < 25%

Contraindications for Destination Therapy

Heart failure due to uncorrected thyroid disease, obstructive or restrictive cardiomyopathy

Technical obstacles, which pose an inordinately high surgical risk

Body mass index (BMI) > 40 kg/m²

Positive pregnancy test

Platelet count < 50,000

Untreated aortic aneurysm > 5 cm

Psychiatric disease, irreversible cognitive dysfunction or psychosocial issues

Presence of active, uncontrolled infection

Intolerance to anticoagulant or antiplatelet therapies

International normalized ratio (INR) > 2.5, which is not due to anti-coagulant therapy, or Plavix (clopidogrel)

Evidence of intrinsic hepatic disease

Severe chronic obstructive pulmonary disease (COPD) or severe restrictive lung disease

Fixed pulmonary hypertension with a pulmonary vascular resistance (PVR) > 8 Wood units that is unresponsive to pharmacological intervention

cerebrovascular accidents (CVA) within 90 d

Creatinine > 3.5 mg/dL or the need for chronic renal replacement therapy

Significant peripheral vascular disease accompanied by rest pain or extremity ulceration

Any condition, other than heart failure, that could limit survival to < 3 y

relieving symptoms, and further controlled clinical trials are needed to determine survival benefit with the newest devices. Even though DT with an LVAD represents an expensive treatment for end-stage heart failure, there is already a precedent for managing patients with end-stage disease using a mechanical device. Hemodialysis is used extensively in renal failure patients irrespective of age to achieve 60% 2-year survival. As newer devices promise improved outcomes, we are entering an era when LVAD therapy may exceed these outcomes and become the staple in management of end-stage heart failure.

MANAGEMENT OF PATIENTS ON LONG-TERM LVAD SUPPORT

Unloading of the failing left ventricle with an LVAD often improves native cardiac function.[26] There is regression of myocyte hypertrophy, improved cytosolic calcium transients, upregulation of apoptosis inhibiting genes, improved mitochondrial function, and normalization of myocardial phenotype expression. These changes are associated with enhanced inotropic response to β-agonists and reversal of degenerative changes in cytoskeletal proteins and dystrophin.

These effects on the native heart partly explain the sustained improvement and excellent quality of life experienced by some DT patients. The best results have been achieved when the LVAD was implanted electively into NYHA class IV dilated cardiomyopathy patients who failed medical therapy but had not deteriorated into cardiogenic shock. For these patients, mechanical unloading results in a symbiotic relationship between the blood pump and the native heart. In contrast, terminally ill ischemic cardiomyopathy patients who are inotrope or balloon pump dependent tend not to improve to the same extent.

Medical management plays a particularly important part in patients with newer-generation continuous-flow devices. Both axial-flow and centrifugal blood pumps are particularly sensitive to the differential pressure across the device (afterload). Patients with these pumps benefit from continuous afterload reduction (ACE inhibition and β-blockade) with a mean systemic blood pressure of 60 to 70 mm Hg and little more than 10 to 20 mm Hg pulse pressure in the circulation. An increase in peripheral vascular resistance may reduce pump flow dramatically with failure to unload the left ventricle and renewed symptoms of breathlessness.

Reduction in preload does not alter the flow rate of a rotary blood pump. Hypovolemia or pulmonary hypertension may result in negative left ventricular pressure throughout the whole native cardiac cycle. Septal shift may then occur and produce an hourglass-shaped left ventricle. This impairs right ventricular function and decreases blood flow through the lungs. Thus, cardiac filling must be balanced with pump speed. This is most challenging in the immediate postoperative period when bleeding or elevated pulmonary vascular resistance (in response to transfusion) may impair blood flow to the left atrium. Care must be taken not to disrupt the native cardiac cycle. At low or medium pump speed, cardiac output is derived partly through the apical conduit but is boosted by stroke volume ejection

through the aortic valve. The optimal situation is when about 30% of systemic flow is provided antegrade by the unloaded left ventricle while the LVAD delivers 3 to 5 L/min blood flow through the apex. Whether this strategy improves recovery better than complete unloading, remain to be seen. Although complete unloading can lead to atrophy, this state may be required before the left ventricular pressure work index is reduced sufficiently to promote reverse remodeling.

With axial-flow pumps, the native heart is often able to respond to increased physiologic demand by increasing cardiac output. Our long-term Jarvik FlowMaker patients with idiopathic dilated cardiomyopathy have virtually normal exercise tolerance (NYHA I) without changing their pump speed from 10,000 rpm (revolutions per minutes). There is little point in incorporating heart rate–responsive or pulse pressure–sensitive technology when the patient's own heart provides this function.

While mechanical reliability has increased and the infection risk substantially decreased with second-generation pumps, the problems of thrombus formation and thromboembolism persist. Many thromboembolic events have occurred within the first 4 weeks of LVAD implantation and may derive from preexisting cardiac thrombi or thrombosis in the aortic root if the aortic valve does not open. Detailed anticoagulation management is an imperative for these patients. Most devices are maintained on warfarin within an international normalized ratio (INR) between 2.0 and 3.0. Many centers also add aspirin to this regime though the combination comes at the cost of an added risk for gastrointestinal or cerebral hemorrhage.

SUMMARY

Heart failure treatment strategies can now be tailored to the patient's requirements. Clearly, the very restricted number of donor hearts should be reserved for those patients most likely to benefit in life expectancy and quality of life. Those with potentially recoverable myocardium could be offered a trial mechanical unloading with adjuvant medical treatment while holding transplant in reserve. Those with irreversible myocardial injury and little residual function can be offered an LVAD for symptomatic relief either permanently or pending transplant.

The prospects for community-based lifetime mechanical circulatory support as a widespread treatment for advanced heart failure have improved substantially since the REMATCH trial. Prolonged clinical experience has established the safety of diminished pulse pressure circulation, and mechanical unloading appears to promote recovery of the failing left ventricle. To achieve reproducible success, intervention must be brought forward out of the end-stage arena. The mechanical reliability, user-friendly nature, and freedom from infection in the smaller continuous-flow devices facilitate this approach while detailed medical management improves long-term outcome. In the future, prolonged circulatory support may be used to reverse the heart failure syndrome while the myocardium is regenerated by stem cell therapy.[27]

REFERENCES

1. Redfield MM. Heart failure: an epidemic of uncertain proportions. *N Engl J Med*. 2009;347(18):1442-1444.

2. McMurray JJ, Stewart S. Epidemiology, aetiology, and prognosis of heart failure. *Heart*. 2000;83(5):596-602.

3. Hunt SA. ACC/AHA 2005 guideline update for the diagnosis and management of chronic heart failure in the adult: a report of the American College of Cardiology/American Heart Association Task Force on Practice Guidelines (Writing Committee to update the 2001 Guidelines for the Evaluation and Management of Heart Failure). *J Am Coll Cardiol*. 2005;46(6):e1-e82.

4. Westaby S. Coronary revascularization in ischemic cardiomyopathy. *Surg Clin North Am*. 2004;84(1):179-199.

5. Hosenpud JD, Bennett LE, Keck BM, Boucek MM, Novick RJ. The Registry of the International Society for Heart and Lung Transplantation: eighteenth Official Report—2001. *J Heart Lung Transplant*. 2001;20(8):805-815.

6. Deng MC. Orthotopic heart transplantation: highlights and limitations. *Surg Clin North Am*. 2004;84(1):243-255.

7. Deng MC, De Meester JM, Smits JM, Heinecke J, Scheld HH. Effect of receiving a heart transplant: analysis of a national cohort entered on to a waiting list, stratified by heart failure severity. Comparative Outcome and Clinical Profiles in Transplantation (COCPIT) study group. *BMJ*. 2000;321(7260):540-545.

8. Shah NR, Rogers JG, Ewald GA, et al. Survival of patients removed from the heart transplant waiting list. *J Thorac Cardiovasc Surg*. 2004;127(5):1481-1485.

9. Westaby S. Non-transplant surgery for heart failure. *Heart*. 2000;83(5):603-610.

10. Beltrami AP, Urbanek K, Kajstura J, et al. Evidence that human cardiac myocytes divide after myocardial infarction. *N Engl J Med*. 2001;344(23):1750-1757.

11. Britten MB, Abolmaali ND, Assmus B, et al. Infarct remodeling after intracoronary progenitor cell treatment in patients with acute myocardial infarction (TOPCARE-AMI): mechanistic insights from serial contrast-enhanced magnetic resonance imaging. *Circulation*. 2003;108(18):2212-2218.

12. Dor V. Surgical remodeling of left ventricle. *Surg Clin North Am*. 2004;84(1):27-43.

13. Westaby S. Ventricular assist devices as destination therapy. *Surg Clin North Am*. 2004;84(1):91-123.

14. Frazier OH. Mechanical cardiac assistance: historical perspectives. *Semin Thorac Cardiovasc Surg*. 2000;12(3):207-219.

15. Arabia FA, Copeland JG, Smith RG, et al. International experience with the CardioWest total artificial heart as a bridge to heart transplantation. *Eur J Cardiothorac Surg*. 1997;11(Suppl):S5-S10.

16. Muller J, Wallukat G, Weng YG, et al. Weaning from mechanical cardiac support in patients with idiopathic dilated cardiomyopathy. *Circulation*. 1997;96(2):542-549.

17. Goldstein DJ, Oz MC, Rose EA. Implantable left ventricular assist devices. *N Engl J Med*. 1998;339(21):1522-1533.

18. Navia JL, McCarthy PM, Hoercher KJ, et al. Do left ventricular assist device (LVAD) bridge-to-transplantation outcomes predict the results of permanent LVAD implantation? *Ann Thorac Surg*. 2002;74(6):2051-2062.

19. Frazier OH, Rose EA, McCarthy P, et al. Improved mortality and rehabilitation of transplant candidates treated with a long-term implantable left ventricular assist system. *Ann Surg*. 1995;222(3):327-336.

20. Pasque MK, Rogers JG. Adverse events in the use of HeartMate vented electric and Novacor left ventricular assist devices: comparing apples and oranges. *J Thorac Cardiovasc Surg*. 2002;124(6):1063-1067.

21. Rose EA, Gelijns AC, Moskowitz AJ, et al. Long-term mechanical left ventricular assistance for end-stage heart failure. *N Engl J Med*. 2001; 345(20):1435-1443.

22. Westaby S, Banning AP, Saito S, et al. Circulatory support for long-term treatment of heart failure: experience with an intraventricular continuous flow pump. *Circulation*. 2002;105(22):2588-2591.

23. Frazier OH, Myers TJ, Westaby S, Gregoric ID. Clinical experience with an implantable, intracardiac, continuous flow circulatory support device: physiologic implications and their relationship to patient selection. *Ann Thorac Surg*. 2004;77(1):133-142.

24. Westaby S, Siegenthaler M, Beyersdorf F, et al. Destination therapy with a rotary blood pump and novel power delivery. *Eur J Cardiothorac Surg*. 2010;37(2):350-356.

25. Slaughter MS, Rogers JG, Milano CA, et al. Advanced heart failure treated with continuous-flow left ventricular assist device. *N Engl J Med*. 2009;361(23):2241-2251.

26. Zhang J, Narula J. Molecular biology of myocardial recovery. *Surg Clin North Am*. 2004;84(1):223-242.

27. Flugelman MY, Lewis BS. The promise of myocardial repair—towards a better understanding. *Eur Heart J*. 2004;25(17):1483-1485.

CHAPTER 7
BRIDGE-TO-TRANSPLANTATION

Lyle D. Joyce

BACKGROUND

Ventricular assist devices (VADs) were initially developed as a means of supporting the left ventricle during failure to wean from cardiopulmonary bypass. The hope was that this support would be short term, giving the myocardium time to recover, and that the device would be able to be explanted. In contrast, the first total artificial hearts (TAHs) were developed as a permanent therapy (even though the first two implants actually served as a bridge-to-transplantation [BTT]).[1,2] The Jarvik-7 TAH was the first mechanical device to be implanted as a permanent therapy for a patient who had been declared a nontransplant candidate by three transplant centers.[3] This landmark case provided enough optimism to the medical community to stimulate swamping the US Food and Drug Administration (FDA) with requests from multiple US centers for not only approval of using the Jarvik TAH but also a variety of left ventricular assist devices (LVADs) as destination therapy (DT). In 1984, the FDA attempted to slow the pace of clinical implants by not approving any more centers for permanent implantation, limiting their use to bridging end-stage heart failure patients to transplant. At the time, many anticipated that this move would signal the end of long-term mechanical circulatory support, since the thought of carelessly using donor organs in such high-risk patients was considered unfathomable. To the contrary, several devices emerged with clinical outcomes that demonstrated patients on VADs could actually become superior candidates to those intensive care unit (ICU)–bound patients being treated medically.

This chapter will discuss the use of long-term mechanical circulatory support devices. The use of the intra-aortic balloon pump (IABP) and outcomes of short-term ventricular support devices such as Impella, TandemHeart, and the Circulite pumps are less well-documented but show promise as BTT devices where donor availability makes it feasible to use such devices for short periods of time when full cardiac support is not necessary.

INDICATIONS FOR BRIDGE-TO-TRANSPLANT

In general, a patient should be considered for LVAD therapy as a bridge-to-transplant (BTT) when he or she meet the criteria for congestive heart failure and is eligible for cardiac transplant according to standard United Network for Organ Sharing (UNOS) guidelines (Table 7–1). Assessment of cardiac function is often based on hemodynamic criteria such as systolic blood pressure less than 80 mm Hg (or mean arterial pressure , 65 mm Hg), pulmonary capillary wedge pressure (PCWP) more than 20 mm Hg, systemic vascular resistance more than 2100 dynes/s/cm², urine output less than 20 mL/h (in adults) despite diuretics, and a cardiac index less than 2 L/min/m² despite maximal inotropic or IABP support.[4] A list of the criteria to consider when selecting a patient for LVAD support as BTT is given in Table 7–2. In addition to the clinical parameters that guide patient selection, one must also consider the anticipated waiting time, which is a function of patient size, blood type, UNOS region, and status.

DEVICE SELECTION

■ FIRST-GENERATION DEVICES

Investigators initially believed that the human body would require pulsatile flow. For that reason the first-generation pumps were all volume displacement pumps. Cardiac support was excellent, but there were numerous reasons for desiring an alternative. The devices were large and some were not implantable. Infection became a major source of morbidity and mortality. The stiff drivelines required for such devices provide irritation to the skin which often leads to a break in the skin/lead seal and vulnerability to ascending infections.[5] Durability[6] and noise were issues with some implants. Thromboembolic complications were not uncommon. The size of pulsatile devices limited their use in smaller patients and increased the likelihood of pocket infections and bleeding difficulties.[7] The REMATCH (Randomized Evaluation of Mechanical Assistance for the Treatment of Congestive Heart Failure) randomized trial[8] documented the clinical value of such devices, but the future would demand devices that were more durable and user-friendly with lower complication rates. In addition to the first-generation LVADs, use of a TAH has been successful in bridging patients with biventricular failure to transplantation. In Copeland's series from the University of Arizona, 81 patients underwent implantation of a CardioWest TAH device with a survival to transplantation of 79%, compared with 46% survival among 35 control patients who met the same entry criteria but did not receive the artificial heart.[9] TAH patients also experienced an increase in posttransplant survival relative to medical controls, suggesting that bridging with device may be the optimal treatment for patients with irreversible biventricular failure that are candidates for cardiac transplantation.

■ SECOND-GENERATION DEVICES

It may have been primarily the cost of the first-generation devices that led to the clinical experience which provided the recognition that nonpulsatile flow may be tolerated by the human body. For many years, VADs and TAHs were not FDA approved for marketing. Therefore, financial coverage for patient care with an assist device was not available. Few centers had the financial strength to support large investigative numbers. Meanwhile, surgeons were experiencing situations where patients could not be weaned from the cardiopulmonary bypass pump after cardiac surgery. Rather than allowing the patient to

TABLE 7–1. Current Prioritization System for Cardiac Transplantation as Directed by the UNOS

Status 1A

    Patients who must stay in hospital and require IV drugs, a heart assist device, a ventilator, or who have a life expectancy of a week or less without a transplant

Status 1B

    Patients who are not confined to hospital but require a heart assist device or continuous IV medications

Status 2

    A patient of any age who does not meet the criteria for status 1A or 1B

UNOS, United Network for Organ Sharing.

die on the operating room table, several surgeons began using a "poor man's" LVAD, right VAD (RVAD), or bientricular assist devices (BiVAD) by simply keeping the patient on centrifugal pumps for a few days in hopes that the patient's myocardium might recover to the point of being able to explant the devices. As experience increased, physicians learned that not only did many patients survive, but that other organ systems seemed to flourish on continuous flow.[10] Perhaps this observation should not have been a surprise had we believed what we were taught in our medical physiology classes in that only the major blood vessels in the human body possess pulsatile blood flow. At the capillary level where actual tissue interchange takes place, there is no pulsatility.[11] Don Olsen and others conducted animal studies to further verify the feasibility of providing acceptable blood flow to end organs without pulsatility.[12-15]

Axial-flow pumps provide many potential advantages over their pulsatile predecessors. The small size provides promise for use even in small children. The low noise level provides the opportunity for patients to anomalously attend events such as church services, orchestra concerts, and other quiet activities without annoying those who sit next to them. The lack of need for a compliance chamber allows the driveline to be smaller in diameter and much more pliable, reducing the weight and irritation on the skin exit site. This appears to be responsible for a lower rate of driveline infection. While axial-flow pumps may be fraught with a higher rate of pump thrombosis, it appears that there will be a significantly lower rate of embolic phenomenon.

TABLE 7–2. Patient Selection for BTT

Indications for BTT

    New York Heart Association (NYHA) class IV

    Inotropic support, if tolerated

    No contraindication for listing as status 1A or status 1B meet the following:

    • Pulmonary Capillary Wedge Pressure (PCWP) or PAD > 20 mm Hg

    • Cardiac Index < 2.2 L/min/m^2 or systolic blood pressure < 90 mm Hg

    Body surface area (BSA) > 1.2 m^2

Contraindications to BTT

    Heart failure due to uncorrected thyroid disease, obstructive or restrictive cardiomyopathy

    Technical obstacles, which pose an inordinately high surgical risk

    Body mass index (BMI) > 40 kg/m^2

    Positive pregnancy test

    Platelet count < 50,000

    Untreated aortic aneurysm > 5 cm

    Psychiatric disease, irreversible cognitive dysfunction, or psychosocial issues

    Presence of active, uncontrolled infection

    Intolerance to anticoagulant or antiplatelet therapies

    International normalized ratio (INR) > 2.5, which is not due to anticoagulant therapy, or Plavix (clopidogrel)

    Evidence of intrinsic hepatic disease

    Severe chronic obstructive pulmonary disease (COPD) or severe restrictive lung disease

    Fixed pulmonary hypertension with a pulmonary vascular resistance (PVR) > 6 Wood units that is unresponsive to pharmacologic intervention

    CVA within 90 d

    Creatinine > 3.5 mg/dL or the need for chronic renal replacement therapy

    Significant peripheral vascular disease accompanied by rest pain or extremity ulceration

    Any other contraindication to transplantation

Unless the emboli are pumped out through the aortic valve in an unloaded left ventricle, the low clearances within the axial-flow pumps will not allow passage of significant-sized emboli to cause end-organ damage. D. Olsen (oral communication, 2003) studied this effect by injecting clot into the left ventricle in the animal and found that the clot was pulverized to such a degree that there were no end-organ embolic detrimental effects. This was pushed all the way to pump occlusion by "wash-in" thrombus.

All presently available axial-flow pumps have the same principle effect on cardiac function although there is some question as to whether the Jarvik intraventricular pump will differ from the other extraventricular pumps. Each system is implanted with the expectation of needing both Coumadin (warfarin) as well as antiplatelet therapy. Learning curves are being worked out in the clinical trials with each device. The unique unanswered questions with each device in comparison to the pulsatile devices include what changes are required in the implantation techniques as well as changes that are required in post-op management, including fluid management and anticoagulation. General consensus suggests that axial-flow pumps will not unload the left ventricle as completely as pulsatile pumps. For BTT, this does not seem to be an issue. In fact, space issues at the time of transplant may be improved since some preserved cardiac dilatation provides greater flexibility in donor size acceptance.

Goldstein et al studied the impact of pump speed on end-organ function with the DeBakey VAD and its relationship to patient size.[16] There was no statistically significant difference with respect to pump speed, but larger patients had statistically significant higher pump flows. There was no difference in renal function, but larger patients had lower postoperative total bilirubin levels. The larger flow in larger patients with similar pump speeds likely is a result of increased blood return to the left ventricle. The resultant increase in left ventricular end-diastolic pressure (LVEDP) is directly proportional to the pressure difference across the pump. LVAD pump flow in axial-flow pumps is equal to the LVEDP—aortic diastolic pressure. The ability to offer variable pump speeds may become an issue in the younger BTT population. These individuals are able to regain health to the point that they want to resume the extreme sport type activities in which healthy people of the same age engage. The University of Vienna[17] has evaluated the safety and feasibility of a physiologically responsive controller. As the patient's heart rate increased, there was some increase in pump flow. When the heart rate algorithm was activated, the patient's rise in heart rate was detected by the controller which triggered a rise in pump speed. This in turn resulted in a dramatic increase in pump flow. Then as exercise stopped, the heart rate returned to baseline and pump speed and pump flow were appropriately reduced. The system was stable up to rates of 220 beats/min.

■ THIRD-GENERATION DEVICES

Once continuous flow had been established as a viable mechanism for device miniaturization, several companies began investigating the use of even smaller VADs that were based on the concept of centrifugal flow. By replacing mechanical bearings with magnetically levitated rotor systems, these devices improve

durability. Although clinical experience with these third-generation pumps is just getting under way, early data suggest they may play an important role in the BTT population.[18]

CURRENT DEVICE AVAILABILITY

LVADs that are currently FDA approved for BTT include the following:

1. Thoratec HeartMate XVE (Thoratec Corporation, Pleasanton, CA)—The HeartMate XVE is a first-generation pulsatile fully implantable VAD that was used for patients enrolled in the REMATCH trial. It has been FDA approved for BTT but has largely been supplanted by newer-generation technology.

2. Thoratec pVAD (Thoratec corporation, Pleasanton, California)—These external first-generation pulsatile pumps are FDA approved for BTT indications. Clinical implants started in 1984 and the results have been widely published. This pump can be used as LVAD, RVAD, or BiVAD according to the clinical need. An implantable VAD (iVAD) version is also available.

3. Thoratec HeartMate II—This pump was first implanted clinically in 2000. After initial studies in Europe, the pump was redesigned and the first US use of the new version was reported in 2004.[19] This pump is FDA approved as DT and BTT.

In addition to those devices that have already been approved, there are a number of LVADs that are under clinical investigation for BTT:

1. HeartAssist 5 VAD System (Micromed Cardiovascular, Inc. Houston, TX) This device is a modification of the original Micromed DeBakey VAD introduced by Dr Michael DeBakey in 1999.[20] Its features are described in Chapter 33. The first clinical implant of the DeBakey MicroMed VAD was in November 1998 by Wieselthaler et al.[17] The device has extensive experience in Europe,[16,21-23] and there were two clinical trials started in the United States: DT and BTT. The studies were interrupted for some design changes and application has been resubmitted to the FDA to begin clinical studies in the United States. A clinical trial is under way in Europe.

2. Jarvik-2000 (FlowMaker) (company privately owned by Rob Jarvik)—The first implant occurred in 2000.[24,25] The Jarvik-2000 (FlowMaker) is unique in that the motor is located within the inflow cannula and therefore is an intraventricular pump. The goal is to provide partial ventricular support, reducing the left ventricular size and end-diastolic pressure. This gives the native ventricle an opportunity to remodel itself. The technology is best for patients who require only true left ventricular assistance rather than total left ventricular output replacement. Jarvik Heart received FDA approval in July 2005 to begin a pivotal trial as BTT. The study was approved for up to 25 centers in the United States and is scheduled to enroll up to 160 patients. Its pilot study enrolled 63 patients at eight medical centers. There were no reported device failures during that trial. Modifications have been made to its bearing design also (described in Chapter 34).

3. Berlin Heart INCOR—The first pump was implanted on June 17, 2002 at the German Heart Institute in Berlin. The

INCOR axial-flow pump is unique in its design in that the impeller is magnetically suspended. Thus there are no contact points. Europe has had a significant clinical experience with 200 implants as of July 11, 2005. Little clinical data have been published, but reported results are comparable to the other axial-flow systems.[26]

4. HeartWare—The HVAD pump (HeartWare Inc, Framingham, MA), is a third-generation device with a hydromagnetically levitated rotor. It was first used clinically in 2006 and has completed enrollment for FDA approval under the BTT indication.

5. Therumo DuraHeart—This device is also a centrifugal flow third-generation pump. An FDA-approved BTT trial is under way at this time.

6. Levacor—This device is a third-generation centrifugal pump that is presently undergoing clinical studies in the United States under an FDA-approved pilot trial.

7. EvaHeart—This device has undergone preliminary clinical studies in Japan and a proposal for a US trial is now being submitted to the FDA.

CLINICAL EXPERIENCE

Success in bridging a patient to transplantation is improving with newer devices, better patient selection, and more experience with perioperative care. Although each of these factors makes BTT success a moving target, there is a clear benefit in younger patients (Fig. 7–1).[27] The largest published BTT series using second-generation technology comes from the HeartMate II prospective multicenter study enrolling 133 patients. In this group of patients, 75% achieved the principal outcome of transplantation, recovery, or ongoing support at 180 days.[28] Experience in the third-generation BTT patient population is limited, but early data from 23 patients who underwent implantation of a HeartWare HVAD demonstrated 86% survival at 1 year with two patients' successful BTT.[29] Data on the completed pivotal trial are forthcoming.

There are conflicting data on the impact of LVAD support on posttransplant survival. Several studies have demonstrated an increase in the panel reactive antibody (PRA) among patients who are bridged with a device, but the impact this has on rejection and survival remains controversial.[30,31] Experience with second-generation LVADs suggests that posttransplant survival is not adversely affected by LVAD implantation.[32,33] In fact, data are beginning to emerge that support the idea that bridging a patient to transplant with a VAD may actually improve posttransplant outcomes.[34,35] A number of factors may contribute to improved transplant outcomes when a VAD is used to support a patient on the waiting list. End-organ perfusion is improved with LVAD implantation, which may impact the overall substrate for a patient undergoing cardiac transplantation.[36] Recent data suggests that reversal of pulmonary hypertension can be achieved with mechanical unloading, even in instances of what was previously thought to be "fixed" pulmonary hypertension.[37,38]

One of the common dilemmas involved in LVAD implantation for BTT is the impact of this therapy on the failing right heart. Ventricular suction can create a shift in the ventricular septum which in turn has a major impact on right heart function. Suction can often be provoked by coughing or a Valsalva maneuver when the patient is relatively hypovolemic or if the pump speed is excessive. Excessive suction carries the risk of air embolization in the open-chest situation; however, transcranial Doppler analysis has failed to detect microthrombi or bubbles from cavitation effects in the postsurgical state.[39] Wieselthaler

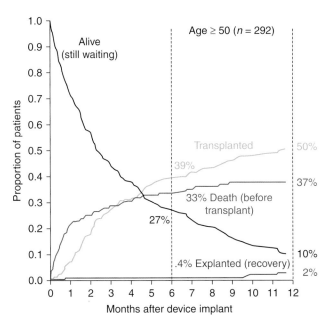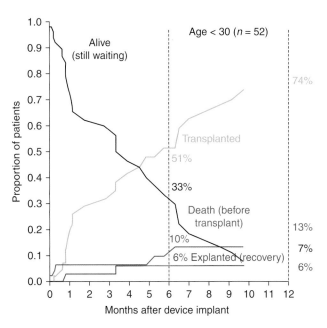

FIGURE 7–1. Competing outcomes after device implantation for BTT. The International Society for Heart and Lung Transplantation/Mechanical Circulatory Support Device analysis, January 2002 to December 2004. (Reproduced with permission from Deng et al.[27] Copyright Elsevier.)

found a need for inotropic support to augment right heart function in all patients. Conscious effort was made to not exceed flows of 2.5 L/min/m^2 for the first 24 to 48 hours after implantation and to maintain a mixed venous saturation of greater than 60% for adequate tissue perfusion. After the first implant phase, the pump was ramped up to provide mixed venous oxygen saturations of greater than 70% with mean arterial pressures greater than 65 mm Hg. OH Frazier (personal communication, 2010) does not use this slow startup process and does not feel there is a detrimental effect on the right heart.

Sudden pump stoppage in second- and third-generation pumps carries the potential of sudden hemodynamic deterioration similar to what one would see with sudden onset of aortic valve insufficiency. Measured flow reversal through the pumps appears to be in the range of 1.5 L/min. Although this degree of regurgitation may be tolerated in a normal heart, a cardiomyopathic heart may fail quickly. This may require emergent return to the operating room to occlude the outflow graft or replace the pump. The author has developed an emergency snare technique that will allow rescue at the bedside or in the emergency room, giving the team time to assess the patient's ability to be managed medically (if there has been reversed remodeling with resultant improved myocardial function after LVAD support) or the convenience of going back to the operating room under a more controlled setting; however, experience has shown such a maneuver rarely to be needed.

Another pitfall of bridging to transplant with an LVAD involves a propensity toward thrombotic events. Pump stoppage from pump thrombus is a small but documented risk with axial-flow pumps.[40,41] Anticoagulation protocols are being developed to optimize the critical zone between pump thrombosis and spontaneous hemorrhage. Pump thrombus is suspected when pump power and current requirements increase and pump flow decreases. This can occur gradually over a period of time with little hemodynamic impact (most likely with primary pump thrombus formation) or can occur precipitously (likely thrombus "wash-in"). If the pump manages to mince the clot and pass it on through, the patient may have no clinical effects. If the pump cannot mince the clot, it may stop or result in prolonged elevation of pump current demands with or without significant decrease in pump flow but increased hemolysis.[42] Most device centers now attempt to recognize the early signs of pump thrombus formation of whatever etiology and treat the problem with platelet inhibitors, heparin infusion, or instillation of systemic recombinant tissue plasminogen activators to lyse the thrombus.[43]

SUMMARY

LVAD therapy as BTT has evolved from a desperate bailout measure in the sickest patients to become a standard treatment option in properly selected patients. The decision of when to bridge with a device is complex and must take into account the surgical team's experience, a patient's clinical risk, anticipated waiting time, and the latest data on outcomes with newer devices.

REFERENCES

1. Cooley DA, Liotta D, Hallman GL, Bloodwell RD, Leachman RD, Milam JD. Orthotopic cardiac prosthesis for two-staged cardiac replacement. *Am J Cardiol.* 1969 Nov;24(5):723-730.
2. Cooley DA, Akutsu T, Norman JC, Serrato MA, Frazier OH. Total artificial heart in two-staged cardiac transplantation. *Cardiovasc Dis.* 1981 Sep;8(3):305-319.
3. DeVries WC, Anderson JL, Joyce LD, et al. Clinical use of the total artificial heart. *N Engl J Med.* 1984 Feb 2;310(5):273-278.
4. Williams MR, Oz MC. Indications and patient selection for mechanical ventricular assistance. *Ann Thorac Surg.* 2001 Mar;71(3 Suppl):S86-S91.
5. Holman WL, Skinner JL, Waites KB, Benza RL, McGiffin DC, Kirklin JK. Infection during circulatory support with ventricular assist devices. *Ann Thorac Surg.* 1999 Aug;68(2):711-716.
6. Dowling RD, Park SJ, Pagani FD, et al. HeartMate VE LVAS design enhancements and its impact on device reliability. *Eur J Cardiothorac Surg.* 2004;25(6):958-963.
7. John R, Kamdar F, Liao K, Colvin-Adams M, Boyle A, Joyce L. Improved survival and decreasing incidence of adverse events with the HeartMate II left ventricular assist device as bridge-to-transplant therapy. *Ann Thorac Surg.* 2008 Oct;86(4):1227-1234.
8. Rose EA, Gelijns AC, Moskowitz AJ, et al. Long-term mechanical left ventricular assistance for end-stage heart failure. *N Engl J Med.* 2001 Nov 15;345(20):1435-1443.
9. Copeland JG, Smith RG, Arabia FA, et al. Cardiac replacement with a total artificial heart as a bridge to transplantation. *N Engl J Med.* 2004 Aug 26;351(9):859-867.
10. Joyce LD, Kiser JC, Eales F, King RM, Overton JW, Jr, Toninato CJ. Experience with generally accepted centrifugal pumps: personal and collective experience. *Ann Thorac Surg.* 1996;61(1):287-290.
11. Guyton AC HJ. Textbook of Medical Physiology. 9th Edition, 161-169. 2010. Philadelphia, PA, WB Saunders.
12. Fossum TW, Morley D, Benkowski R, et al. Chronic survival of calves implanted with the DeBakey ventricular assist device. *Artif Organs.* 1999; 23(8):802-806.
13. Fossum TW, Morley D, Olsen DB, et al. Complications common to ventricular assist device support are rare with 90 days of DeBakey VAD support in calves. *ASAIO J.* 2001 May;47(3):288-292.
14. Macha M, Litwak P, Yamazaki K, et al. Survival for up to six months in calves supported with an implantable axial flow ventricular assist device. *ASAIO J.* 1997 Jul;43(4):311-315.
15. Konishi H, Antaki JF, Litwak P, et al. Long-term animal survival with an implantable axial flow pump as a left ventricular assist device. *Artif Organs.* 1996;20(2):124-127.
16. Goldstein DJ. Worldwide experience with the MicroMed DeBakey Ventricular Assist Device as a bridge to transplantation. *Circulation.* 2003 Sep 9; 108(Suppl 1):II272-II277.
17. Wieselthaler GM, Schima H, Hiesmayr M, et al. First clinical experience with the DeBakey VAD continuous-axial-flow pump for bridge to transplantation. *Circulation.* 2000 Feb 1;101(4):356-359.
18. Esmore D, Kaye D, Spratt P, et al. A prospective, multicenter trial of the VentrAssist left ventricular assist device for bridge to transplant: safety and efficacy. *J Heart Lung Transplant.* 2008;27(6):579-588.
19. Frazier OH, Delgado RM, III, Kar B, Patel V, Gregoric ID, Myers TJ. First clinical use of the redesigned HeartMate II left ventricular assist system in the United States: a case report. *Tex Heart Inst J.* 2004;31(2):157-159.
20. DeBakey ME. A miniature implantable axial flow ventricular assist device. *Ann Thorac Surg* 1999 Aug;68(2):637-640.
21. Noon GP, Morley DL, Irwin S, Abdelsayed SV, Benkowski RJ, Lynch BE. Clinical experience with the MicroMed DeBakey ventricular assist device. *Ann Thorac Surg.* 2001 Mar;71(3 Suppl):S133-S138.
22. Wieselthaler GM, Schima H, Dworschak M, et al. First experiences with outpatient care of patients with implanted axial flow pumps. *Artif Organs.* 2001;25(5):331-335.
23. Hetzer R, Potapov EV, Weng Y, et al. Implantation of MicroMed DeBakey VAD through left thoracotomy after previous median sternotomy operations. *Ann Thorac Surg.* 2004;77(1):347-350.
24. Westaby S, Banning AP, Jarvik R, et al. First permanent implant of the Jarvik 2000 Heart. *Lancet.* 2000 Sept 9;356(9233):900-903.

25. Frazier OH, Myers TJ, Westaby S, Gregoric ID. Use of the Jarvik 2000 left ventricular assist system as a bridge to heart transplantation or as destination therapy for patients with chronic heart failure. *Ann Surg.* 2003;237(5):631-636.

26. Schmid C, Tjan TD, Etz C, et al. First clinical experience with the Incor left ventricular assist device. *J Heart Lung Transplant.* 2005;24(9):1188-1194.

27. Deng MC, Edwards LB, Hertz MI, et al. Mechanical circulatory support device database of the International Society for Heart and Lung Transplantation: third annual report—2005. *J Heart Lung Transplant.* 2005; 24(9):1182-1187.

28. Miller LW, Pagani FD, Russell SD, et al. Use of a continuous-flow device in patients awaiting heart transplantation. *N Engl J Med.* 2007 Aug 30;357(9): 885-896.

29. Wieselthaler GM, Driscoll O, Jansz P, Khaghani A, Strueber M. Initial clinical experience with a novel left ventricular assist device with a magnetically levitated rotor in a multi-institutional trial. *J Heart Lung Transplant.* 2010 June 18.

30. Bull DA, Reid BB, Selzman CH, et al. The impact of bridge-to-transplant ventricular assist device support on survival after cardiac transplantation. *J Thorac Cardiovasc Surg.* 2010 Jul;140(1):169-173.

31. Joyce DL, Southard RE, Torre-Amione G, Noon GP, Land GA, Loebe M. Impact of left ventricular assist device (LVAD)-mediated humoral sensitization on post-transplant outcomes. *J Heart Lung Transplant.* 2005;24(12):2054-2059.

32. Russo MJ, Hong KN, Davies RR, et al. Posttransplant survival is not diminished in heart transplant recipients bridged with implantable left ventricular assist devices. *J Thorac Cardiovasc Surg.* 2009 Dec;138(6):1425-1432.

33. John R, Pagani FD, Naka Y, et al. Post-cardiac transplant survival after support with a continuous-flow left ventricular assist device: impact of duration of left ventricular assist device support and other variables. *J Thorac Cardiovasc Surg.* 2010 Jul;140(1):174-181.

34. Smedira NG, Hoercher KJ, Yoon DY, et al. Bridge to transplant experience: factors influencing survival to and after cardiac transplant. *J Thorac Cardiovasc Surg.* 2010;139(5):1295-1305, 1305.

35. Pal JD, Piacentino V, Cuevas AD, et al. Impact of left ventricular assist device bridging on posttransplant outcomes. *Ann Thorac Surg.* 2009 Nov; 88(5):1457-1461.

36. Russell SD, Rogers JG, Milano CA, et al. Renal and hepatic function improve in advanced heart failure patients during continuous-flow support with the HeartMate II left ventricular assist device. *Circulation.* 2009 Dec 8; 120(23):2352-2357.

37. Alba AC, Rao V, Ross HJ, et al. Impact of fixed pulmonary hypertension on post-heart transplant outcomes in bridge-to-transplant patients. *J Heart Lung Transplant.* 2010 July 8.

38. John R, Liao K, Kamdar F, Eckman P, Boyle A, Colvin-Adams M. Effects on pre- and posttransplant pulmonary hemodynamics in patients with continuous-flow left ventricular assist devices. *J Thorac Cardiovasc Surg.* 2010 Aug;140(2):447-452.

39. Potapov EV, Nasseri BA, Loebe M, et al. Transcranial detection of micro-embolic signals in patients with a novel nonpulsatile implantable LVAD. *ASAIO J.* 2001 May;47(3):249-253.

40. Miller LW, Pagani FD, Russell SD, et al. Use of a continuous-flow device in patients awaiting heart transplantation. *N Engl J Med.* 2007 Aug 30; 357(9):885-896.

41. Slaughter MS, Rogers JG, Milano CA, et al. Advanced heart failure treated with continuous-flow left ventricular assist device. *N Engl J Med.* 2009 Dec 3; 361(23):2241-2251.

42. Christiansen S, Van Aken H, Breithardt GG, Scheld HH, Hammel D. Successful cardiac transplantation after 4 cases of DeBakey left ventricular assist device failure. *J Heart Lung Transplant.* 2002;21(6):706-709.

43. Potapov EV, Loebe M, Abdul-Khaliq H, et al. Postoperative course of S-100B protein and neuron-specific enolase in patients after implantation of continuous and pulsatile flow LVADs. *J Heart Lung Transplant.* 2001;20(12):1310-1316.

CHAPTER 8
BRIDGE TO RECOVERY

Magdi H. Yacoub and Emma J. Birks

INTRODUCTION

Left ventricular assist devices (LVADs) are being increasingly used in patients with severe heart failure resistant to optimal medical therapy. Implantable pumps have evolved to become an extremely useful modality and their design and flow characteristics continue to evolve further. The pulsatile pumps are described as the first-generation pumps; they are efficient and provide good cardiac output and offloading. The axial-flow pumps are the second-generation devices, they are relatively simple in design and are intended to be small, easy to implant, and reliable and might be associated with fewer complications than the larger pulsatile devices. The smaller surface area of foreign material, minimal movement of the device inside the body, and the small driveline may also reduce device-related infection. The third-generation devices currently being introduced are the centrifugal magnetic levitation pumps (also continuous-flow pumps) which are likely to have longer durability and require less anticoagulation.

Historically, LVADs were primarily used to bridge such patients to heart transplant,[1] but the extreme shortage of donor organs worldwide resulted in a pressing need to develop alternative forms of therapy for these patients. Results from the destination therapy trials demonstrate a survival and quality-of-life advantage for LVADs,[2] and destination therapy with LVADs may increase as an expanding option in the future. However, a current and exciting use for these devices is as a bridge-to-recovery. There is now evidence that prolonged near-complete unloading of the left ventricle (LV) using an LVAD is associated with a significant amount of structural reverse remodeling, which is usually associated with functional improvement.[3,4] Sufficient recovery to allow explantation of the device can occur and has been observed in some patients.[5-7] However, the proportion of patients in whom recovery occurs sufficiently to allow explantation of the device has generally been small and in most units has been reported to occur in only around 5% of patients.[8,9] In these patients normal or near-normal cardiac function can occur for as long as 10 years or more.[10] In an attempt to enhance the incidence of recovery, we have previously developed a protocol using the pulsatile HeartMate I LVAD combined with drugs known to enhance reverse remodeling followed by the use of the β_2-adrenoceptor agonist, clenbuterol.[11,12] This drug has been shown to produce physiologic hypertrophy and other beneficial effects on excitation-contraction (EC) coupling and myocardial metabolism in several experimental models of normal and diseased myocardium.[14-18] The rationale for using this form of therapy has been previously described.[11] Using this combination

therapy, we have achieved recovery sufficient to allow explantation of the device in more than 70% of patients with dilated cardiomyopathy.[12] These patients have maintained good ventricular function for long periods of time.

PATIENT SELECTION FOR BRIDGE-TO-RECOVERY

Predicting which patients are likely to recover to a degree that would permit device explantation has been a challenge that has generated considerable research and debate. Currently, there are no clear indications that have been established for bridge-to-recovery. However, a number of clinical markers have been used to guide this decision process. Factors that have been shown to be associated with successful recovery include pre-explantation left ventricular ejection fraction (LVEF) of greater than 45%, left ventricular end-diastolic diameter less than 55 mm, stability of unloading-induced cardiac recovery, duration of LVAD support, and heart failure duration.[13] In general, patients with nonischemic cardiomyopathy are considered for weaning and recovery whereas ischemic patients are not.

THE HAREFIELD PROTOCOL

The weaning protocol established at the Harefield Hospital consists of pharmacologic management divided into two stages. The first stage is geared toward enhancing reverse remodeling and involves treatment with four drugs immediately post-op after weaning from inotropic therapy: lisinopril 40 mg daily, carvedilol 50 mg twice daily, spironolactone 25 mg daily, and losartan 100 mg daily.[14] The second stage of pharmacologic therapy is initiated after a constant left ventricular size has been maintained for at least 2 weeks, based on echocardiographic assessment. Carvedilol is replaced by a selective β_1-blocker (bisoprolol), and clenbuterol is given at an initial dose of 40 µg twice daily, followed by 40 µg three times daily, and finally 700 µg three times daily. Resting heart rate is maintained at a level below 100 beats/min.

Transthoracic echocardiography (TTE) is performed prior to LVAD insertion and weekly after implantation for the first month, then every 2 weeks for 6 months, and every month thereafter. For the first 4 weeks, measurements are made on full device support. However, after week 4, measurements are obtained with the device turned on and off. Parameters that are assessed include left ventricular diameter during systole and diastole, ejection fraction, and left atrial diameter. Based on the patient's tolerance of stopping the device over a 20-minute period, a 6-minute walk test is performed with repeat TTE measurements after exertion. A patient was considered for explantation based on the following measurements taken 15 minutes after stopping the device: a left ventricular end-diastolic diameter of less than 60 mm, a left ventricular end-systolic diameter of less than 50 mm, and an LVEF of more than 45%; a left ventricular end-diastolic pressure (or pulmonary-capillary wedge pressure) of less than 12 mm Hg; a resting cardiac index of more than 2.8 L/min/m² of body surface area; and maximal oxygen consumption (Vo₂ max) with exercise of more than

16 mL/kg of body weight per minute and an increase in minute ventilation (VE) relative to the production of carbon dioxide (Vco$_2$) (VE/Vco$_2$ slope) of less than 34.[14]

OUTCOMES

In our series, a total of 15 patients were enrolled in a prospective evaluation for bridge-to-Recovery. Eleven of these patients met criteria for explantation. Of the patients who were explanted, one died of intractable arrhythmias 24 hours after explantation and another died of carcinoma of the lung 27 months after explantation. Freedom from recurrent heart failure among the survivors was 100% and 88.9% at 1 and 4 years after explantation, respectively. Quality of life improved after explantation, as did hemodynamic status measured by TTE. At measurements taken 59 months after explantation, the mean LVEF was 64 ± 12%, the mean left ventricular end-diastolic diameter was 59.4 ± 12.1 mm, the mean left ventricular end-systolic diameter was 42.5 ± 13.2 mm, and the mean maximal oxygen uptake with exercise was 26.3 ± 6.0 mL/kg of body weight per minute (Fig. 8–1).[14]

POTENTIAL INFLUENCE OF PULSATILE VERSUS CONTINUOUS FLOW PUMPS ON RECOVERY

As device technology continues to evolve, there are a number of important implications for using an LVAD for bridge-to-recovery.

Because of their inherent design characteristics, first-generation VADs are thought to more completely unload the ventricle relative to their axial-and centrifugal-flow counterparts. Although all of the current VADs are designed to pump blood from the apex of the left ventricle to the ascending or descending aorta, there are fundamental differences in the mode of action of the devices and the pattern of flow and/or pressure generation which can influence the degree and timing of unloading, the instantaneous flow in the left ventricle, and coronary arteries and aortic root. All those factors, at least in theory, could have an important effect on "recovery."

DEGREE AND TIMING OF UNLOADING

Pulsatile devices have been shown to be extremely effective in unloading the LV both during systole and diastole,[19] resulting in diminution in both end-systolic and end-diastolic volumes within a relatively short period of time. This is thought to be important in inducing recovery. There is experimental evidence that in-vitro stretching cardiac muscle, particularly during diastole, results in induction of atrial natriuretic peptide (ANP) and brain natriuretic peptide (BNP) expression,[20] which is thought to be a marker of pathologic hypertrophy. We have timed pulsatile device (HeartMate I) ejection by phonocardiography and related that to native left ventricular contraction and/or ejection (Fig. 8–2). As expected, there was asynchrony between these events with intermittent cardiac ejection occurring infrequently but always coinciding with device ejection (see Fig. 8–2). This results in a marked

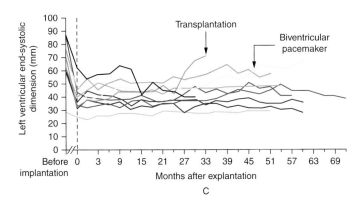

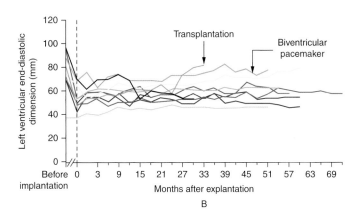

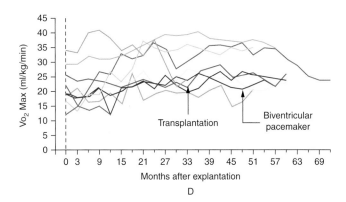

FIGURE 8–1. Preserved hemodynamics after LVAD explantation. (Reproduced with permission from Birks et al.[14] Copyright Massachusetts Medical Society. All rights reserved.)

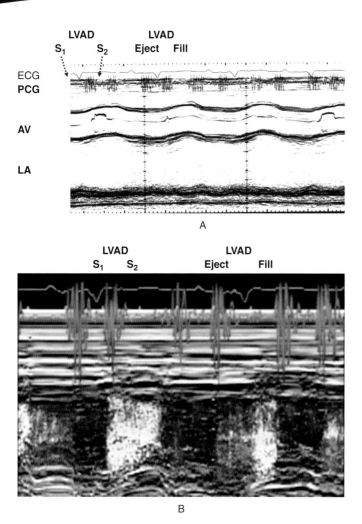

FIGURE 8–2. A. M-mode echocardiogram showing aortic valve opening to occur during LVAD ejection when native ventricular systole coincides with LVAD ejection, indicated by the period between LVAD inflow valve closure (LVAD S₁) and LVAD outflow closure (LVAD S₂). **B.** Simultaneous native ventricular and VAD ejection occurs in this patient shown by color flow mapping of the LV apex. (Reproduced with permission from Yacoub MH, Birks EJ, Tansley P, Henein MY, Bowles CT. Bridge to recovery: the Harefield approach. *J Congest Heart Failure Circ Support.* 2001;2(Suppl 1):27-30.)

increase in afterload during these cardiac cycles and can be tolerated by the recovering ventricle only if peak systolic pressure is not excessively high. This latter objective is achieved in the Harefield protocol by using angiotensin-converting enzyme (ACE) and angiotensin type 1 (AT1) receptor antagonists. Although, at least in theory continuous-flow pumps are designed to unload the LV during systole and diastole, in clinical practice incomplete loading has been reported.[21] This might be due to the fact that the software used does not allow the pump to run too fast because of concerns regarding sucking the ventricle flat and inducing arrhythmias.

PATTERN OF FLOW IN AND SHAPE OF THE LEFT VENTRICLE

The asynchrony of action of the device with the LV coupled with the particular mode and timing of filling of pulsatile devices

results in a complex series of changes in the pattern of flow in and shape of the left ventricle. The filling of pulsatile devices occurs passively with minimal or no suction force. This results in intermittent laminar flow in the LV (see Fig. 8–2B), which acts as a conduit. However, in the presence of inflow valve regurgitation, a strong backward (regurgitant) jet produces varying degrees of distension of the LV and LA, depending on the degree of regurgitation and timing in relation to the cardiac cycle. In contrast, in the presence of a normally functioning inflow valve, the shape of the LV cavity assumes a tubular form during diastole with varying degrees of distension, depending on how much of the previous diastole has coincided with a closed inflow valve and on the amount of pulmonary venous return which is a function of RV output. The degree of filling of the LV determines the level of peak systolic pressure generated by ventricular contraction (Fig. 8–3). When and if the peak systolic pressure in the LV exceeds that in the aorta, the aortic valve opens—at that point two additional factors can influence the pressure in the LV: systemic vascular resistance and whether the device is ejecting simultaneously, which is usually the case (see Fig. 8–2).

Continuous-flow pumps produce a specific pattern of flow in the left ventricle which depends on the speed of the pump[22] and influences the shape of the LV. With a relatively slow speed (9600 rpm [revolutions per minute]), flow through the LV is essentially continuous with short periods of interrupted flow during isometric ventricular systole (Fig. 8–4) and early ventricular diastole (see Fig. 8–4). When pumps speed is increased, the flow in the LV gets greatly disturbed particularly during early diastole which could result in large gradients detected by continuous wave (CW) Doppler (Fig. 8–5). This is usually accompanied by hour glass deformation of the LV and could be associated with multiple ventricular ectopics. The changes in flow and pressure in the LV cavity can produce changes in wall tension as well as ventricular deformation which in turn can affect myocardial oxygen demand and stimulation of mechanoreceptors on the myocardial and other cells as well as the extracellular matrix. These changes could potentially affect several aspects of recovery.

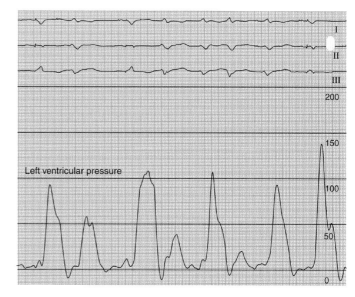

FIGURE 8–3. LV pressure trace of a patient on a HeartMate I device.

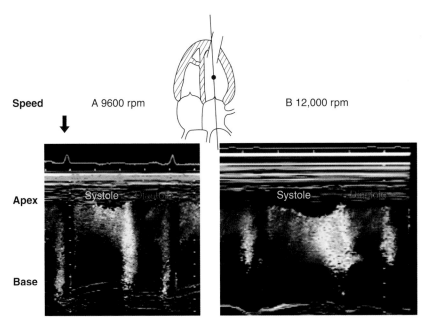

Speed   A 9600 rpm   B 12,000 rpm

Apex

Base

FIGURE 8–4. Color M-mode recording of the left ventricle showing continuous systolic and diastolic flow at the apex at a speed of 9600 rpm **(A)** and 12,000 rpm **(B)**. (Reproduced with permission from Henein et al.[21] Copyright Wolters Kluwer Health.)

INFLUENCE ON CORONARY FLOW

Although the coronary circulation is tightly regulated by a variety of mechanical, biochemical, metabolic, and neural mechanisms, mechanical factors relating to interaction between intravascular flow and the native heart could influence different aspects of coronary flow relevant to the process of recovery. In spite of the fact that the major part of coronary flow occurs during diastole, systolic coronary flow accounts for at least a third of the total coronary flow and is thought to be important for myocardial viability/recovery. Systolic coronary flow is influenced by several factors which include a higher perfusion pressure during systole to perfuse all parts of the contracting myocardium. When compared to continuous-flow pumps, pulsatile devices appear to produce a higher intravascular pressure particularly during ejection by the device. This could enhance both systolic and diastolic coronary flow albeit intermittently. Coronary flow, particularly during systole, can be affected by the flow dynamics in the aortic root, as is explained later.

Another factor which could influence coronary flow is endothelial generation of nitric oxide (NO) in response to the shear stress produced by pulsatility.[23,24] This could in theory reduce the local coronary vascular resistance, platelet adhesiveness, as well as protect against the development of coronary atherosclerosis.

Although maintenance of coronary flow to the LV is important for recovery, a frequently neglected topic is flow to the right ventricle which is arguably just as important for the process of recovery both in the longer term and also during device support by maintaining an adequate cardiac output. The drop in pulmonary arterial pressure and RV afterload produced by a drop in LA pressure with mechanical support helps to improve RV function and lower its myocardial oxygen demand. In addition the drop in

RV end-diastolic pressure could enhance coronary flow to the RV. However, the sudden increase in cardiac output and systemic venous return imposes a large diastolic overload on the right ventricle with increases in myocardial oxygen consumption which required a higher coronary flow. A higher pulsatile pressure in the right coronary system could help to achieve this goal.

AORTIC ROOT DYNAMICS

The aortic root is located in a strategic position "inside" the heart in proximity to many vital structures, including the LV, the coronary ostia, the conducting tissue, the fibrous network of the heart, and all cardiac valves. The aortic root is formed of several components, which have very specific geometric, cellular, and molecular structures that perform extremely sophisticated functions described as a "tale of dynamism and cross talk."[25] Many of these functions are linked to coronary flow and LV function and therefore could be relevant to "recovery."

During LV ejection, the sinotubular junction produces a vortex which redirects blood into the sinuses of Valsalva which enhances systolic coronary flow[24] and "washes" the sinuses both during systole and diastole. When the outflow graft of a pulsatile device pump is anastomosed to the ascending aorta, the periodic reversal of flow into the aortic sinuses recreates some of these vortices, whereas when the outflow graft is anastomosed to the descending aorta, many of these forces are blunted when they reach the aortic root.

Continuous-flow pumps, particularly when anastomosed to the descending aorta, may produce stagnant conditions in the aortic root which can interfere with coronary flow and increase the chances of formation (buildup) of clot in the aortic root and left ventricular outflow tract (LVOT) with an adverse effect on recovery and long-term results.

ASSESSMENT OF RECOVERY

Although some inferences can be drawn by monitoring changes in left ventricular size and function during device support, a structured protocol of assessing recovery with the pump switched off or effectively off is considered essential for the success of bridge-to-recovery programs.[12] Assessment of left ventricular function is more difficult with a continuous-flow pump compared to a pulsatile device as cessation of a continuous-flow pump leads to backflow through the device which loads the left ventricle. Off-pump testing would therefore not accurately reflect unsupported left ventricular function but a stressed heart. We have assessed flow through the HeartMate II and Jarvik-2000 axial-flow pumps in the catheter laboratory by running them at progressively slower speeds until no net forward and no backward flow through the device occurred. For the Jarvik-2000, the manufacturers produced a controller which runs the pump at lower speeds than normal,

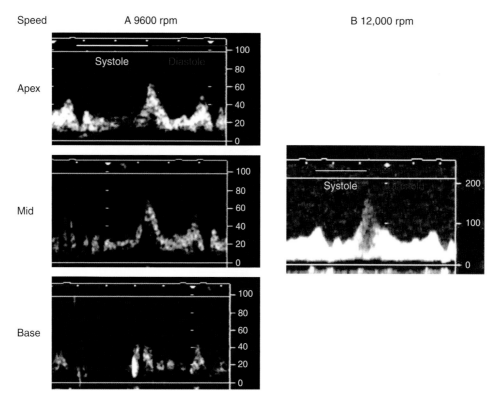

FIGURE 8–5. A. Pulsed wave velocities of left ventricular diastolic velocities at 9600 rpm taken at three levels: base, midcavity, and apex. **B.** Continuous wave Doppler with a pump speed of 12,000 rpm. Note the significant increase in early diastolic velocities. (Reproduced with permission from Henein et al.[21] Copyright Wolters Kluwer Health.)

down to 6000 rpm. We have shown that during cardiac catheterization a pump speed of 6000 produces no net forward and backward flow.

Patients on axial-flow pumps are taking warfarin; therefore provided the international normalized ratio (INR) is greater than 2.5, no additional anticoagulation is required when the pump is turned down for short periods to assess recovery whereas HeartMate I patients are only on aspirin and require full heparinization before cessation of the pump.

EXPLANTATION

When myocardial recovery occurs, explantation of pulsatile ventricular assist devices has traditionally comprised median sternotomy and laparotomy with associated extensive dissection of adhesions that can increase morbidity and mortality. We have developed minimally invasive techniques for the removal of both left[25] and right[26] pulsatile ventricular assist devices which appear to be safe with a low complication rate. We have also successfully used a similar technique for explantation of the HeartMate II axial-flow LVAD. For the Jarvik-2000 axial-flow pump "explantation" can be achieved by ligating the outflow graft, disconnecting the device, and removing the driveline leaving the device in situ (Khaghani, personal communication). This avoids any surgical damage to the heart and is a relatively

minor procedure for the patient to undergo. The effect of leaving the pump inside the ventricle is not known, but to date with follow-up of up to 10 months there have been no complications and in particular no thromboembolism with the patients being anticoagulated.[26] The Berlin group have explanted two patients from the Incor continuous-flow pump leaving the transected apical cannula, occluding it with a self-expanding plug.[27]

CLINICAL EXPERIENCE AND THE FUTURE

To date the experience with recovering patients on axial-flow pumps has been small but encouraging. The longest follow-up (to our knowledge) is one of our patients who received a HeartMate II and recovered 5 months later, and he has remained well (for over 3 years). In addition, three patients on a Jarvik have recovered well and are being followed up. We also have several more Jarvik-2000 patients showing goods signs of recovery. The Berlin group[19] have explanted two patients from the Incor continuous-flow pump after 6 and 7 months of support and they are reported to be well after 4 and 6 months, respectively.

These results are very early and the numbers still small. The role of continuous-flow pumps in recovery is an exciting area and needs further evaluation, and the only way to make a true comparison with the pulsatile pumps may be to directly compare their effect on recovery in a randomized trial.

REFERENCES

1. Birks EJ, Yacoub MH, Banner NR, Khaghani A. The role of bridge to transplantation and whether LVAD patients should be transplanted. *Curr Opin Cardiol*. 2004;19:148-153.

2. Rose EA, Gelijns AC, Moskowitz AJ, et al. Randomized Evaluation of Mechanical Assistance for the Treatment of Congestive Heart Failure (REMATCH) study group. Long-term mechanical left ventricular assistance for end-stage heart failure. *N Engl J Med*. 2001;345(20):1435-1443.

3. Dipla K, Mattiello JA, Jeevanandam V, Houser SR, Margulies KB. Myocyte recovery after mechanical circulatory support in humans with end-stage heart failure. *Circulation*. 1998;97(23):2316-2322

4. Terracciano CMN, Harding SE, Tansley PT, Birks EJ, Barton PJR, Yacoub MH. Changes in sarcolemmal Ca entry and sarcoplasmic reticulum Ca content in ventricular myocytes from patients with end-stage heart failure following myocardial recovery after combined pharmacological and ventricular assist device therapy. *Eur Heart J*. 2003;24:1329-1339.

5. Frazier OH, Myers TJ. Left ventricular assist system as a bridge to myocardial recovery. *Ann Thorac Surg*. 1999;68(2):734-741.

6. Frazier OH, Delgado RM, 3rd, Scroggins N, Odegaard P, Kar B. Mechanical bridging to improvement in severe acute "nonischemic, nonmyocarditis" heart failure. *Congest Heart Fail*. 2004;10(2):109-113.

7. Hetzer R, Muller JH, Weng YG, Loebe M, Wallukat G. Midterm follow-up of patients who underwent removal of a left ventricular assist device after cardiac recovery from end-stage dilated cardiomyopathy. *J Thorac Cardiovasc Surg*. 2000;120(5):843-853.

8. Mancini DM, Beniaminovitz A, Levin H, et al. Low incidence of myocardial recovery after left ventricular assist device implantation in patients with chronic heart failure. *Circulation*. 1998;98:2383-2389.

9. Mann DL, Willerson JT. Left ventricular assist devices and the failing heart: a bridge to recovery, a permanent assist device, or a bridge too far? *Circulation*. 1998;98:2367-2369.

10. Farrar DJ, Holman WR, McBride LR, et al. Long-term follow-up of Thoratec ventricular assist device bridge-to-recovery patients successfully removed from support after recovery of ventricular function. *J Heart Lung Transplant*. 2002;21(5):516-521.

11. Yacoub MH. A novel strategy to maximize the efficacy of left ventricular assist devices as a bridge to recovery. *Eur Heart J*. 2001;22(7):534-540.

12. Birks EJ, Tansley PD, Hardy J, et al. Reversal of end stage heart failure using a combination of left ventricular assist device (LVAD) and pharmacologic therapy. *New Engl J Med*. Submitted.

13. Dandel M, Weng Y, Siniawski H, et al. Prediction of cardiac stability after weaning from left ventricular assist devices in patients with idiopathic dilated cardiomyopathy. *Circulation*. 2008;118(14 Suppl):S94-S105.

14. Birks EJ, Tansley PD, Hardy J, et al. Left ventricular assist device and drug therapy for the reversal of heart failure. *N Engl J Med*. 2006;355(18):1873-1884.

15. Wong K, Boheler KR, Bishop J, Petrou M, Yacoub, MH. Clenbuterol induces cardiac hypertrophy with normal functional, morphological and molecular features. *Cardiovasc Res*. 1998;37:115-122.

16. Wong K, Boheler KR, Petrou M, Yacoub MH. Pharmacological modulation pressure overload cardiac hypertrophy changes in ventricular function, extracellular matrix, and gene expression. *Circulation*. 1997;96:2239-2246.

17. Petrou M, Clarke S, Morrison K, Bowles C, Dunn M, Yacoub M. Clenbuterol increases stroke power and contractile speed of skeletal muscle for cardiac assist. *Circulation*. 1999;99(5):713-720.

18. Soppa GKR, Smolenski RT, Latif N, et al. Effects of chronic administration of clenbuterol on function and metabolism of adult rat cardiac muscle. *Am J Physiol Heart Circ Physiol*. 2005;288:H1468-H1476.

19. Thohan V, Stetson SJ, Nagueh SF, et al. Cellular and hemodynamics responses of failing myocardium to continuous flow mechanical circulatory support using the DeBakey-Noon left ventricular assist device: a comparative analysis with pulsatile-type devices. *J Heart Lung Transplant*. 2005 May;24(5):566-575.

20. Wiese SD, Breyer T, Dragu A, et al. Gene expression of brain natriuretic peptide in isolated atrial and ventricular human myocardium—influence of angiotensin II and diastolic fiber length. *Circulation*. 2000 Dec;102:3074-3079.

21. Henein M, Birks EJ, Tansley PDT, Bowles CT, Yacoub MH. Temporal and spacial changes in LV pattern of flow during continuous assist device "Heartmate II." *Circulation*. 2002;105(19):2324-2325.

22. Yacoub MH, Kilner PJ, Birks EJ, Misfeld M. The aortic outflow and root: a tale of dynamism and crosstalk. *Ann Thorac Surg*. 1999;68:S37-S43.

23. Casey PJ, Dattilo JB, Dai G, et al. The effect of combined arterial hemodynamics on saphenous venous endothelial nitric oxide production. *J Vasc Surg*. 2001 Jun;33(6):1199-1205.

24. Bellhouse BJ, Bellhouse FH. Fluid mechanics of the mitral valve. *Nature*. 1969 Nov 8;224(219):615-616.

25. Tansley P, Yacoub M. Minimally invasive explantation of implantable left ventricular assist devices. *J Thorac Cardiovasc Surg*. 2002;124(1):189-191.

26. Haj-Yahya S, Birks EJ, Hardy J, Yacoub MH, Khaghani A. A minimally invasive technique for explantation of right ventricular assist devices. *Ann Thorac Surg*. In Press.

27. Hetzer R, Weng Y, Potapov EV, et al. First experiences with a novel magnetically suspended axial flow left ventricular assist device. *Eur J Cardiothorac Surg*. 2004 Jun;25(6):964-970.

CHAPTER 9
ANESTHETIC CONSIDERATIONS DURING LVAD SURGERY

Thomas P. Laberge, Michael K. Loushin, and Michael F. Sweeney

PREOPERATIVE CONSIDERATIONS

Patients requiring general anesthesia (GA) for placement of a left ventricular assist device (LVAD) present challenges to the anesthesiologist during the perioperative period. This is major surgery which presents anesthetic risks which may not be present for other surgeries. These patients are critically ill and frequently managed preoperatively in an intensive care unit (ICU). Typical American Society of Anesthesiology (ASA) physical status is 4 (Table 9–1) or 4E (indicating an emergency procedure).[1]

Such patients require multiple hemodynamic monitors. Besides the ASA standard monitors, an invasive arterial line is required prior to induction of anesthesia. The timing for placement of a central venous pressure (CVP) and/or a pulmonary artery (PA) catheter depends on the critical illness and hemodynamic instability of the patient.[2] In hemodynamically unstable patients, an intra-aortic balloon pump (IABP),[3] for afterload reduction and to assist coronary and systemic perfusion, may be placed prior to the operation.

Pharmacologic support of the failing ventricle is almost always required to maintain an adequate systemic arterial blood pressure (SBP). The commonly administered vasopressors/inotropes include calcium, dopamine, epinephrine, milrinone, dobutamine, and vasopressin. A single agent or a combination of the above agents may be required to maintain an adequate SBP. Continuous intravenous (IV) infusions must not be discontinued, as this may result in acute hemodynamic decompensation. Therefore some form of reliable IV access must be in place. Emergency drugs such as epinephrine, calcium, vasopressin, and phenylephrine should be available during transport of the patient to the operating room (OR).

Critically ill patients requiring a VAD rapidly develop multiorgan dysfunction, involving the respiratory, renal, hepatic, and endocrine systems. With multiorgan dysfunction, pulmonary edema often occurs further compromising systemic oxygen delivery. Cardiogenic pulmonary edema often requires a high concentration of inspired oxygen. Mechanically ventilated patients frequently require significant positive end expiratory pressure (PEEP) to improve ventilation and oxygenation. When transporting ventilated patients to the OR, a PEEP valve on the ventilation bag is essential.

With the combination of renal and heart failure, assessment of intravascular volume status is difficult without invasive monitors such as a PA catheter. If renal or hepatic failures are present, choice of anesthetic agents should be tailored to account for that particular organ dysfunction. Knowing the interactions of anesthetic agents with certain dysfunctions will allow careful titration of anesthesia in critically ill cardiac patients. For example, cisatracurium, a muscle relaxant, does not require metabolism and excretion by the renal or hepatic systems and may be more appropriate in patients with renal dysfunction.

When transporting these patients from the ICU to the OR, monitoring electrocardiogram (ECG), pulse oximetry, and SBP is essential. Any existing invasive monitors must also be displayed on the transport monitor. If the patient is not endotracheally intubated, supplemental oxygen should be utilized during transport. Patients may require assisted ventilation or endotracheal intubation prior to transport, if their respiratory status is unstable.

Also, the patient's blood must be typed and crossmatched for packed red blood cells (PRBCs) and perhaps fresh frozen plasma. There is potential for massive blood loss in these cases, sometimes prior to going on cardiopulmonary bypass (CPB). Blood should be available in the OR prior to induction of GA.

The potential for awareness during induction and maintenance of GA is another concern. Even small amounts of anesthesia can cause further hemodynamic instability, though smaller amounts of drug can increase the risk of intraoperative awareness. Administration of medications such as midazolam or scopolamine can decrease the chance of intraoperative awareness. Scopolamine is an excellent amnestic agent which has minimal hemodynamic effects.

One of the challenges of these critically ill patients is to plan for an induction of GA that will ensure adequate anesthesia and avoid acute hemodynamic decompensation. Knowing the interactions of commonly administered inotropes and vasopressors with anesthetic agents along with an in-depth understanding of the patient's pathophysiology can guide careful titration of GA.[4]

INTRAOPERATIVE MANAGEMENT

Induction of GA varies depending on the presence or absence of an IABP or prior placement of a VAD.[5] A patient with one of these devices functioning is usually more stable on induction of GA than one without. Patients without one of these devices may be relatively stable on heart failure medications at one extreme or may be in cardiogenic shock. Prior to OR entrance, appropriate IV inotropic and vasoactive drugs should be prepared, along

TABLE 9–1. ASA Physical Status Classification System

ASA Physical Status Classification System	
1	A normal healthy patient
2	A patient with mild systemic disease
3	A patient with severe systemic disease that limits function but is not incapacitating
4	A patient with severe systemic disease that is a constant threat to life
5	A moribund patient who is not expected to survive without the operation
6	A declared brain-dead patient whose organs are being removed for donor purposes

ASA, American Society of Anesthesiology.

with the standard monitoring devices and airway equipment. Additional monitoring equipment that is needed includes invasive PA and SBP monitoring apparatuses and a transesophageal echocardiogram (TEE) machine. Before induction, at least one large-bore IV line and an arterial line are placed with the assistance of local anesthetic and judicious anxiolytic. After full preoxygenation, anesthesia is induced IV with a cardiovascular-friendly medication such as etomidate. Muscle relaxation is achieved in a rapid fashion, usually with a large nondepolarizing muscle-relaxant dose. Our preference here is rocuronium. Cricoid cartilage pressure prior to intubation is prudent in most patients, even if adequate NPO status is met. This is because of the effects of marginal cardiac output on gastric emptying times. If tracheal intubation is perceived to be difficult, airway establishment prior to GA and muscle relaxant is the safest method, usually via the fiberoptic approach. After successful induction and tracheal intubation, maintenance of GA is achieved with a balanced combination of inhalation agent such as isoflurane, narcotic such as fentanyl, amnestic, and muscle relaxant dosed with attention to preoperative renal function. Depending on the response to GA, inotropic/vasoactive agents may need to be increased or started before CPB.

Next, a PA catheter is passed, usually via the right internal jugular vein, and a TEE probe is placed. The ability to transcutaneously pace and perform cardioversion/defibrillation is attained by placing external pads, after implanted devices, if any, have been appropriately reprogrammed for the OR setting. Additional large-bore IV access is also established at this time. Reasonable urine output is maintained with loop and/or osmotic diuretics. Last, an antifibrinolytic such as ε-aminocaproic acid is started[6] and prophylactic antimicrobial(s) given.

Upon surgical incision blood loss is the major concern. Patients are often on preoperative anticoagulants as well as antiplatelet drugs, which can potentiate bleeding. The patient's heart failure may have led to liver congestion and hepatic coagulopathies. Finally, many patients receiving an LVAD have had prior sternotomies and are at an increased risk of massive blood loss during repeat sternotomy and mediastinal dissection.

As noted earlier, a TEE probe was placed prior to surgical incision for evaluation of certain specific cardiac areas. The first structure that needs to be evaluated is the aortic valve (AV). Significant AV insufficiency cannot be present after LVAD placement. If the AV is insufficient, forward flow cannot occur efficiently and pulmonary edema will result. If more than trace AV insufficiency is noted during TEE evaluation, the surgical team can oversew the valve closed, thereby ensuring cardiac decompression.[7] The second structure that should be assessed prior to bypass is the atrial septum. A patent foramen ovale (PFO) or atrial septal defect can result in a postbypass shunt, which is usually right-to-left, and causes systemic arterial desaturation. If the shunt should be left-to-right and large enough, it will additionally stress the right ventricle (RV). Intactness of the atrial septum is determined by color flow imaging and performing a "bubble" study (Fig. 9–1). This contrast echocardiogram is most sensitive when performed with a 30-cm H_2O airway pressure release maneuver, using the ME four-chamber or bicaval view. A two-person technique works best for this.[8] The ascending aorta is interrogated for calcification, and the left ventricular (LV) apex inspected for thrombus, since these are the future LVAD cannulation sites.

Standard heparin dosing for CPB is used (3-4 mg/kg, initial dose). Acquired antithrombin III deficiency should be suspected if the patient doesn't anticoagulate adequately and appropriate amounts of AT III concentrate or fresh frozen plasma given. Ventilation is discontinued, and mediastinal carbon dioxide insufflation begun. Placement of the LVAD and perhaps AV and PFO closure then proceeds. During CPB the anesthesiologist ensures that the aforementioned inotropic/vasoactive infusions are ready and appropriate blood products available for post–CPB use. After the aortic cross clamp is removed, drug infusions are started as deemed necessary following a reasonable reperfusion period. It is best to avoid generalized vasoconstrictors, or catecholamines at vasoconstrictor doses, to minimize cardiac afterload. Prior to termination of CPB several issues need to be settled. First, ventilation with 100% oxygen is initiated. Then, TEE reevaluation proceeds. TEE confirms the absence of gas bubbles within the cardiac chambers as well as reconfirming the competency of the AV. Other routine factors are also addressed prior to CPB discontinuance.

After CPB separation, TEE is used to determine appropriate placement of the LV outflow cannula (attention to ventricular septal abutment), as well as to evaluate the effectiveness of LV decompression, with attention to the degree of mitral valve insufficiency. Excellent hemodynamic condition following LVAD placement largely depends upon RV performance. Reasonable heart rate and rhythm and optimal preload are essential. RV afterload is minimized with optimization of acid-base balance favoring alkalosis, avoidance of alveolar hypoxia, and pulmonary vasodilators such as nitroprusside, nitroglycerine, milrinone, nitric oxide, and/or prostacyclin. Bleeding after CPB is usually multifactorial and may include residual anticoagulation, prior liver dysfunction with resultant cofactor deficiency, CPB and prior renal insufficiency–induced platelet

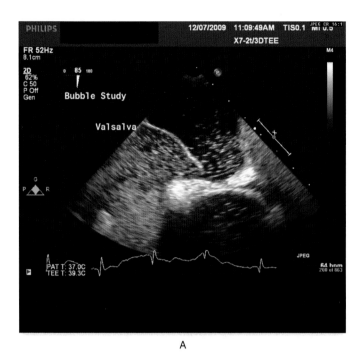

A

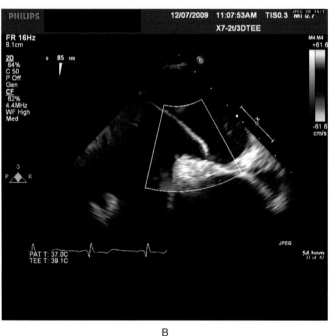

B

FIGURE 9-1. Bubble study positive for PFO with bubbles passing from the right atrium (RA) to the left atrium (LA). (Courtesy of Dr. Ingela Schnittger, Stanford University Medical Center, Stanford, CA.)

dysfunction, thrombocytopenia, and ongoing surgical blood loss. Bleeding is managed with one or a combination of the following: scavenged red blood cells (RBCs), blood bank products, IV desmopressin.[9] Efficacy and safety of recombinant factor VIIa has yet to be established in this group of patients; therefore its use cannot routinely be recommended. Sedation and analgesia are maintained for transport of the patient to the ICU using one or a combination of the following drug regimens: bolus or infusions of narcotic and benzodiazepine, or propofol or dexmedetomidine infusions.

POSTOPERATIVE INTENSIVE CARE

After a short period of transition and settling in to ICU care, close attention is paid to the magnitude of blood loss via chest tubes. The exploration rate for bleeding postoperatively is fairly high for any type or combination of VAD placements. Appropriate blood product replacement is given. The use of initial or repeat doses of vitamin K is controversial, since subsequent coumadin dosing will eventually be needed. Antifibrinolytic therapy with ε-aminocaproic acid is generally continued for 4 to 6 hours after hemorrhage has abated to an acceptable level. It is important to stress that true patient stability is impossible to attain in the face of ongoing brisk bleeding, since the preload of native and mechanical pumps is never optimal for very long. Also, chest tube blood loss levels which dramatically drop might indicate clot that is diminishing the ability of the thoracic cavity to be evacuated. Tamponade syndrome may then ensue. If filling pressures are rising, echocardiography (transthoracic and/or TEE) is useful for demonstration of impaired cardiac filling.[10]

Cardiac rhythm can also be problematic. Epicardial DDD pacing at a rate of 90 to 110 is best for slow rhythms.[11] Maintaining a normal blood pH, potassium level, and core temperature while providing for adequate patient comfort will all help with arrhythmia control. Also, keeping plasma magnesium levels in the high normal range can prevent and even terminate problematic heart rhythms, most notable of which is atrial fibrillation.[12] Medical therapy with amiodarone, among others, will be needed in some patients.[13] Cardioversion and defibrillation are most safely accomplished after the LVAD is disconnected from AC wall power and allowed to run off of its batteries. Cardiopulmonary resuscitation performance is otherwise unchanged. Older-generation technologies have specific hand-pumping options for these types of situations. Acute LVAD failure of an electronic nature is initially managed by AC power disconnect and battery reinsertion and/or change. If this doesn't work, controller modification as directed by written instruction is undertaken and the VAD coordinator contacted.

Since the newer-generation LVADs pump continuously and with variable pulsatility, systolic and diastolic SBP will be different only if there is LV preload and significant efficient systolic LV function. Therefore cuff blood pressures and pulse oximetry may not be reliable. Lack of pulsatility is associated with impaired LV filling, inadequate LV decompression, and/or MV insufficiency. Assessing CVP and PA pressures will help to sort this out. If an LVAD only has been inserted, the RV must be watched carefully for decompensation. A rising CVP and possibly a narrow PA pulse pressure in the face of a low PA wedge pressure can mean acute RV decompensation. Echocardiography should be repeated to look for RV dilation and degree of tricuspid valve insufficiency. If pulmonary vascular resistance elevation is suspected, a trial of a pulmonary vasodilator such as nitric oxide or nebulized prostacyclin is indicated. An "inodilator" such as milrinone is almost always useful and synergistic.[14] It is important to remember that pulmonary causes of elevated pulmonary vascular resistance such as atelectasis, edema, or pleural effusion cannot be successfully managed with medicines. Only the proper titration of positive airway pressure or fluid evacuation will result in a decrease of the stress on the RV.

Mean SBP is best maintained in the 65 to 85 torr range. This is to ensure that adequate blood flow to certain vital organs, especially brain and kidneys, in the face of possibly impaired vascular autoregulation. Blood flow is adjusted and monitored via the LVAD and can be compared to the usual indicators of flow such as PA catheter thermodilution and true mixed venous oximetry. Intermittent monitoring for evolution of metabolic acidosis and a rising lactate level is also a useful adjunctive maneuver.

Maintaining lung volumes at around a normal functional residual capacity is one of the main goals of postoperative respiratory therapy.[15] A PEEP level of 5- to 10-cm H_2O is almost always needed in the early postoperative setting. Weaning from deep mechanical ventilator breaths, while utilizing a pressure support (PS) of 4- to 6-cm H_2O is promptly undertaken. When this level of PS over physiologic PEEP and an Fio_2 of less than or equal to 0.5 are tolerated, extubation can be entertained—from a purely respiratory standpoint. Additional requirements for extubation are acceptable heart rate/rhythm and hemodynamics on low-to-moderate CV support, an adequate level of consciousness and normal strength, near normothermia, absence of significant anemia, absence of ongoing bleeding, and metabolic stability (acid-base, electrolytes, and fluid balance).[16] Hopefully, extubation might occur within 6 hours of operation termination, but many patients will not be good candidates for this "fast-track" approach, due to preoperative status and procedural duration. Nonetheless, the anesthetic should always be designed so that early extubation is an option. After extubation, continuance and possibly escalation of preoperative respiratory therapy should be the baseline upon which modalities such as incentive spirometry, semirecumbent position, and thoughtful mobilization are superimposed. If atelectasis ensues, noninvasive mechanical ventilation with bilevel positive airway pressure (BiPAP) can frequently obviate the need for reintubation. Nosocomial pneumonia is always a concern. If not aggressively treated, the offending microbes may spread into the bloodstream and possibly the LVAD. The appearance of fever, increasing blood neutrophil count, and cough with or without purulent sputum should alert the clinician. Obtaining a sample of sputum via bronchoscopic lavage and suction of a radiologically affected lung region is the preferred method for microbe identification. Empiric antimicrobial therapy is then begun and fine-tuned upon reception of culture and sensitivity results. The duration of therapy is controversial, though at least 1 week postextubation is reasonable. If the blood culture is found to be positive, 2 weeks duration is prudent. If blood cultures are persistently positive, vegetations or clots should be sought. If seen, the patient should receive appropriate therapy for 6 weeks IV, (ie, the subacute endocarditic approach).

Urine output of 50 to 100 cc/h is desirable in most adult patients postoperatively. Judicious diuretic dosing will be needed in many patients to ensure this. Acute renal failure is most commonly related to preoperative creatinine clearance and postoperative hemodynamics. Minimizing nephrotoxic medications, renal vasoconstrictor levels, and maintaining a renal perfusion pressure of 60 torr or greater will help to keep the kidneys in the game. Urine which turns red after initially clearing might indicate intravascular hemolysis, which is many times related to evolving thrombus in the bloodstream. If the red urine is from hemoglobinemia (ie, little or no RBCs on urine analysis), a peripheral blood smear to look for RBC fragments and a plasma-free hemoglobin (Hgb) are obtained. Regular dosing of an osmotic diuretic such as mannitol is indicated if the plasma-free Hgb level is 50 mg/dL or greater. Most episodes of this type of hemolysis will resolve spontaneously.

Pain control is also important, since inadequately managed pain can have many deleterious effects on patient outcome. Narcotic analgesics remain the mainstay of pain control, though a few useful adjuncts are available. Blood narcotic levels adequate for postoperative analgesia are best maintained with a constant IV infusion and frequent miniboluses via nursing and possibly patient-controlled analgesia (PCA) pumps. Patients with significant prior proximate narcotic experience may need more, and not benefit from agonist-antagonist drugs such as nalbuphine. This type of patient may also accrue substantial narcotic efficacy with the use of alpha 2 agonists such as clonidine or dexmedetomidine.[17] Medications which act via altering prostaglandin metabolism (acetaminophen or nonsteroidal anti-inflammatory drug [NSAIDs]) are most useful when used on a regular schedule. Caution must be used with the NSAID drugs, though they remain relatively underutilized.[18] If renal function is decent and upper gastrointestinal issues quiescent, a medication such as intravenous ketorolac may be used for up to 72 hours, commencing on postoperative day 1, as long as some form of antacid therapy is under way. A judicious, as needed, dosing regimen with a benzodiazepine such as midazolam or lorazepam should be considered in the tense patient, as anxiety is well known to accentuate pain perception. Finally, attempts should be made to assess whether or not any periods of sleep are occurring. Sleep deprivation has numerous negative effects on patient well-being, both psychologic and physiologic.[19] If a "quiet as is reasonable" setting and minimization of spatial intrusion are not working, a light sedative such as diphenhydramine or zolpidem can be helpful. A purported advantage of zolpidem is less aberration of normal sleep stage progression. No doubt, the quiet nature of the newer-generation devices will help with patient sleep. Regional anesthetic techniques are not routinely used on patients who have had VAD placement, owing to anticoagulation proximity. Fortunately, most patients will be getting a lot more comfortable by postoperative days 5 to 7, especially as "hardware" (catheters, chest tubes, etc) is removed.

Close neurologic observation of these patients is also warranted, since a major cause of morbidity and mortality is related to cerebrovascular accident (CVA) or cerebral edema. Head CT scanning should be ordered, even when the index of suspicion is low. Magnetic resonance imaging (MRI) is not feasible with currently available LVAD technology. Inappropriately decreased level of consciousness with systemic hypertension can indicate cerebral hyperperfusion syndrome (HPS). Conservative medical therapy of intracranial hypertension, in conjunction with a judicious decrease in LVAD flow should result in rapid cerebral edema abatement. If a CVA is appreciated, thromboemboli must be considered. Evidence for thromboemboli may appear on the skin or in a concealed region such as the abdomen. Unexplainable decreasing renal function with or without red urine, abdominal distension with a rising lactate level, or elevating hepatic enzyme levels can all indicate thromboemboli to mesenteric or renal vessels. Ultrasound or CT studies can help to clarify the situation. For acute clot, escalation of anticoagulation is usually in order. Additionally, persistence or emergence of hypercoagulability should be considered. Thrombolytic therapy is sometimes undertaken, though risky since intracranial hemorrhage can occur. Electroencephalography (EEG) should be intermittently or continuously performed in the patient who is on a neuromuscular blocker or who is inappropriately obtunded, since nonconvulsive abnormal electrical activity (seizures) may be occurring, and an anticonvulsant indicated.[20]

Finally, aggressive nutritional rehabilitation provides one of the keys to full and prompt patient recovery, especially in the cachectic individual with preoperative protein losing enteropathy. The second- and third-generation devices are ideally suited for this approach. This is due to its compact configuration and lack of intraperitoneal placement. Hence, paralytic ileus, pancreatitis, mechanical obstruction, and perforation risks should be diminished greatly. When enteral (PO, NG, or NJ) food is not tolerated in spite of proper tube placement and/or medications which augment gut motility, (metoclopramide, erythromycin, or enteral naloxone), total parenteral nutrition should not be delayed. Our approach is to provide for full nutrition by days 2 to 4 postoperatively, preferably via the enteral route. This route is most desirable for purposes of restoring gut mucosal integrity and ameliorating cholestatic liver dysfunction.[21]

Using a fairly standard and well-executed perioperative management plan, successful implantation and maintenance of an LVAD will result in more patients being able to "cross the bridge" to well-being, arriving at the other side intact.

REFERENCES

1. Schmid C, Wilhelm M, Dietl K, et al. Noncardiac surgery in patients with left ventricular assist devices. *Surgery.* 2001;129:440-444.
2. Practice guidelines for pulmonary artery catheterization. A report by the ASA Task Force on pulmonary artery catheterization. *Anesthesiology.* 1993;78:380-394.
3. Melhorn U, Kroner A, de Vivie ER. 30 years clinical intra-aortic balloon pumping: facts and figures. *Thorac Cardiovasc Surg.* 1999;47(Suppl):298-303.
4. Slogoff S, Keats AS, Dear WE, et al. Steal-prone coronary anatomy and myocardial ischemia associated with four primary anesthetic agents in humans. *Anesth Analg.* 1991;72:22-27.
5. Mahmood AK, Courtney JM, Westaby S, et al. Critical review of left ventricular assist devices. *Perfusion.* 2000;15:399-420.
6. Levi M, Cromheecke ME, de Jonge E, et al. Pharmacologic strategies to decrease excessive blood loss in cardiac surgery: a meta-analysis of clinically relevant endpoints. *Lancet.* 1999;354:1940-1947.
7. Tribouilloy CM, Enriquez-Sarano M, Bailey KR, et al. Assessment of severity of aortic regurgitation using the width of the vena contracta: a clinical color Doppler imaging study. *Circulation.* 2000;102:558-564.
8. Konstadt SN, Louie EK, Black S, et al. Intraoperative detection of patent foramen ovale by transesophageal echocardiography. *Anesthesiology.* 1991;74:212.
9. Despotis GJ, Levine V, Saleem R, et al. Use of point-of-care test in identification of patients who can benefit from desmopressin during cardiac surgery: a randomized controlled trial. *Lancet.* 1999;354:106-110.
10. Tsang TSM, Oh JK, Seward JM. Diagnosis and management of cardiac tamponade in the era of echocardiography. *Clin Cardiol.* 1999;22:446-452.
11. Kusomoto FM, Goldschlager N. Cardiac pacing. *N Engl J Med.* 1996;334:89-98.
12. England MR, Gordon G, Salem M, et al. Magnesium administration and dysrhythmias after cardiac surgery. *JAMA.* 1992;268:2395-2402.
13. Daoud EG, Strickberger A, Man C, et al. Preoperative amiodarone as prophylaxis against atrial fibrillation after heart surgery. *N Engl J Med.* 1997;337:1785-1791.
14. Levy JH, Bailey JM, Deeb M. Intravenous milrinone in cardiac surgery. *Ann Thorne Surg.* 2002;73:325-330.
15. Van Belle AF, Wesseling GJ, Penn OC, et al. Postoperative pulmonary function abnormalities after coronary artery bypass surgery. *Respir Med.* 1992;86:195-199.
16. Yang KL, Tobin MJ. A prospective study of indices predicting the outcome of trials of weaning from mechanical ventilation. *N Engl J Med.* 1991;324:1445-1450.
17. Bovile JG. Update on opioid and analgesic pharmacology. *Anesth Analg.* 2001;92:51-55.
18. Myles P, Power I. Does ketorolac cause postoperative renal failure? *Br J Anaesth.* 1998;80:420-421.
19. Oates H. Non-pharmacologic pain control for the CABG patient. *Dimen Crit Care Nursing.* 1993;12:296-304.
20. Arrowsmith JE, Grocott H, Reves JG, et al. Central nervous system complications of cardiac surgery. *Br J Anaesth.* 2000;84:378-393.
21. Kehlet H. Manipulation of the metabolic response in clinical practice. *World J Surg.* 2000;24:690-695.

CHAPTER 10
LVAD IMPLANTATION TECHNIQUE

George Dimeling and Phil Oyer

INTRODUCTION

As with any cardiac surgical procedure, the technical precision with which a device is inserted can have a profound impact on the short- and long-term outcomes associated with the intervention. Subtle nuances in technique can affect postoperative bleeding risks, pump function, and standard surgical complications like infection and stroke. With the rapid evolution in left ventricular assist device (LVAD) technology, there is no "one-size-fits-all" approach to device insertion. Different engineering characteristics of newer devices mandate an individualized approach to implantation. However, there are a number of basic principles that apply to the field of LVAD surgery regardless of the device that is being implanted. This chapter will address the fundamental principles of LVAD implantation.

BASIC IMPLANTATION TECHNIQUE

While there are many variations on the basic theme, there is a basic system that the surgeon typically follows when implanting a device. Prior to making an incision, the surgeon must carefully review the transesophageal echocardiogram (TEE) in order to determine presence of any mitral, tricuspid, or aortic valvular dysfunction; presence of mural thrombi; or presence of patent foramen ovale (PFO), which could potentially impair device function and may need to be addressed surgically before device insertion. Although minimally invasive or alternative approaches have been described and employed, typically, the operation begins with a full median sternotomy. This provides excellent exposure for initiating cardiopulmonary bypass (CPB), elevating the heart for inflow cannula insertion and clamping the aorta for outflow graft anastomosis. A pericardial cradle is created by placing sutures into the pericardium and looping them around the retractor in manner that applies tension to the pericardium, thereby elevating the heart. This maneuver allows for better visualization and access to the structures of interest during device insertion.

Prior to administering heparin, a pump pocket is created in order to create a space for the device to sit in after anastomosis to the left ventricular (LV) apex. This step of the operation represents the point at which there is the most variability between the different device types. First-generation pulsatile LVADs often require extensive pocket dissection or intraperitoneal access in order to create enough space for these large devices

(Fig. 10–1). Second-generation axial-flow pumps are smaller and require much less dissection in order to permit intracorporeal implantation. These devices characteristically avoid the pitfalls of intraperitoneal insertion. With a newer third generation of LVAD technology (and some second-generation technology) accomplishing even smaller pump size, pump pocket dissection has been avoided altogether in some cases by placing the device inside the pericardium. For an implantable first-generation device, the pump pocket location depends on the presence of lung disease or previous abdominal surgery. The options for pump placement include extraperitoneal (with a pocket formed below the rectus abdominus and internal oblique muscles and above the posterior rectus sheath) and intraperitoneal. There are advantages and disadvantages to each strategy.[1] Extraperitoneal insertion poses a greater infection risk due to bleeding complications of pocket dissection. On the other hand, intraperitoneal insertion exposes the device to the abdominal viscera. In patients likely to be transplanted, the intra-abdominal placement is often avoided due to complications explanting the device. Others have described an approach that utilizes an intraperitoneal pocket using Gore® Dualmesh® Plus Biomaterial to shield the LVAD from the abdominal contents.[2]

In a virgin chest (and in newer-generation devices) an extraperitoneal pocket is the preferred approach. The inferior aspect of the midline incision is extended deep through the linea alba and can be continued above the posterior rectus sheath and peritoneum (Fig. 10–2). Once the desired tissue plane has been accessed, the pocket is extended laterally to the left with blunt dissection and hemostasis is achieved with electrocautery and clip placement. For implantation of larger devices, the diaphragm is incised either laterally at the level of the LV apex or medially. Experience has shown that either diaphragmatic incision will not impair respiratory mechanics. Many devices come with a mock pump that can be positioned inside the pocket in order to verify adequate dissection.

After the pump pocket has been prepared, heparin is administered and CPB is instituted once cannulation has been performed. The VAD is simultaneously prepared on a back table according to the manufacturer's instructions and transferred to the operative field. Inflow cannula insertion is usually performed first by selecting a site in the LV apex that is lateral to the left anterior descending (LAD) artery. Inflow cannulation stitches can be placed either before or after apical coring. Apical coring is accomplished either via a cruciate incision with circumferential tissue removal or with a coring device (provided by many device companies). Great care must be taken when implanting a continuous-flow device to position the inflow cannula in such a way that it is directed away from the septum in the direction of the mitral valve. Once apical coring has been performed, the left ventricle is then inspected for thrombus and debrided of calcium. Trabeculae that might obstruct the flow into the cannula are divided. There is often a tendency to not resect enough trabeculae. As long as the papillary muscles are preserved, generous resection is preferred. Ten to twelve pledgetted horizontal mattress sutures are then placed in a ringlike fashion around the ventriculotomy in an everting fashion (epicardium to endocardium, as shown in Fig. 10–3). It is essential to get good bites of

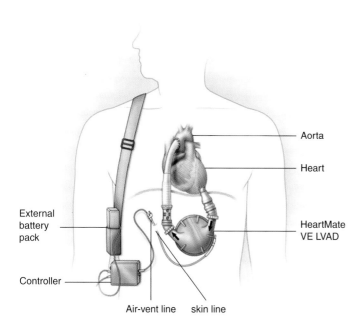

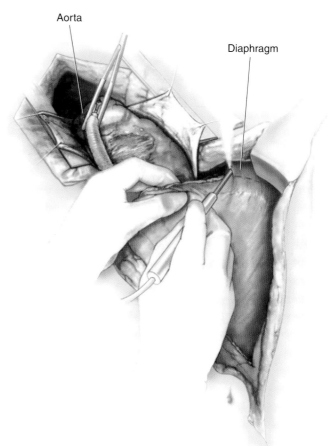

FIGURE 10–1. First-generation pulsatile LVADs are characterized by their large size, relative to newer devices. The implantable pumps require either extensive pocket dissection or intraperitoneal insertion in order to accommodate the large device. (Reproduced with permission from Rose EA, Gelijns AC, Moskowitz AJ, et al. Randomized Evaluation of Mechanical Assistance for the Treatment of Congestive Heart Failure (REMATCH) study group. *N Engl J Med.* 2001 Nov 15;345(20):1435-1443. Copyright © Massachusetts Medical Society. All rights reserved.)

FIGURE 10–2. Dissection of the pump pocket. (Reproduced with permission from Pennington DG, Lohmann DP, (eds). Novacor LVAS implantation technique. *Operative Techniques in Thoracic and Cardiovascular Surgery: A Comparative Atlas,* Vol. 4, No. 4.; 1999, Nov:318-329. Copyright © Elsevier.)

tissue, and this may be more easily accomplished by using Tevdek sutures with a longer needle. In friable ventricular tissue, small pledgets may actually pull through the muscle during the process of securing the device. Some centers have utilized a felt ring in place of pledgets to avoid this complication. These techniques will redistribute the tension away from the (often friable infarcted) tissue and provide the added benefit of reducing air entry.

After securing the inflow cannula to the LV apex, the device is de-aired, with a clamp placed across the vented outflow graft. With many pumps, the outflow graft is connected after the distal anastomosis is completed to allow better, continuous venting of the pump. The pump is placed within the abdominal pocket, and the length of the outflow graft is measured and trimmed. Ideally, the graft should lie under the right sternal border and out of harm's way in the event of a redo (particularly in cases where transplant is anticipated). Driveline positioning is performed, with two simple concepts employed to prevent late infection: maintaining adequate distance between the cutaneous incision and the device and developing a long tunnel that gradually rises through the preperitoneal plane to the skin. In first-generation implants, the pocket is often extended laterally to the right of the linea alba approximately 10 cm at the level of the umbilicus (Fig. 10–4). The tunneling device is typically placed through a skin incision to the right of the umbilicus and tunneled to the device pocket. Most devices utilize a system whereby the driveline is attached to the tunneling device and pulled through the tract and the skin where it is secured.

Placement of the outflow cannula can often be performed by placing a partial occlusion clamp across the ascending aorta. A longitudinal aortotomy is made with an 11 blade knife and extended with a Potts scissors. To perform an end-to-side anastomosis 4-0 or 5-0 Prolene suture is used (Fig. 10–5). After completion of the anastomosis, de-airing can be performed by temporarily releasing the partial occlusion clamp, filling the graft with blood, and allowing air to escape via an 18-gauge needle placed in the most superior portion os the graft. Any aortic regurgitation greater than mild on TEE findings is repaired prior to the insertion of the cannula by arresting the heart and oversewing the aortic valve. If a PFO is identified with the intraoperative TEE, it should be closed even if there is no shunt preoperatively. The shifts in atrial pressures with a single VAD in place can lead to unwanted desaturation postoperatively. The need for repair or replacement of the mitral and/or tricuspid valves in the setting of regurgitant disease remains controversial. In a non–bridge-to-recovery setting, mitral regurgitation is likely less problematic although in the face of significant pulmonary hypertension preoperatively, providing a competent valve may provide earlier and more complete reversal. If only an LVAD is being placed in the face of poor right ventricular (RV)

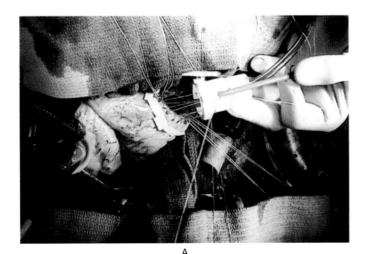

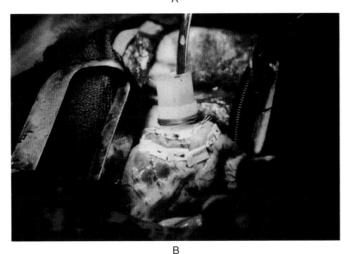

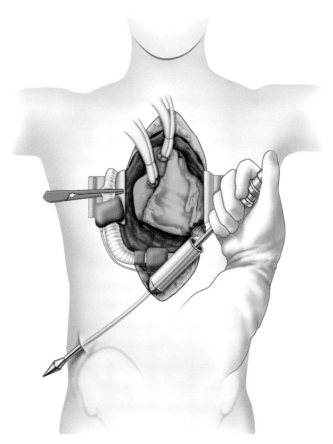

FIGURE 10–4. Positioning of the driveline. (Reproduced with permission Noon GP, Loebe M, Irwin S, et al. Implantation of the MicroMed DeBakey VAD. *Operative Techniques in Thoracic and Cardiovascular Surgery: A Comparative Atlas*, Vol 7, No. 3; 2002:111-170. Copyright © Elsevier.)

FIGURE 10–3. Inflow cannula insertion is performed by placing 10 to 12 pledgetted sutures around the ventriculotomy site. (Reproduced with permission from Slater JP, Williams M, Oz MC, et al. Implantation techniques for the TCI HeartMate left ventricular assist systems. *Operative Techniques in Thoracic and Cardiovascular Surgery: A Comparative Atlas*, Vol 4, No. 4; 1999. Copyright © Elsevier.)

function, dealing with tricuspid valve pathology may be beneficial in handling the right side in the postoperative setting.

After de-airing is complete, the patient is weaned from CPB and the device is activated according to the manufacturer's instructions. Cannulae are removed and hemostasis is achieved. There are several techniques of draining the surgical site, but the important concept is one of ensuring minimal areas where a hematoma can reside with its increased risk of pump pocket infection. The authors' approach is to place one or two chest tubes in the mediastinum, and a Blake drain is attached to a Jackson Pratt bulb suction device to evacuate the pump pocket. The pericardial contents can be covered with a number of commercially available devices to facilitate ease of reentry when the device is implanted as a bridge-to-transplantation. The sternum and incisions are closed in the usual fashion, and the driveline is secured with sutures.

SPECIAL CONSIDERATIONS

■ REDO STERNOTOMY

Quite frequently, patients have undergone previous cardiac surgery and the LVAD implantation occurs as either a first or multiple-time redo procedure. Therefore, careful dissection using an oscillating saw to divide the sternum is required to prevent hemorrhagic complications of reentry. External defibrillation pads are placed to permit treatment of arrhythmogenic complications. In cases of severe adherence of the dilated right ventricle (RV) to the sternum, the patient may require peripheral cannulation and/or cooling prior to dividing the sternum. In addition, virtually every LVAD insertion must be performed with the expectation that the patient will require another sternotomy, either for transplant or device changeout (although the latter represents a much less frequent event with newer device technology). A number of strategies have been employed to minimize the danger of reentering the previous sternotomy incision. Perhaps the most commonly reported approach involves inserting the device via a left thoracotomy.[3] In this technique, the patient is positioned in the right lateral decubitus position (with the left side up) in a similar fashion to positioning for a

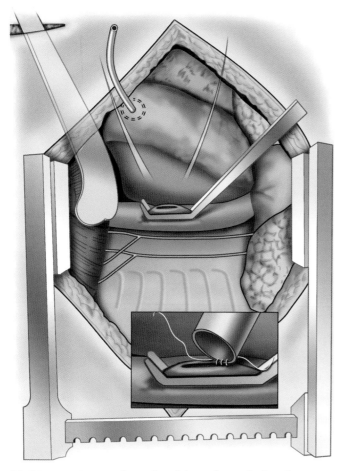

FIGURE 10–5. Exposure for sewing of the outflow graft when the LVAD is placed via left thoracotomy. (Reproduced with permission fom Pierson et al.[3] Copyright © Elsevier.)

thoracoabdominal aneurysm repair (both groins exposed by rotating the hips at 45 degrees). Lung isolation is achieved with a double lumen endotracheal tube, and cannulation is performed through the groin. A generous posterolateral thoracotomy incision is made to permit access to the descending aorta and LV apex through the pericardium. Implantation proceeds in the same sequence as through a sternotomy once CPB is initiated, with positioning of the inflow cannula followed by placement of a side-biter clamp on the descending aorta to permit anastomosis of the outflow graft. There is some suggestion that a descending aortic anastomosis reduces recirculatory flow that may create stagnation at the aortic root, based on computer flow modeling.[4]

■ OFF-PUMP INSERTION

Several different strategies have been utilized to facilitate LVAD insertion without the use of CPB. The off-pump approach to LVAD surgery carries many advantages in redo surgery, where a prolonged pump run may be associated with worsening end-organ function, atherosclerosis may limit access to the groin for cannulation, and excessive manipulation of the heart during dissection may be poorly tolerated. Frazier and colleagues have

described a nonthoracic, extraperitoneal, off-pump insertion technique that permits LVAD implantation without the use of CPB and extensive mediastinal dissection.[5] Using this technique, exposure to the LV apex was gained through a left subcostal incision (similar to what one would use for placement of epicardial pacemaker leads) that also permits access to the supraceliac aorta for outflow graft anastomosis. Alternatively, transdiaphragmatic insertion of the LV inflow cannula can be achieved via a left upper quadrant subcostal incision without entering the peritoneal cavity, mediastinum, or left chest.[6] Off-pump LVAD insertion has also been described via a redo sternotomy to expose the ascending aorta for outflow graft anastomosis and left anterior thoracotomy to minimize manipulation of the heart during inflow cannula insertion.[7]

■ CHALLENGES OF ABERRANT ANATOMY

In addition to the challenges posed by a redo sternotomy, many anatomic challenges may be present at the time of LVAD insertion. Many patients with end-stage heart failure undergo surgical ventricular restoration (SVR) as a strategy for improving cardiac function. However, some of these patients will suffer from progression of their cardiomyopathy such that LVAD therapy is required. Williams and Conte have described the challenges of VAD insertion under these conditions, whereby the suture line of the reconstructed anterior wall is identified to guide the surgeon to the apex.[8] In these cases, the new "functional" apex is typically more inferolateral to the natural apex, and the surgeon must be cognizant of this in order to properly direct the inflow cannula toward the mitral valve.[8] Difficulty in achieving proper inflow cannula placement can also be seen in cases of cardiomyopathy secondary to conotruncal abnormalities. These patients typically have a morphologic RV supplying their systemic circulation, and inflow cannula positioning can be compromised by the presence of a bulky moderator band. Joyce et al have promoted the use of epicardial ultrasound imaging to properly position the device in a way that promotes flow through the mitral valve.[9]

CONCLUSION

There are currently a number of strategies for safely inserting an LVAD utilizing a variety of different approaches. In the current era, the default approach for most long-term intracorporeal devices involves accessing the mediastinum through a sternotomy, followed by implantation assisted by CPB. Future application of newer technology will undoubtedly permit an increasing use of off-pump and minimally invasive approaches.

REFERENCES

1. Wasler A, Springer WE, Radovancevic B, Myers TJ, Stutts LA, Frazier OH. A comparison between intraperitoneal and extraperitoneal left ventricular assist system placement. *ASAIO J.* 1996;42(5):M573-M576.
2. Icenogle T, Sandler D, Puhlman M, Himley S, Sato DJ, Schaefer S. Intraperitoneal pocket for left ventricular assist device placement. *J Heart Lung Transplant.* 2003;22(7):818-821.
3. Pierson RN, III, Howser R, Donaldson T, et al. Left ventricular assist device implantation via left thoracotomy: alternative to repeat sternotomy. *Ann Thorac Surg.* 2002;73(3):997-999.

4. Kar B, Delgado RM, III, Frazier OH, et al. The effect of LVAD aortic out-flow-graft placement on hemodynamics and flow: implantation technique and computer flow modeling. *Tex Heart Inst J*. 2005;32(3):294-298.

5. Frazier OH, Gregoric ID, Cohn WE. Initial experience with non-thoracic, extraperitoneal, off-pump insertion of the Jarvik 2000 Heart in patients with previous median sternotomy. *J Heart Lung Transplant*. 2006;25(5):499-503.

6. Cohn WE, Frazier OH. Off-pump insertion of an extracorporeal LVAD through a left upper-quadrant incision. *Tex Heart Inst J*. 2006;33(1):48-50.

7. Collart F, Feier H, Metras D, Mesana TG. A safe, alternative technique for off-pump left ventricular assist device implantation in high-risk reoperative cases. *Interact Cardiovasc Thorac Surg*. 2004;3(2):286-288.

8. Williams J, Conte J. Ventricular assist device placement following surgical ventricular restoration. *Interact Cardiovasc Thorac Surg*. 2006;5(2):90-91.

9. Joyce DL, Crow SS, John R, et al. Mechanical circulatory support in patients with heart failure secondary to transposition of the great arteries. *J Heart Lung Transplant*. 2010;29(11):1302-1305.

CHAPTER 11

ANTICOAGULATION FOR VENTRICULAR ASSIST DEVICES

Ettore Vitali, Alessandro Barbone, Filippo Milazzo, and Marco Lanfranconi

INTRODUCTION

Bleeding and neurologic events are well-known major postoperative complications following implantation of mechanical circulatory support (MCS). Bleeding can occur either as an early surgical complication or later due to anticoagulation therapy and coagulation system impairment. Thromboembolism mainly occurs in the subacute or chronic phase because of the thrombogenicity of the blood-contacting surfaces within the devices. Bleeding and thromboembolic events are linked because they are two sides of the same issue: managing hemostasis. Over the years coagulation management protocols have changed, thanks to improving experience, improving knowledge, and evolution of the available devices. Historically, we have implemented three distinct coagulation management protocols: (1) a "conventional" protocol from 1998 to 1992; (2) a multisystem protocol A from 1993 to 2000; (3) a multisystem protocol B from 2000 to the present. Although the bleeding and thrombotic complications after left ventricular assist device (LVAD) surgery remain a concern, the new generation of devices (available since 2005) has helped address this problem, being much more "forgiving" with respect to anticoagulation management.

GENERAL CONSIDERATIONS

Coagulation is a physiologic activity of the formed elements of the blood, clotting factors, and endothelial tissue. Normally it is finely regulated by multiple interactive molecular pathways, some from the blood itself, some from other cell types, and some from foreign bodies. A detailed description of the system is beyond the scope of this discussion, but a practical and functional explanation has been provided since the late 19th century in Virchow's triad: activation of the coagulation system is determined by the interaction of three main factors:

- Blood coagulability: a balance between clotting factors that function in activating and deactivating the system
- Blood flow: stasis and turbulence favor coagulation
- Endothelial injury: in the normal state, endothelium generates an antithrombotic milieu

Put simply, in patients who are supported with MCS, the endothelium is missing; thus the system can be "rebalanced" only by impacting on the other two remaining categories. It is also intuitive that by limiting stasis\turbulence within the device at an engineering level, less is required to correct the coagulable state in the clinical setting. It should be noted that a considerable effort has been made to reduce shearing stress and stasis within the devices and facilitate the homing of endothelial cell progenitors to within the device, with mixed results. In this chapter we present a historical perspective in order to better describe the current status of the field. As an example we will report the experience in the Niguarda Ca' Granda Center in Milan throughout the device era, describing the strategies for managing anticoagulation during each phase of this evolution.

"CONVENTIONAL" PROTOCOL

At the very beginning, anticoagulation was based on intravenous heparin in the early postoperative period (target: partial thromboplastin time [PTT] > 1.5-2, to be started when drainage output was significantly reduced) and oral warfarin in the chronic phase (target: international normalized ratio [INR] value = 2.5-3). In Milan 46% of patients (6/13) had early bleeding requiring one or more surgical revision for hemostasis, a low rate of late bleeding (1/13 patients), and thromboembolic events in 3/13 patients. It should be noted that during this early phase the mean length of support was 13 days (range: 2-46 days).

MULTISYSTEM PROTOCOL A

In 1993, a new coagulation management and anticoagulation treatment protocol was proposed by the group at the "La Pitié–Salpetrière" Hospital in Paris that obtained excellent results in the control of biological bleeding and thromboembolic complications in patients assisted with MCS.[1] MCS implantation strongly stimulates the coagulation and fibrinolytic systems, as well as platelet activation. The bridging period can be considered an example of prolonged period of contact activation.[2] The "La Pitié" protocol in patients assisted with MCS considers that hemostatic disturbances are primarily a consequence of disseminated intravascular coagulation (DIC). DIC is a multifaceted syndrome and often is underappreciated in the early phase of its evolution. Indeed some studies documented the presence of sustained thrombin generation and fibrinolysis in patients with MCS despite normal values on routine coagulation tests or even when thromboembolic or bleeding complications are not clinically evident.[1,2] So, even if overt bleeding or thromboembolic events do not occur, DIC can evolve and become clinically evident with severe complications if not recognized and treated in its early phase. Therefore, using the protocol of La Pitié enables early recognition of the four interconnected stages of DIC: (1) procoagulant activation featuring compensated thrombophilia; (2) fibrinolytic activation with clot kinetic-structure dissociation and consumption of platelets, coagulation factors, and their inhibitors; (3) generalized hypocoagulability associated with localized hypercoagulability due to the reduction in coagulation factors, platelets, and inhibitory systems; (4) secondary (hyper) fibrinolysis with exhaustion of all inhibitory system factors. The resultant control and treatment of hemostatic systems, called "multisystem therapy,"[3] has three major objectives: (1) to stabilize the platelet system; (2) to balance the procoagulant system and its regulation (particularly the ATIII system)[3]; (3) to control the activation of the fibrinolytic system.

■ LABORATORY TESTS

To monitor the coagulation status and the effectiveness of the treatment, a simplified multisystem approach is used based on routine laboratory tests supplemented by other specific tests.

- Platelet count, prothrombin time (PT), partial thromboplastin time (PTT), and fibrinogen are common laboratory tests useful to evaluate coagulative alterations with or without treatment.

- D-dimer is an indicator of procoagulant activation as are the fibrinogen/fibrin degradation products (FDPs); the latter can also indicate fibrinolytic activation.

- α_2-Antiplasmin is the most powerful inhibitor of fibrinolysis and its decrease represents the degree of its consumption during a pathologic activation of the fibrinolytic system.

- Antithrombin III (ATIII) activity, both in plasma (pATIII) and in serum (sATIII), is a very useful and specific test. ATIII is a natural thrombin inhibitor and is activated by heparin. pATIII indicates the potential capacity to combine with thrombin; sATIII indicates the remaining ATIII potential for combination in the blood after clot formation. The difference between pATIII and sATIII is the antithrombin potential index (API). API variations, together with other coagulation parameters, are a marker of the state of global coagulability. The depletion of ATIII or its failure to adapt is reflected by a decrease in pATIII and an increase in sATIII, resulting in a reduction in API (Szefner calls this situation the "pinching" phenomenon that is biologically evident as hypocoagulability with bleeding but with underlying hypercoagulability because the decrease of API corresponds to serious decrease in antithrombinic activity that can therefore lead to thrombosis).[4]

- Thromboelastography (TEG) is performed both on native whole blood and with heparinase to check the effect of minimal heparin doses (Fig. 11–1). TEG is the only sensitive test that explores the whole coagulation system studying different phases and characteristics of clot formation. TEG studies the kinetics and dynamics of clot formation, the platelet activity, and the presence of fibrinolysis. From TEG the thrombodynamic potential index (TPI) is obtained (Table 11–1). The TPI defines a biological state of hypocoagulability (TPI < 6), normocoagulability (TPI of 6-15), or hypercoagulability (TPI > 15). Another parameter from TEG, the maximal amplitude (MA), is useful to assess platelet dysfunction (MA < 50) or a probable platelet-related hypercoagulability (MA > 68). TEG data coupled with the blood tests required by this approach are essential to check the coagulation state throughout its evolution and guide in pharmacologic intervention.

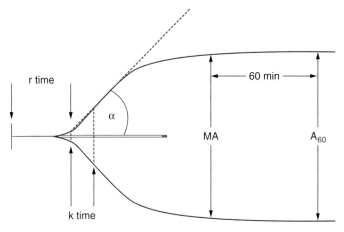

FIGURE 11–1. The normal thromboelastogram (TEG).

■ PHARMACOLOGICAL THERAPY

The aim of pharmacological therapy is to preserve platelet function, avoid thrombosis, and control fibrinolysis. Unfortunately, this requires a multipharmacological approach. Achieving balanced hemostasis can occur by utilizing a combination of the following drugs:

- Dipyridamole at high dosages (800 mg/d) can be administered intravenously at the time of implant immediately after anesthesia induction. The aim is to protect the platelets by maintaining their resting state. Platelets treated with high-dose dipyridamole become less sensitive to external proaggregant factors (platelet activation by cardiopulmonary bypass [CPB] or ventricular assist device [VAD]), thereby preserving their hemostatic capacity.[5,6]

- Anticoagulation during CPB is managed with standard dose of heparin (300 IU/kg). To reach and maintain the anticoagulation target by heparin, a normal ATIII activity is needed; in cases where this does not occur, 1000 IU of ATIII or more can be administered.[3] The dose of heparin is then adjusted to maintain an activated coagulation time (ACT) more than 420 to 450 seconds. Complete reversal of CPB heparinization is obtained by protamine usually at a ratio of protamine/heparin = 0.5 and accordingly to the ACT at the end of CPB. Some degree of residual heparinization can almost always be

TABLE 11–1. Main Parameters of Thromboelastography

Reaction time	r	Normal value: 12-15 mm
Coagulation time	k	Normal value: 9-13 mm
Maximal amplitude	MA	Normal value: 59-68 mm
Elasticity constant	ε	$\dfrac{100 \times MA}{100 - MA}$
Thrombodynamic potential index	TPI	$\dfrac{\varepsilon}{k}$ Normal value: 6-15

revealed by performing a TEG with heparinase. Nevertheless, this is typically well tolerated and corrected only when there is concern for hemorrhagic effects.

- Tranexamic acid can be administered intraoperatively at doses of 15 to 50 mg/kg according to the preoperative value of α_2-antiplasmin, CPB time, and the degree of post–CPB bleeding. The aim is to counterbalance the primary hyperfibrinolysis induced by CPB. Sometimes, tranexamic acid is used in the early postoperative period at dose of 250 to 500 mg until the α_2-antiplasmin levels are normalized in order to correct residual primary hyperfibrinolysis.

- Aspirin at a low dose (100 mg/d) is given postoperatively after 2 to 4 days in most devices when platelet count is more than 100,000/mm^3. At this dose aspirin never leaves the portal circulation, thus irreversibly inhibits platelet cyclooxygenase impairing platelet activation but leaving the endothelial Prostaglandin I2 (Prostacyclin) (PGI2) PGI2 system intact.[7]

- Ticlopidine at a relatively low dose (250 mg/d) is added in certain devices that are known to require more aggressive anticoagulation, and in instances in which TEG demonstrates thrombocytosis or platelet-related hypercoagulability (platelet antiadhesive activity).

- Pentoxifylline at a dose of 800 mg/d is given to improve hemorheology when fibrinogen levels begin to increase in the postoperative period.

- Low-dose heparin (100-300 IU/h) is administered postoperatively after recovery of normal hemostatic capacity as indicated by clinical findings (chest drain output), laboratory tests, and TEG (TPI > 6).

The targets of this therapy are (1) TPI value between 6 and 15 and (2) API value between 35 and 45.

Reaching and maintaining these targets is generally not difficult unless septic DIC or multiple organ system failure (MOSF) appears in the clinical course. Achieving these targets means that "low-dose" heparin provides efficient antithrombin and prophylactic effects, while retaining adequate function of the inhibitory system and thrombin formation sufficient for satisfactory hemostasis but insufficient for a state of hypercoagulabilty.[4]

After the early postoperative period, low-dose heparin is replaced by warfarin to reach a standard and therapeutic INR value once again depending on the device-patient characteristics. Low-molecular-weight heparin (LMWH) is administered only on demand when the INR is not at the desired level, although its role is anecdotal and dosages are more experience than evidence based. A limitation of LMWH is the absence of a laboratory test that is capable of testing blood levels and the clinical effect of the

TABLE 11–2. Bleeding Complication With Multisystem Protocol A Compared to "Conventional" Protocol

	Reoperation for Bleeding	Reoperation for Late Bleeding
"Conventional" protocol (1988-1992)	6/13 (46%)	1/13 (8%)
Multisystem protocol A (1993-2000)	5/34 (15%)	4/34 (12%)

drug, thereby impeding a dose-response use. Oral anticoagulation therapy decreases the level of coagulation factor X but is not able to antagonize its activated form because it does not act on the ATIII system and therefore fails to prevent the formation of thrombin microdoses which are a potential risk for thrombosis.[4] This situation is evidenced by hypercoagulability as seen in some cases with TEG. In this case, to counterbalance this potentially unfavorable situation, oral anticoagulation therapy must be increased (INR value > 3.5 up to 4), ticlopidine must be added, and higher doses of LMWH must be administered.

This multisystem protocol A was used in Milan until the year 2000; compared to the initial phase there was a reduction in early bleeding with some increase in late bleeding complications (Table 11–2). These were associated with an increase in nonseptic DIC or multiple-organ failure (MOF)–related thromboembolic events (with the caveat that during this period the average length of support dramatically increased, as shown in Table 11–3). A representative case is a male patient, 44 years old, assisted by Novacor LVAD and successfully transplanted after 381 days of support. On postimplant day 14, he suffered a transient ischemic attack (TIA) during what had previously been an uncomplicated clinical course. Laboratory tests showed an elevated TPI despite a therapeutic INR. Consequently, high-dose ticlopidine was added and higher INR values were achieved; nevertheless, the patient suffered two additional TIAs.

TABLE 11–3. Thromboembolic Complication With Multisystem Protocol A Compared to "Conventional" Protocol

		Length of Support
"Conventional" protocol (13 patients)	1 pulmonary embolism	13 ± 12 d (range 2-46)
	1 perioperative stroke	
	1 TIA	
Multisystem protocol A (34 patients)	2 strokes (MOSF, sepsis)	109 ± 208 d (range 4-1142)
	1 stroke (low compliance)	
	9 TIAs (1.6/patient)	

MOSF, multiple organ system failure; TIA, transient ischemic attack.

MULTISYSTEM PROTOCOL B

After 2000, a newer generation of assist devices became available. The revolution of introducing the axial-flow pump was not simply limited to the smaller pump size and continuous-flow physiology. The absence of a compliance chamber or prosthetic valves combined with the reduced blood-contacting surface of the newer-generation devices highly impacted on the incidence of thromboembolic events. However, the axial-flow devices unexpectedly produced high shearing stresses on platelets due to the elevated rpm (revolutions per minute) required by the impeller, resulting in platelet damage and activation.[8] Thus anticoagulation therapy for second-generation devices focuses much more on platelet activation and preservation, compared with the previous era. The platelet moves from being an "innocent bystander" of the phenomenon to becoming the activating and promoting agent. Therapy is therefore focused not on higher INR levels or heparin administration, but on a more complete and accurate control of platelet activation. The parallel research on coronary stents further enhances understanding of the platelet physiology and provides new powerful drugs that are rapidly being introduced in MCS therapy. During this transition, important studies (that resulted from many of the adverse events during early axial-flow use) were conducted on device fluid dynamics and performance. In addition, early attempts to introduce heparin-bonded surface within the new devices to reduce drug dependency led to major disasters. On a practical standpoint, the warfarin requirement was reduced (target INR: 2-2.5), and the objective of maintaining a low rate of early bleeding complications along with a decrease in late bleeding complications (Table 11–4) with a parallel reduction in thromboembolic events during lengthy support periods (Table 11–5) was achieved. It should be noted that the four thromboembolic events reported in Milan during the MicroMed DeBakey VAD use occurred in high-risk patients. A TIA occurred in an intubated patient who previously suffered from heavy nasal bleeding that required cessation of anticoagulation in order to control the hemorrhage. A VAD thrombosis, successfully treated with thrombolysis, occurred in a patient who was noted to have suboptimal anticoagulation therapy control during a transient period of illness. Another VAD thrombosis occurred in the course of a urinary tract infection secondary to a permanent indwelling urinary catheter for prostatic disease; this patient was treated with standard doses of intravenous heparin. A retrospective evaluation of ATIII and API trends demonstrated an underlying pathologic activation of his coagulation cascade. Subsequently, the patient suffered from severe DIC

TABLE 11–4. Bleeding Complications With Multisystem Protocol A Compared to Multisystem Protocol B

	Reoperation for Early Bleeding	Reoperation for Late Bleeding
Multisystem therapy A	5/34 (15%)	4/34 (12%)
Multisystem therapy B	4/35 (11%)	1/35 (3%)

during emergency heart transplant, which was successfully treated with the multisystem therapy.

THIRD GENERATION OF DEVICES

Currently, a third generation of devices has reached the assist device market. With these centrifugal flow pumps, the impeller is no longer longitudinal to the blood flow (axial flow) but perpendicular (centrifugal flow). This not only influences the shape of the device that is once again smaller and more compact, but increases the hemodynamic efficiency. A direct consequence of these design features is a lower rpm rate to maintain systemic perfusion, further reducing the shearing stress on the platelet. Furthermore, engineers have developed strategies to avoid stagnation within the device. Magnetic levitation has completely removed bearings from these devices, thereby minimizing heat production and consequently limiting thrombus formation. Experience has shown that even a microscopically insignificant thrombus can be the substrate for a more aggressive and dangerous thrombosis. Consequently, anticoagulation with the third generation of devices is reduced to minimal levels, comparable to those of a mechanical aortic valve. Finally, after years of center-based complex algorithms, a standardized and reproducible anticoagulation protocol has become available, permitting this technology to be implemented in widespread use with large clinical trials to determine outcomes. Implantable or paracorporeal devices that employ this technology require a

TABLE 11–5. Thromboembolic Events With Multisystem Protocol A Compared to Multisystem Protocol B

		Length of Support
Multisystem protocol A (34 patients)	2 strokes (MOF, sepsis)	109 ± 208 d (range 4-1142)
	1 stroke (low compliance)	
	9 TIAs (1.6/patient)	
Multisystem protocol B (range 1-453)	1 stroke (67 years old)	88 ± 110 d (range 4-1142)
	1 TIA (after bleeding)	
	2 VAD thrombosis	

MOF, multiple organ failure; TIA, transient ischemic attack; VAD, ventricular assist device.

modest anticoagulation regimen with IV heparin to be initiated when clinically feasible (usually chest drain output < 30 mL for several hours) and to be held at 50% of normal level for CPB (standard ACT 180-200 seconds or a PTT of 50-60 seconds). This is transitioned to oral warfarin for an INR of 1.7 to 2.0 whenever the patient can start oral medications. Typically, a single dose of 100 mg of aspirin per day is administered to maintain platelet aggregation levels at a low level. The data available worldwide are still relatively limited, but the experience accumulated to date at the Istituto Clinico Humanitas in Milan remains promising. Although anecdotal, our early experience with the HeartWare HVAD is notable for the absence of a single cerebrovascular accident or thromboembolic event despite very little anticoagulation therapy (in several cases even none and for up to 6 months). With more experience using these types of devices, it may become possible to relax the anticoagulation and antiplatelet requirement even further.

CONCLUSION

In our clinical experience treating patients on MCS, the multisystem anticoagulation protocol proved to be effective in reducing the incidence of bleeding and thromboembolic events either with the first- or second-generation devices.[9,10] After the introduction of the multisystem protocol B in 2000, the incidence of late bleeding, as well as the rate of thromboembolic event, decreased due to improved coagulation control in the chronic phase. Four thromboembolic events were registered and all of them happened in patients who were at high risk for thrombosis. It should be pointed out that the number of thromboembolic events has been favorably low without relying on heavy antiplatelet therapy. Hopes are high that the third generation of VADs will usher in an era of therapy in which thromboembolic and bleeding complications will occur in only a small minority of patients. While limited in volume, our experience in managing the anticoagulation and antiplatelet therapy of assist device patients over the years is illustrative of the evolution that has taken place within the field with the development of new devices and patient management strategies. The need for multicenter prospective randomized studies remains a worthy but difficult goal to achieve in light of the current financial restrictions on the global economy. Fortunately, the need to definitively elucidate the best pharmacological approach and minimize hemorrhagic and thromboembolic complications during MCS may have been overcome in part by the outcomes associated with the third generation of devices.

REFERENCES

1. Spanier T, Oz M, Levin H, et al. Activation of coagulation and fibrinolytic pathways in patients with left ventricular assist devices. *J Thorac Cardiovasc Surg.* 1996 Oct;112(4):1090-1097.
2. Tanaka K, Wada K, Morimoto T, et al. Hemostatic alterations caused by ventricular assist devices for postcardiotomy heart failure. *Artif Organs.* 1991 Feb;15(1):59-65.
3. Williams MR, D'Ambra AB, Beck JR, et al. A randomized trial of antithrombin concentrate for treatment of heparin resistance. *Ann Thorac Surg.* 2000 Sep;70(3):873-877.
4. Szefner J. Control and treatment of hemostasis in cardiovascular surgery. The experience of La Pitie Hospital with patients on total artificial heart. *Int J Artif Organs.* 1995;18(10):633-648.
5. Teoh KH, Christakis GT, Weisel RD, et al. Dipyridamole preserved platelets and reduced blood loss after cardiopulmonary bypass. *J Thorac Cardiovasc Surg.* 1988 Aug;96(2):332-341.
6. Zilla P, Fasol R, Groscurth P, Klepetko W, Reichenspurner H, Wolner E. Blood platelets in cardiopulmonary bypass operations. Recovery occurs after initial stimulation, rather than continual activation. *J Thorac Cardiovasc Surg.* 1989;97(3):379-388.
7. Pedersen AK, FitzGerald GA. Dose-related kinetics of aspirin. Presystemic acetylation of platelet cyclooxygenase. *N Engl J Med.* 1984 Nov 8;311(19): 1206-1211.
8. Koster A, Loebe M, Hansen R, et al. Alterations in coagulation after implantation of a pulsatile Novacor LVAD and the axial flow MicroMed DeBakey LVAD. *Ann Thorac Surg.* 2000 Aug;70(2):533-537.
9. Vitali E, Lanfranconi M, Ribera E, et al. Successful experience in bridging patients to heart transplantation with the MicroMed DeBakey ventricular assist device. *Ann Thorac Surg.* 2003;75(4):1200-1204.
10. Vitali E, Lanfranconi M, Bruschi G, Russo C, Colombo T, Ribera E. Left ventricular assist devices as bridge to heart transplantation: the Niguarda experience. *J Card Surg.* 2003 March;18(2):107-113.

CHAPTER 12
LYSIS THERAPY FOR VAD THROMBOSIS

Christof Schmid and Hans H. Scheld

Left ventricular assist device (LVAD) technology has evolved from the first-generation devices that included large pump chambers and implantation via a separate pump pocket in the posterior rectus sheath to continuous-flow pumps that lack the conduits and valves that were prone to thrombus formation and deposition. In the early devices, cerebral and systemic embolism occurred not infrequently, because despite aggressive anticoagulation there was no mechanism preventing the displacement of thrombotic material.[1] Continuous-flow pumps emerged with the assumption that the thromboembolic hazard was much lower in these pumps due to their smaller size and freedom from areas of blood stasis within the pump.[2]

Nevertheless, thromboembolic complications have become a leading problem in ventricular assist device (VAD) therapy as perioperative bleeding complications and device infection have been minimized in the current era. Despite all advances in device technology, thrombus formation and the rate of embolic events could not be lowered to a negligible percentage.[1] In the bulky first-generation devices, thrombotic material became adherent to the Dacron grafts and biological valves, and was rarely seen inside the pump chamber. In the first-generation axial-flow pumps, thrombus formation developed around and inside the inflow conduit, whereas the impeller housing was only rarely affected (Figs. 12–1 and 12–2).

After the initial implants with second-generation axial-flow devices, several centers reported on patients who presented with a declined pump flow and an increased current consumption (power demand) suspicious of thrombus formation or dislodgement inside the pump. In a few cases, current consumption declined to a degree that suggested thrombotic obstruction ahead of the impeller. Other patients experienced pump stoppage, either momentarily or permanently. These events led to regurgitant flow across the device with consequent severe hemodynamic compromise. As in second-generation devices a large mass of thrombotic material has only rarely been observed inside the pump housing, there is currently a large debate whether a thrombus develops within the device at all or is typically dislodged into it. Theoretically, thrombus formation may also occur inside the left atrium or ventricle, or may be already present prior to surgery and loosen during long-term anticoagulation (Fig. 12–3).

Lysis therapy is considered if there is a significant decline of pump output or an ongoing pump stoppage which proves irreversible following augmentation of heparin treatment and a bolus treatment with antiaggregant drugs like aspirin.[3] An imminent low output syndrome is a strong indicator for urgent therapy. Contraindications to lysis therapy include conditions that would lead to deleterious bleeding complications. Diseases like gastric ulcers or sigmoid diverticulae are usually an exclusion criterion for VAD implantation and play only a minor role in this context. More often, the question that emerges is at what time interval postoperatively lysis therapy can be attempted with an acceptable risk. Since a large experience with mechanical support devices is lacking, investigators have turned their attention to the use of lysis therapy in patients with other diseases, such as pulmonary embolism. In our own experience, patients successfully underwent lysis therapy within 4 days following open-heart surgery without significant bleeding complications. Nevertheless, a general recommendation cannot be made, and the decision toward lysis therapy has always been based on individual considerations.

Lysis therapy may be performed with different drugs, including streptokinase, urokinase, and recombinant tissue plasminogen activator (rtPA). In our own experience, we always used rtPA-lysis for its simplicity and its well-known indications such as stroke, pulmonary embolism, left or right ventricular thrombi, and acute myocardial infarction. Patients are initially treated with 25 to 50 mg given as IV bolus. If the bleeding risk is considered low or the acuity of the situation is high, another 50 mg should be added as a continuous infusion over a period of 1 to 2 hours. Since partial thromboplastin time (PTT) may increase during lysis, the dosing of IV heparin can be temporarily lowered. Coagulation parameters must be surveyed in short intervals. Following lysis, the PTT should be augmented to or kept at levels of 80 to 100 seconds, and antiplatelet therapy intensified.

Our experience includes eight patients with a total of 10 episodes suspicious of thrombus formation and consecutive rtPA-lysis. All patients survived lysis therapy and normalized pump flow and power demand within 3 hours. No severe bleeding complications were seen, and there was no evidence of intracranial hemorrhage. Four patients suffered from a brief period of epistaxis while could be easily controlled by nasal tamponade. Repeat thrombolysis, which was necessary in two patients, was as successful as the initial procedures.[4] Therefore, in our experience lysis therapy has been found to be highly efficacious. If the pump does not stop, the (reduced) blood flow through the inflow conduit (still) allows the lytic drug to be delivered to the thrombotic mass. The thrombus decreases in size and is finally split into tiny pieces by the rotation of the impeller. Thus, the rate of clinically evident thromboembolism is low in these cases.

rtPA was the drug of choice in our institution, but alternative treatment modalities are present. The first lysis therapy in a LVAD patient ever was done by intra-atrial urokinase

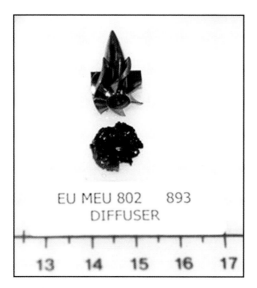

FIGURE 12-1. Thrombus removed from the pump chamber. (Reproduced with permission from Rothenburger et al.[4] Copyright © Wolters Kluwer Health.)

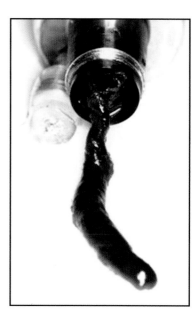

FIGURE 12-3. Large thrombus in the inflow cannula, which looks like being dislodged into it.

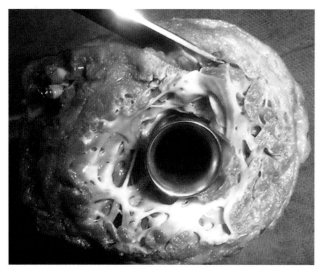

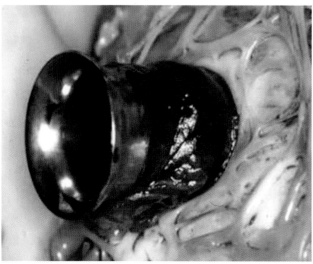

FIGURE 12-2. Intraventricular thrombus around the inflow cannula.

administration. This Novacor patient demonstrated complete resolution of his neurologic findings and proofed the feasibility of lysis therapy in patients with long-term mechanical support systems.[5] Accordingly, it can be presumed that most currently available lytic drugs may be beneficial in these situations.

In conclusion, lysis therapy is well justified in case of thrombus-related continuous-flow pump dysfunction. The risk is certainly lower as compared to a surgical pump exchange on an emergency basis, and pump flow is usually fully restored.

REFERENCES

1. Schmid C, Weyand M, Nabavi DG, et al. Cerebral and systemic embolization during left ventricular support with the Novacor N100 device. *Ann Thorac Surg.* 1998;65:1703-1710.
2. Noon GP, Hetzer R, Loebe M, et al. Clinical experience with the DeBakey VAD axial flow pump. *Cardiovasc Engineering.* 2000;5:30-32.
3. Schmid C, Wilhelm M, Rothenburger M, et al. Effect of high dose platelet inhibitor treatment on thromboembolism in Novacor patients. *Eur J Cardiothorac Surg.* 2000;17:331-335.
4. Rothenburger M, Wilhelm MJ, Hammel D, et al. Treatment of thrombus formation associated with the MicroMed DeBakey VAD using recombinant tissue plasminogen activator. *Circulation.* 2002;106:I189-I192.
5. Kasirajan V, Smedira NG, Perl J, II, McCarthy PM. Cerebral embolism associated with left ventricular assist device support and successful therapy with intraarterial urokinase. *Ann Thorac Surg.* 1999;67:1148-1150.

CHAPTER 13

INFECTIOUS COMPLICATIONS OF MECHANICAL CIRCULATORY SUPPORT

Joyce L. Sanchez and Dora Y. Ho

INTRODUCTION

Infections are a well-known complication of ventricular assist devices (VADs). They are more often than not difficult to treat and can cause significant morbidity and mortality in patients. VAD-related infections are associated with VAD malfunction, rehospitalization, thromboembolic events, and delay in transplantation. This carries heavy implications for both transplant candidates as well as patients who undergo destination therapy. The literature of these device-related infections is an actively growing area of investigation. This chapter aims to define various types of VAD-associated infections and the breadth of these infections, and discusses the following topics: host factors, defining types of infection, the associated microbiology, management, and prevention of VAD-related infections.

HOST FACTORS

Most infectious disease consultants' approach to any infection begins with examination of the host. Breakdown in host defenses allowing organism entry puts patients at risk for infections. The most obvious anatomic factor in VAD patients is the presence of a foreign body with entry and exit sites through the skin giving pathogens a portal of entry.

One could extrapolate that host factors associated with infections in patients with other foreign bodies (such as hemodialysis catheters, central venous catheters, external fixators, etc) could be applied to patients with VADs. One observational study by Herrmann et al,[1] following 32 left ventricular assist device (LVAD) recipients, found that there were higher numbers of LVAD-related infections in patients who were older, had longer ventilator support, and underwent surgical device revision. Larger, more recent studies have not found this to be the case. One cohort study by Simon et al investigated age, sex, type of cardiomyopathy, diabetes, prior sternotomy, length of hospitalization before VAD implantation, type of VAD, operative time, driveline site, and duration of VAD support. They initially found no statistically significant variable. On subgroup analysis they did find that patients with VAD-associated infections were

more likely to have diabetes, suggesting that diabetes was a risk factor.[2] Another study by Malani et al showed that need for hemodialysis was a risk factor for surgical site infections.[3] By their analysis there was no statistically significant difference between patients with and without surgical site infections regarding age, sex, duration of VAD support or cardiopulmonary bypass, or presence of cardiovascular disease. Diabetes mellitus was not evaluated in this study. Poston et al[4] performed a retrospective review of VAD patients and in their multivariate analysis found that reoperation during VAD support and longer intensive care unit (ICU) stay were predictors of VAD-related bloodstream infections. Interestingly, they found that biventricular support was a protective factor in VAD-related infection.

More recently, studies have investigated risk factors for fungal infections. This is of particular interest as systemic fungal infections have been associated with increased risk of all-cause mortality.[5] A retrospective chart review by Darouchiche et al compared demographic and clinical characteristics of patients with bacterial versus fungal infections. In multivariate analysis they found that preoperative use of total parenteral nutrition (TPN) was the only statistically significant factor associated with VAD-related fungal infection.[5]

Defects in cellular and humoral immunity have not traditionally been thought to be contributing factors in VAD-associated infections. Indeed these patients are, for the most part, considered immunocompetent; at least until patients whose VADs are implanted as a bridge undergo heart transplant. In a study by Ankersmit et al, T-cell function, apoptosis, and presence of *Candida* infection were analyzed in patients with New York Heart Association (NYHA) class IV heart failure who received an LVAD versus medical therapy.[6] Serum samples between the two groups showed lowered T-cell proliferative responses and a higher rate of spontaneous apoptosis in patients who received LVADs compared with controls. Furthermore, the risk of developing a *Candida* infection was 28% in LVAD recipients compared with 3% in the controls ($P < 0.001$). How well the LVAD versus control patients were matched was unclear, however. A later review by Itescu and John also outlined this phenomenon pointing toward LVAD patients developing progressive defects in cellular immunity due to selective loss of Th1 cytokine producing CD4 T cells through activation-induced cell death as well as unopposed activation of Th2 cytokine producing CD4 T cells resulting in B-cell hyperreactivity and dysregulated immunoglobulin synthesis.[7]

TYPES OF INFECTIONS/DIAGNOSTICS

The definition of VAD-related infections has not been standardized. However, most of the literature does agree on the spectrum of disease and on most key aspects used to define the types of these infections. There are two portals of organism entry: the first being the driveline exit site, the second being from hematogenous source. Most authors distinguish localized infection from more severe, systemic infection. Local infections include driveline site infections and VAD pocket infections. Systemic infections include VAD-related bloodstream infections and VAD-related endocarditis. For the purposes of this chapter,

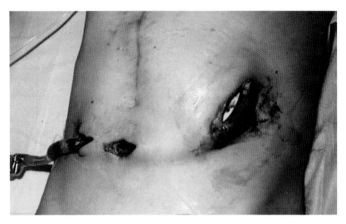

FIGURE 13-1. Severe wound infection of the lateral wall uncovering the pump chamber and driveline. (Reproduced with permission from Tjan et al.[8] Copyright © Elsevier.)

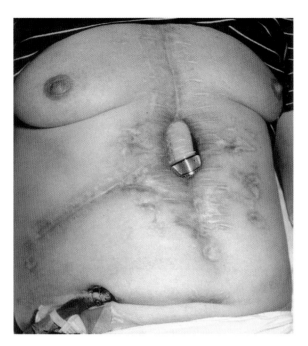

FIGURE 13-2. Severe median wound infection with a visible outflow conduit. (Reproduced with permission from Tjan et al.[8] Copyright © Elsevier.)

four types of infection are described: driveline site infection, VAD pocket infection, VAD-related bloodstream infection, and VAD-related infective endocarditis. As with any postsurgical patient in the ICU, other primary infections including ventilator associated pneumonia and urinary tract infections do occur, but these are beyond the scope of this chapter's discussion.

Localized driveline site infection is defined as cellulitis and/or purulent drainage from the driveline exit site. Some investigators also required isolation of at least one pathogen from the site[2,5] to meet the definition of driveline site infection, while others do not. Pocket infections are defined as the presence of a fluid collection and/or localized purulence in the pocket where the VAD is placed along with the isolation of at least one pathogen. In older pulsatile models, the device would be placed in the peritoneum. Continuous-flow pumps are placed in the subcutaneous space of the abdominal wall, while newer models are implanted in the pericardial space. Severity of pocket infections is variable but can be very serious (Figs. 13–1 and 13–2).[8]

VAD-related bloodstream infection is defined by isolation of the same organism from more than one blood culture as well as from the driveline site and/or VAD pocket though it is also implicated when there is more than one positive blood culture with the same organism and no other identifiable source.[2,5] VAD-related infective endocarditis is defined as by isolation of the same organism from more than one positive blood culture and association with one or more embolic events. Some studies required histopathologic evidence of infection of the inflow/outflow conduits of an explanted device[3] though this may not always be applicable for patients whose VADs are destination therapy. Signs and symptoms for VAD-related endocarditis are variable, from very mildly raised body temperature to the more obvious presentation similar to infective endocarditis and endarteritis.[9,10]

MICROBIOLOGY

As with intravascular devices in general, the most commonly seen pathogens in VAD-related infections are from gram-positive organisms, especially *Staphylococcus* species. In Host Factors section the

retrospective study by Simon et al, *Staphylococcus epidermitis* was isolated in 38% and *Staphylococcus aureus* in 24% of LVAD-related bloodstream infections.[2] The specific factor possessed by *S. aureus* making it especially opportunistic and pathogenic is an area of active investigation. In particular, the relationship of bacterial adherence proteins to VAD membranes has been suggested to be a component contributing to the aggressive pattern of infection by this pathogen.[11] Other less commonly seen gram-positive organisms include *Enterococcus* and *Corynebacterium* species, which more often are seen in local infection. Deng et al isolated enterococci from 18% of driveline and VAD pocket infections.[12]

Gram negatives consist of the next most common group of organisms implicated in VAD-related infections. Sivaratnam and Duggan suggest that gram-negative rods tend to involve the VAD devices directly and are associated with poor outcomes in their retrospective review of the literature.[13] In a review by Gandelman et al, 29% of LVAD patients with nosocomial bloodstream infections had gram-negative organisms isolated—the two most common being *Pseudomonas aeruginosa* and *Enterobacter* species.[14] Other less commonly seen pathogens include *Klebsiella, Acinetobacter, Citrobacter, Serratia, Escherichia coli,* and *Proteus* species.[13,14] These organisms have also been seen in local infection. In a retrospective review by Zierer and colleagues following LVAD patients with late-onset local driveline infections, gram negatives (*Enterobacter faecalis* and *Klebsiella pneumonia*) were implicated in local infections, second to gram positives.[15]

Fungal infections in VAD patients have gained importance in recent years. In a retrospective study by Gordon et al, 38% of bloodstream infections were found to be LVAD associated. When stratified by pathogens, fungemia had the highest hazard ratio for death (10.9) over gram-negative bacteremia (5.1) and gram-positive bacteremia (2.2). In this study, the cases of fungemia were from *Candida*.[16] In a subsequent retrospective chart review by Aslam and collegues,[5] *Candida albicans* was the most common fungal pathogen responsible for VAD-related infections. These were mostly implicated in invasive infections of the bloodstream (65% of the fungal infections). Nurozler et al prospectively looked at LVAD patients with fungal infections and also found the majority associated with *Candida* species. They also reported two infections with *Aspergillus* and one with *Syncephalastrum*.[17]

TREATMENT

No head-to-head randomized controlled trials exist comparing different antibiotic regimens in the treatment of VAD-related infections. Indeed it would be difficult to conduct such studies as there are several factors influencing choice of antibiotic therapy. Important considerations include type of infection, severity of illness, prior antibiotic use, current antibiotics, prior culture results (when applicable), antibiogram of the patient care unit or hospital, allergies, and renal and liver function.[18,19] Whenever possible, blood cultures from at least two different sites should be collected before initiation of antibiotics to increase the likelihood of isolating a pathogen. A full diagnostic workup should be initiated as soon as possible.

Despite advances in microbiological technology, in most clinical laboratories isolation and identification of pathogens from patient specimens still require traditional culture techniques, which routinely take up to several days. Thus, when a VAD-related infection is suspected, antibiotic selection is almost always empiric and based on the aforementioned factors. Treatment of local driveline site infections in stable patients can usually be limited to gram-positive coverage, while broader gram-positive and gram-negative coverage should be initiated when systemic infection is suspected.[19] Intravenous vancomycin is generally included in empiric regimens given the frequency of staphylococcal infections, methicillin-resistant *Staphylococcus aureus* (MRSA) in particular.[10] Rare exceptions in this recommendation include patients with vancomycin intolerance or known presence of vancomycin-resistant enterococci (VRE). In these cases, other agents such as linezolid, quinupristin/dalfopristin, and daptomycin are suitable alternatives.[20] A newer antibiotic, telavancin, which is FDA-approved for treatment of complicated skin and skin structure infections, also has activity against MRSA, but the clinical experience with its use for device-related infections is limited. Antibiotic coverage should subsequently be narrowed once culture identification and sensitivity results become available to prevent emergence of multidrug-resistant organisms and to minimize side effects from broad-spectrum antibiotics. This approach also allows longevity of the antibiotic armamentarium for the patient, should relapses or other infections arise.[18]

When infections are confined to the driveline site, antibiotics, local wound care, and immobilization of the device are mainstays of treatment.[2,21,18] While most local infections are successfully treated with less than 14 days of antibiotics, there have been cases when relapses occurred requiring chronic suppressive antibiotics until the device is removed with transplantation.[16] Thus, after diagnosis and treatment of a driveline site infection, the patient should be followed closely for any signs or symptoms of relapse. Deeper VAD pocket infections, being more serious, require aggressive measures with hospitalization and surgical debridement with irrigation and drainage, in addition to antibiotic treatment.

In many cases, the removal of necrotic and infected areas of these wounds leaves a dead space. Some institutions have addressed this with omental and/or muscle flaps to help cover the defect and control infection.[22,23] Other successes have been seen with antibiotic-impregnated bead placement.[24] Since it is very difficult to eradicate organisms when foreign bodies are involved despite these measures, antibiotics are generally administered until either the pump is removed and/or when transplantation occurs.[25] Indeed, VAD patients with active bloodstream infection undergoing bridge-to-transplant are upgraded to United Network for Organ Sharing (UNOS) priority 1A.[26] As outlined by Poston and colleagues, VAD explantation continues to be the only option that decreases mortality in patients with VAD-related bloodstream infections.[4] Finally, it is universally practiced that VAD-related endocarditis be treated with antibiotics and device removal.[10,19]

PREVENTION

No topic regarding infectious diseases is complete without addressing the ultimate goal of prevention. This is especially the case with VAD-related infections, where the morbidity of reoperation can be substantial and device explantation is rarely an option. In VAD patients, the strategies needed to minimize infections should be implemented preoperatively, perioperatively, and post–VAD implantation.

Primary prophylaxis with antibiotics against staphylococci is recommended with placement of VADs. Although there are no randomized controlled clinical trials to support their use, recommendations are extrapolated from studies from both general cardiac surgery and hardware placement in orthopedics.[18] Most experts agree on administration of one dose of a β-lactam, such as cefazolin, approximately 1 hour before placing the device. In patients with β-lactam allergy or known colonization or infection with MRSA, vancomycin should be used.[10] Institutions vary in their protocols. In the REMATCH (Randomized Evaluation of Mechanical Assistance for the Treatment of Congestive Heart Failure) trial, comparing medical versus ventricular assistance in patients ineligible for transplant, antibiotic prophylaxis was very broad including vancomycin, a fluoroquinolone, rifampicin, and fluconazole.[27] There may be variation in antibiotic choice, particularly in the case of patients with known established infections or prolonged hospital course prior to VAD implantation. Antibiotics should be discontinued by 48 hours after closure.

Standard intraoperative infection prevention guidelines should be followed, including aseptic technique and proper operating room (OR) attire. Experience has also specified strategies in VAD implantation. It is imperative to insert the pump chamber in such a way that closure is performed without undue tension.[8] Most also, tunnel the driveline contralateral to the pump pocket, increasing the subcutaneous track that organisms would have to travel before reaching the pocket site.[19] Earlier, larger devices implanted into the abdominal cavity had fewer infections than those implanted into the abdominal wall;[28] however, given the risk of organ injury and advancements in manufacturing smaller devices, this strategy has fallen out of favor.

Appropriate postoperative management is imperative in prevention of VAD-related infections. Once the patient is stable, removal of all tubes and lines is critical in preventing acquisition of other nosocomial infections that may seed the VAD device. Adequate education needs to take place between the patient, nursing staff, and other care providers to address wound care, including dressing change technique, frequency of changes, bathing issues, and so on. Optimization of nutrition early in the post-op course and glucose control in diabetics are also recommended.

SUMMARY

VAD-related infections continue to be a well-established complication of mechanical circulatory support. Though they are associated with morbidity and mortality, early detection and aggressive management can successfully treat these infections, particularly localized infections of the exit site. Bloodstream infections and VAD-related endocarditis are more difficult to treat with medical management alone and, when possible, VAD explantation and/or transplantation improve outcomes. Above all, preventive measures should be implemented preoperatively, perioperatively, and post–VAD implantation.

REFERENCES

1. Herrmann M, Weyand M, Greshake B, et al. Left ventricular assist device infection is associated with increased mortality but is not a contraindication to transplantation. *Circulation*. 1997;95(4):814-817.
2. Simon D, Fischer S, Grossman A, et al. Left ventricular assist device-related infection: treatment and outcome. *Clin Infect Dis*. 2005;40(8):1108-1115.
3. Malani PN, Dyke DBS, Pagani FD, Chenoweth CE. Nosocomial infections in left ventricular assist device recipients. *Clin Infect Dis*. 2002;34(10):1295-1300.
4. Poston RS, Husain S, Sorce D, et al. LVAD bloodstream infections: therapeutic rationale for transplantation after LVAD infection. *J Heart Lung Transplant*. 2003;22(8):914-921.
5. Aslam S, Hernandez M, Thornby J, Zeluff B, Darouiche RO. Risk factors and outcomes of fungal ventricular-assist device infections. *Clin Infect. Dis*. 2010;50(5):664-671.
6. Ankersmit HJ, Tugulea S, Spanier T, et al. Activation-induced T-cell death and immune dysfunction after implantation of left-ventricular assist device. *Lancet*. 1999;354(9178):550-555.
7. Itescu S, John R. Interactions between the recipient immune system and the left ventricular assist device surface: immunological and clinical implications. *Ann Thorac Surg*. 2003;75(6 Suppl):S58-S65.
8. Tjan TD, Asfour B, Hammel D, et al. Wound complications after left ventricular assist device implantation. *Ann Thorac Surg*. 2000;70(2):538-541.
9. Oz MC, Argenziano M, Catanese KA, et al. Bridge experience with long-term implantable left ventricular assist devices. Are they an alternative to transplantation? *Circulation*. 1997;95(7):1844-1852.
10. Baddour LM, Bettmann MA, Bolger AF, et al. Nonvalvular cardiovascular device-related infections. *Circulation*. 2003;108(16):2015-2031.
11. Arrecubieta C, Asai T, Bayern M, et al. The role of *Staphylococcus aureus* adhesins in the pathogenesis of ventricular assist device-related infections. *J Infect Dis*. 2006;193(8):1109-1119.
12. Deng MC, Loebe M, El-Banayosy A, et al. Mechanical circulatory support for advanced heart failure: effect of patient selection on outcome. *Circulation*. 2001;103(2):231-237.
13. Sivaratnam K, Duggan JM. Left ventricular assist device infections: three case reports and a review of the literature. *ASAIO J*. 2002;48(1):2-7.
14. Gandelman G, Frishman WH, Wiese C, et al. Intravascular device infections: epidemiology, diagnosis, and management. *Cardiol Rev*. 2007;15(1):13-23.
15. Zierer A, Melby SJ, Voeller RK, et al. Late-onset driveline infections: the Achilles' heel of prolonged left ventricular assist device support. *Ann Thorac Surg*. 2007;84(2):515-520.
16. Gordon SM, Schmitt SK, Jacobs M, et al. Nosocomial bloodstream infections in patients with implantable left ventricular assist devices. *Ann Thorac Surg*. 2001;72(3):725-730.
17. Nurozler F, Argenziano M, Oz MC, Naka Y. Fungal left ventricular assist device endocarditis. *Ann Thorac Surg*. 2001;71(2):614-618.
18. Chinn R, Dembitsky W, Eaton L, et al. Multicenter experience: prevention and management of left ventricular assist device infections. *ASAIO J*. 2005;51(4):461-470.
19. Gordon RJ, Quagliarello B, Lowy FD. Ventricular assist device-related infections. *Lancet Infect Dis*. 2006;6(7):426-437.
20. Malani PN, Dyke DBS, Pagani FD, Armstrong WS, Chenoweth CE. Successful treatment of vancomycin resistant Enterococcus faecium mediastinitis associated with left ventricular assist devices. *Ann Thorac Surg*. 2003;76(5):1719-1720.
21. Myers TJ, Khan T, Frazier OH. Infectious complications associated with ventricular assist systems. *ASAIO J*. 2000;46(6):S28-36.
22. Sajjadian A, Valerio IL, Acurturk O, et al. Omental transposition flap for salvage of ventricular assist devices. *Plast Reconstr Surg*. 2006;118(4):919-926; discussion 927.
23. Matsumiya G, Nishimura M, Miyamoto Y, Sawa Y, Matsuda H. Successful treatment of Novacor pump pocket infection by omental transposition. *Ann Thorac Surg*. 2003;75(1):287-288.
24. McKellar SH, Allred BD, Marks JD, et al. Treatment of infected left ventricular assist device using antibiotic-impregnated beads. *Ann Thorac Surg*. 1999;67(2):554-555.
25. Sinha P, Chen JM, Flannery M, et al. Infections during left ventricular assist device support do not affect posttransplant outcomes. *Circulation*. 2000;102(19 Suppl 3):III194-III199.
26. United Network for Organ Sharing. Allocation of Thoracic Organs Policy 3.7. Available at: http://optn.transplant.hrsa.gov/PoliciesandBylaws2/policies/pdfs/policy_9.pdf. Accessed September 29, 2010.
27. Rose EA, Gelijns AC, Moskowitz AJ, et al. Long-term use of a left ventricular assist device for end-stage heart failure. *N Engl J Med*. 2001;345(20):1435-1443.
28. Wasler A, Springer WE, Radovancevic B, et al. A comparison between intraperitoneal and extraperitoneal left ventricular assist system placement. *ASAIO J*. 1996;42(5):M573-576.

CHAPTER 14
RIGHT HEART DYSFUNCTION

Walter P. Dembitsky and David L. Joyce

Right heart dysfunction—defined as inotropic/vasodilator support for 14 or more consecutive days post-op, the need for a right ventricular assist device (RVAD), or both—represents a significant limitation to left ventricular assist device (LVAD) implantation and occurs in roughly one-third of patients.[1] Although there is some suggestion that patients who undergo implantation of newer continuous-flow devices may experience this complication with decreasing severity, it is a problem that occurs after both pulsatile and continuous-flow LVAD surgery.[2] Right heart dysfunction impacts on survival, length of intensive care unit (ICU) stay, and hospital stay.[3,4] End-organ function can deteriorate after LVAD implantation, adversely impacting on posttransplant outcomes in patients who are bridged with a device.[5] Early identification of patients who are at risk for right heart dysfunction may allow for concomitant temporary or long-term biventricular support at the time of LVAD implantation, thereby reducing the negative impact of this complication on patient outcomes. Numerous risk calculators have been developed for this purpose. This chapter explores the physiologic basis for right heart dysfunction, the effect this has on outcomes after LVAD surgery, and the techniques for addressing right heart dysfunction both pharmacologically and in the operating room.

RIGHT HEART PHYSIOLOGY

The function of the right ventricle is to maintain a low systemic venous pressure and provide flow to the lungs. In contrast to the systemic circulation, the low pressure, low resistance, and high compliance characteristics of the pulmonary vascular bed with a gradient of 5 mm Hg normally allow almost continuous flow. The right ventricle (RV) is anatomically adapted to generate sustained low pressure perfusion. It is composed of two functionally and anatomically different cavities. The sinus generates the systolic pressure which is attenuated by the cone (Fig. 14–1). Initial systolic pressure is generated in the sinus by the sequential contraction of the papillary muscle, right ventricular free wall, and finally the left ventricle (LV). The pressurized blood is transferred to the more compliant cone region where peak pressure is reduced and prolonged. Experimentally, a pulmonary arterial pulse pressure around 20 mm Hg permits optimum gas exchange. Histologic damage is seen with pressures higher than 20 mm Hg and interstitial edema forms without pulsatility.[6]

The characteristics of the pulmonary vascular bed permit prolonged right ventricular ejection. Acute elevation of the right ventricular afterload alters these ejection characteristics, and the right ventricular pressure volume loop is no longer triangular but resembles that of the left ventricular pressure volume loop (Fig. 14–2).[7] The right ventricle dilates to maintain stroke volume, albeit with a reduced ejection fraction (normal being 40%-60%). The loss of the peristaltic contraction produces an accelerated increase in pulmonary artery pressures and flows. Prolonged isovolumic contraction and ejection time increase myocardial oxygen consumption and the associated demand for increased coronary blood flow. Normally, right ventricular coronary blood flow is equally distributed between diastole and systole. During periods of increased pulmonary artery pressure, the flow becomes similar to the left ventricular coronary blood flow and is almost exclusively diastolic. Diastolic right coronary blood flow becomes increasingly critical to maintenance of right ventricular performance during periods of increased afterload. Reduced systemic blood pressure during periods of acute increases in pulmonary artery pressure produces subendocardial right ventricular ischemia. This is especially true when the right ventricular myocardial tissue perfusion gradient is further compromised by an increased right ventricular end-diastolic pressure and flow restricting coronary arterial occlusive disease.

RIGHT AND LEFT VENTRICULAR INTERACTION

The left and right ventricles necessarily interact since each sequentially pumps blood to the other. In addition to the series effect, the ventricles must directly influence each other's function because the interventricular septum is a common functional wall and because the ventricles share muscle fibers.[8] This ventricular interdependence is influenced by the noncompliant periventricular tissues (usually the pericardium). Numerous studies have defined the beat-to-beat nature of ventricular interdependence and demonstrated that 20% to 70% of right ventricular function is derived from the LV.[9,10] Contractile septal function independent of systolic deformity appears to be an important determinant of systolic right ventricular function.[8,11] In addition, changes in septal position alter right ventricular preload by changing right ventricular volume.[12,13]

INFLUENCE OF LVAD SUPPORT ON RIGHT VENTRICULAR PERFORMANCE

The interactions between the two ventricles are altered by the use of LVADs. During LVAD support global right ventricular contractility is impaired with a leftward septal shifting, but myocardial efficiency and power output are maintained through a decrease in right ventricular afterload and an increase in right ventricular preload.[14,15] The septal shift influence is minimal[14,16,17] compared to that of isolated right ventricular ischemia caused by right coronary occlusion.[16] Isolated right ventricular free wall ischemia during LVAD support appears to be insufficient cause for needing RVAD support.[18] Septal ischemia can result in significant degradation of right ventricular function during LVAD support.[19]

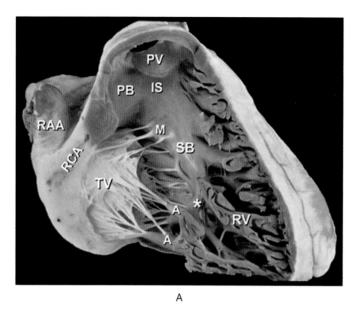

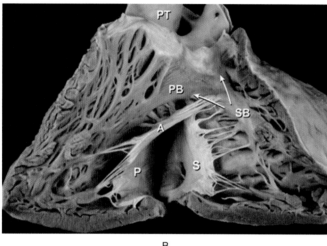

FIGURE 14–1. Anatomy of the right heart. (Reproduced with permission from Fuster V, O'Rourke RA, Walsh RA, Poole-Wilson P. *Hurst's The Heart*, 12th ed. New York, NY: McGraw-Hill, Inc; 2008. Fig 3–33 A and B.)

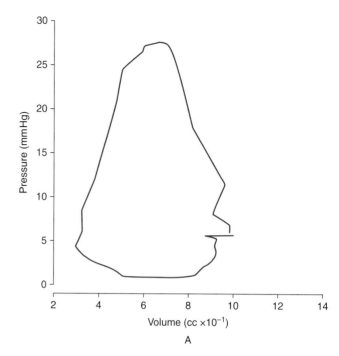

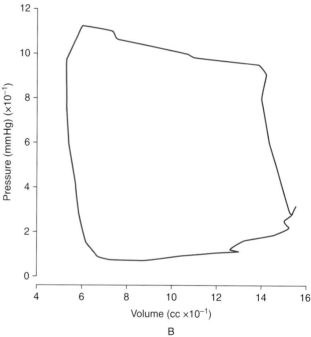

FIGURE 14–2. A. Right ventricle (RV) pressure-volume loop. **B.** Left ventricle (LV) pressure-volume (PV) loop.

Any diminution of right ventricular contractile performance during LVAD support is largely nullified by the reduction in afterload created by reducing the LA contribution to elevated pulmonary artery pressure. Increased systemic blood pressure enhances right coronary blood flow. Increased systemic blood flow increases the sequential return to the right ventricle and requires an increase in right ventricular volume work, potentially exacerbating any preexisting tendency toward tricuspid insufficiency. Three experimental observations which separate mild from severe right ventricular depression during LVAD support are (1) underlying right ventricular dysfunction appears to be necessary; (2) degree of right ventricular afterload reduction is important; and (3) regional ischemia (especially septal) is especially important.[19] These demonstrated conditions have all been observed clinically.[3]

CLINICAL EXPERIENCE WITH RIGHT VENTRICULAR FAILURE DURING LVAD SUPPORT

Left ventricular assist pumps are now accepted therapy for ventricular recovery and chronic circulatory support, both as bridge-to-transplant and as destination therapy. Initial large-scale clinical

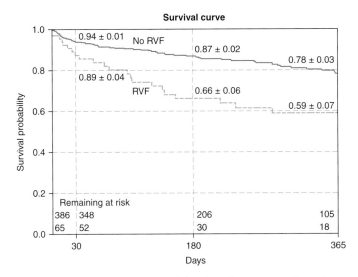

Survival curve

0.94 ± 0.01 No RVF

0.87 ± 0.02

0.78 ± 0.03

0.89 ± 0.04

RVF   0.66 ± 0.06

0.59 ± 0.07

Remaining at risk

386	348	206	105
65	52	30	18

Days

FIGURE 14–3. Kaplan-Meier survival data from the HeartMate II experience demonstrates a trend toward higher survival probability in patients without early right ventricular failure (RVF) relative to those with RVF. (Reproduced with permission from Kormos et al.[22] Copyright © Elsevier.)

use of left ventricular pumps was in patients who failed to be weaned from cardiopulmonary bypass. Temporary short-term roller and centrifugal pumps successfully supported patients' left circulation until the native left ventricle was sufficiently recovered. Right ventricular failure was recognized as an important cause of postcirculatory support LVAD mortality.[5] Clinical series demonstrated that the addition of right ventricular mechanical pumps improved survival for failure to wean patients.

Clinically implantable para- and intracorporeal pulsatile LVAD pumps were successfully used to bridge patients to either recovery or transplant. More recently they have been successfully used to chronically support patients ineligible for transplant.[20] Continuous-flow axial and centrifugal pumps are now being used for chronic support. Early experiences are encouraging, with 2-year survival approaching 60%.[21] Acute right ventricular failure in patients receiving chronic LVADs is associated with a high mortality (Fig. 14–3).[22] This has been significantly reduced by improvements in perioperative management and the application of right ventricular support.

Numerous attempts have been made to define preoperative characteristics that would predict which LVAD recipients might require a biventricular assist device (BiVAD).[23-25] Heart failure patients with compromised hepatic, renal function, requiring preoperative ventilation or circulatory support, who have demonstrated diminished right ventricular pumping capacity most likely will require BiVAD or total artificial heart (TAH) support. A decreased right ventricular stroke work index indicates a diminished capacity of the right ventricular complex to perform and helps define the population needing RVAD support during LVAD implantation.[23] These patients often present with overt right ventricular dysfunction requiring RVAD support to enhance LVAD flow during initial implantation. In other cases, underutilization of RVADs may impair

patient recovery in the early perioperative period by allowing right ventricular pressure and central venous pressure (CVP) to remain high, thereby compromising LVAD flows. The resulting reduction in tissue perfusion gradient limits the extent of hepatic, renal, gastrointestinal, and cerebral recovery.

High preoperative pulmonary artery pressures (and therefore increased right ventricular stroke work index) do not predict the need for RVAD support. The total pulmonary vascular resistance following LVAD implantation is reduced because both the left ventricular end-diastolic pressure and the pulmonary vascular resistance are minimized. The reduced right ventricular afterload permits the hypertrophied right ventricle to function well. Right ventricular exercise hemodynamic studies in patients chronically supported by implantable LVADs have indicated that maximum exercise capacity is primarily limited by the performance of the LV-LVAD complex and not the right ventricle which has been shown to have improved pumping capacity.[26] Histologic and chemical structural changes also demonstrate reverse remodeling in the right ventricles of patients supported by LVADs.[27] Furthermore, reduction in right ventricular pressure reduces the duration of the monophasic right ventricular action potentials and minimizes the chances of generating right ventricular arrhythmias.[28] Therefore, high CVP and low pulmonary artery pressures in patients with left ventricular failure may indicate a failing right ventricle.

At the University of Pennsylvania, a risk score model was established to predict which patients would require RVAD support. Six variables were identified as predictors of RV failure. If a patient met the "high-risk" criteria for that variable, they were given a risk score of "1" for that component. If they were considered "low-risk," they were assigned a score of "0." High-risk criteria for each variable are described in Table 14–1. These scores are then entered into the final risk score equation:

$$18 \times (CI) + 18 \times (RVSWI) + 17 \times (creatinine) + 16 \times (previous\ cardiac\ surgery) + 16 \times (RV\ dysfuction) + 13 \times (SBP)$$

The maximum score using this approach is 98. Applying a cutoff score of 50, whereby a score of less than 50 predicted successful LVAD support and a score of greater than or equal to 50 predicted the need for an RVAD, the authors found a sensitivity

TABLE 14–1. Independent Risk Factors for Right Ventricular Failure after LVAD insertion, as described in the University of Pennsylvania risk score.[23]

Variable	Odds Ratio	Interval	P Value
Cardiac index ≤ 2.2 L/min/m²	5.7	1.3-24.4	0.0192
RVSWI ≤ 0.25 mm Hg · L/m²	5.1	2.1-12.2	0.0002
Severe pre-VAD RV dysfunction	5.0	2.0-12.5	0.0006
Creatinine ≥ 1.9 mg/dL	4.8	1.9-12.0	0.0010
Previous cardiac surgery	4.5	1.7-11.8	0.0023
SBP ≤ 96 mm Hg	2.9	1.2-6.9	0.0162

(Reproduced with permission from Fitzpatrick JR, III, Frederick JR, Hsu VM et al. Risk score derived from pre-operative data analysis predicts the need for biventricular mechanical circulatory support. *J Heart Lung Transplant.* 2008 December;27(12):1286-92. Copyright © Elsevier.)

TABLE 14–2. Right Ventricular Failure Score as described at the University of Michigan.[29]

Risk Score	n	RV Failure (n)	No RV Failure (n)	Likelihood Ratio (95% CI)
≤ 3.0	142	29	113	0.49 (0.37-0.64)
4.0-5.0	25	15	10	2.8 (1.4-5.9)
≥ 5.5	30	24	6	7.6 (3.4-17.1)

Risk score is derived by summing points awarded for the presence of a vasopressor requirement (4 points), AST ≥ 80 IU/L (2 points), bilirubin ≥ 2.0 mg/dL (2.5 points), and creatinine ≥ 2.3 mg/dL (3 points). (Reproduced with permission from Matthews JC, Koelling TM, Pagani FD, Aaronson KD. The right ventricular failure risk score a pre-operative tool for assessing the risk of right ventricular failure in left ventricular assist device candidates. *J Am Coll Cardiol.* 2008 June 3;51(22):2163-72. Copyright © Elsevier.)

and specificity of 83% and 80%, respectively.[23] Investigators at the University of Michigan also established a Right Ventricular Failure Risk Score (RVFRS), described in Table 14–2. The RVFRS can be derived by adding points awarded for the presence of each of the following variables: vasopressor requirement (4 points), aspartate aminotransferase (AST) greater than or equal to 80 IU/L (2 points), bilirubin greater than or equal to 2.0 mg/dL (2.5 points), and creatinine greater than or equal to 2.3 mg/dL (3 points). In this study, patients with an RVFRS greater than or equal to 5.5 were 15-fold greater than those with an RVFRS less than or equal to 3.0 and about 3-fold greater than subjects with an RVFRS of 4.0 to 5.0 to develop RV failure.[29]

IMPLANTATION OF RVADS DURING LVAD SUPPORT

Occasionally, the decision to proceed directly to BiVAD or TAH can be made preoperatively. Systemically compromised patients presenting with multiple organ systems failure may best benefit from biventricular support which provides the highest cardiac outputs with the lowest venous pressures and the least requirement for adrenergic drugs. When the retained natural heart is a persistent liability, full support is best. This occurs in clinical scenarios such as severe arrhythmias, extensive myocarditis, ventricular thrombus, and extensive damage due to infarct ventricular septal defect (VSDs) or other sequelae of ischemic heart disease. Although many patients can be identified preoperatively for RVAD requirement, a significant portion of LVAD recipients will only declare the need for RV support after the device has been implanted.

There are a number of precautions that one should take during LVAD implantation in order to minimize the risk of needing right-sided support. Intraoperative right ventricular function can be optimized in some patients by preoperative reduction in CVP using pharmacologic or mechanical methods, including ultrafiltration.[30] Preoperative oral or intravenous pharmacologic pulmonary vasodilatation is beneficial and can augment the effects of nitric oxide which may be used intraoperatively.[31,32] The fragile nature of the RV myocardium with its dependence on left ventricular function and the influence of RV afterload on RV performance can collectively contribute to right-sided failure over a short period of time. When this occurs, progressive pulmonary circulatory failure proceeds to systemic circulatory failure.

A firm treatment plan will eliminate this undesirable positive feedback mechanism. Pulmonary vascular resistance should be minimized. While being supported with cardiopulmonary bypass following LVAD implantation, patients with chronic vasoactive pulmonary hypertension can be pharmacologically treated with pulmonary vasodilators, including inhaled nitric oxide (iNO), milrinone, dobutamine, prostacyclins, and sildenafil.[31,32] Ventilation is adjusted to reduce the end tidal CO_2 to 24 mm Hg, and oxygen saturation is kept high using appropriate inspired oxygen concentrations. Systemic acidosis is treated, pulmonary effusions are evacuated, and, if necessary, endobronchial obstructions are removed endoscopically. Proper position of the left ventricular or left atrial cannula providing inflow to the LVAD can be determined by use of transesophageal echocardiography and/or epicardial echocardiography with the probe placed on the left ventricle. Left ventricular chamber size should be small. Low pulmonary capillary wedge pressure (PCWP), low pulmonary artery pressure, and high LVAD output all confirm that the left heart is decompressed. The pumping function of the RV should be optimized. Any occlusive disease in the coronaries supplying myocardium contributing to right ventricular function should be bypassed using saphenous vein grafts. Special attention is given to revascularization of the acute marginal branches, posterior descending, and left anterior descending arteries to ensure that blood flow to the free wall and important septal components of the RV pump is assured. Tricuspid valve insufficiency may initially appear to be minimal, but increasing right atrial return from a functioning LVAD and associated septal shift may dramatically increase tricuspid regurgitation in some patients. This effect can be minimized by the incorporation of a tricuspid annuloplasty ring. Elevating the right ventricular heart rate by pacing the right atrium minimizes the diastolic filling time and enhances RV contractility due to the Treppe effect (force-frequency relationship between heart rate and cardiac output). Optimal direct right ventricular pacing is probably best initiated in the sinus and not the conus region of the right ventricle (see Fig. 14–1). Both interventions reduce tricuspid regurgitation. Careful direct inspection must be made to ensure that no patent foramen ovale is present. Our experience indicates that the patent foramen is missed despite the use of a transesophageal echo-guided bubble study in the operating room approximately 20% of the time. Failure to eliminate a right-to-left atrial shunt during LVAD support can result in systemic cyanosis.

Despite these precautions, transient periods of systemic hypotension and low flow associated with elevations in right ventricular filling pressures may occasionally lead to progressive circulatory collapse. The associated acidosis, when this occurs, can provoke a potentiated pulmonary vascular bed to constrict. If intrapulmonary shunting is present, the reduced cardiac output and the resultant lowered systemic venous oxygen saturation create systemic hypoxia which can also incite pulmonary vasoconstriction. Progressive RV failure ensues as its oxygen demand increases, coronary blood flow decreases, and the tricuspid valve begins to leak. To avoid this damaging sequence, we have implemented temporary right heart bypass to allow the right ventricle to recover during these situations. Others have successfully used this approach or a period of right heart and lung bypass.[33-36]

Our current technique evolved from one which we devised in the 1980s using centrifugal pump to support patients who failed to wean from cardiopulmonary bypass. The decision to support the left ventricle, right ventricle, or both was usually made by observing pressures as well as left and right ventricular contractile patterns. A very effective method of determining which ventricle needed support was to use the circulating pump used for cardiopulmonary bypass, usually a roller pump, to temporarily support either a left or right ventricle. The temporary left ventricular support was initiated using a bridge to a left atrial venous line placed into the right superior pulmonary vein. With total venoarterial cardiopulmonary bypass in progress, the systemic venous cannulae were occluded and the right ventricle was allowed to pump blood to the left side where the left atrial cannula captured it. The cardiopulmonary bypass circuit returned blood to the aortic cannula in place, thereby providing left circulatory support. If flows were inadequate, BiVADs were used but the oxygenator was removed. Prolonged support of the circulation using a venoarterial circuit containing an oxygenator was not used because of the bleeding liability presented by the oxygenator and because stasis in the lungs, left ventricle, and right ventricle can cause thrombosis in those structures despite anticoagulation.[37] Patients with low cardiac output with low left atrial pressures or PCWPs and increased CVP were given temporary right circulatory support by placing a cannula in the pulmonary artery through a simple purse string. Using "Y" connector, the arterial flow was then redirected from the aorta into the

pulmonary artery (Fig. 14–4).[38] This allowed the right ventricle to remain decompressed, gradually elevating the systemic pressure and enhancing the important right ventricular coronary blood flow. Increased cardiac output elevates the systemic venous oxygen saturation and the arterial oxygen saturation that occur when intrapulmonary shunting is minimized. Systemic acidosis is more easily adjusted with this approach. During this period of temporary right heart support, the oxygenator gas flow is reduced and the gas exchange function of the natural lung can be assessed. The pulmonary vascular resistance is pharmacologically reduced. Gradually, the temporary pump flow is reduced from the initial flows of 4 to 5 L and the CVP allowed to rise between 10 and 15 mm Hg. If the native right ventricle cannot assume the burden of pulmonary flow within 30 minutes to 1 hour, a short-term device is implanted, heparin is reversed, hemostasis is obtained, and the chest is closed.

PUMP SELECTION FOR RIGHT HEART SUPPORT

Prior to selecting a pump to support the failing right circulation, the duration of support must be estimated. If fewer than 7 days of assistance is needed, widely available short-term pumps may be used. Continuous-flow paracorporeal rotary pumps are well suited for brief use. Generally, they are less expensive than long-term pumps but are more likely to be thrombogenic and/or hemolytic with prolonged use. They are easily inserted because the cannulae required are smaller. Smaller cannulae can be used because flow is continuous and not pulsatile. Furthermore, the pumps generally have a high negative inlet pressure and provide suction to the right atrial venous reservoir. Prolonged use of small catheters with high flows can produce hemolysis as sheer stress on the blood increases, both in the pump and in the cannulae. The positive pressure outflow cannula can be safely and easily used to provide flow for hemodialysis or hemoconcentration. Transmembrane effluent is returned to the systemic venous system through IV tubing and not through the negative pressure side of the pump, to prevent air aspiration. The negative pressure for most pulsatile pumps is far less than it is for roller or fluid dynamic pumps. The risk of air aspiration into the RVAD is that the air can easily be pumped through the lungs and into the systemic circulation with the known dire consequences. Air aspiration is minimized by insulating the potential aspiration site and providing adequate right venous volume and flow access. Percutaneous placement of right atrial cannulae by the femoral veins allows the chest to be closed more easily. If the chest is left open, it should be sealed using adherent plastic drapes. Venous return to the right atrium must be carefully monitored.

Roller pumps can also be used, but, because they are not pressure, limited high negative and positive pressures can be encountered in the ICU when patient motion and blood volume changes alter the resistance to flow. Fluid dynamic, axial, and centrifugal pumps are more easily managed because their flows are limited by pressure. The pumping function can be monitored using flow-measuring devices, usually electromagnetic flow probes. Nonpulsatile flow to the lungs has not proven to be detrimental over the short term in our experience. Paracorporeal

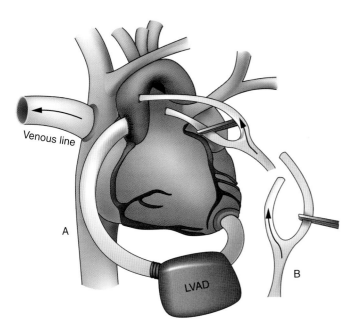

FIGURE 14–4. Cannulation strategy for testing RV function and determining the need for right-sided mechanical circulatory support. (Reproduced with permission from Robert K, Les M, eds. *Mechanical Circulatory Support: A Companion to Braunwald's Heart Disease.* Sept, 2011. Copyright © Elsevier.)

pulsatile pumps have been successfully used to support the right circulation. The episodic characteristics of the flow and the associated intermittent high velocities and flows, coupled with the usually low inlet pressures, require the use of larger-bore cannulae. By the Poiseuille relationship which describes the flow of fluid through a conduit: the resistance is inversely proportional to the fourth power of the radius and directly proportional to the fluid viscosity and velocity as well as the length of the cannula. Therefore, shorter as well as larger internal diameter cannulae are always best when trying to achieve higher flows.

If more than 1 week of support is anticipated or an abbreviated support period is not felt to be beneficial, chronic support is initiated. Traditionally, these have been paracorporeal pulsatile pumps, although newer implantable fluid dynamic pumps may be well suited for this role. A significant disadvantage of short-term paracorporeal pumps is that they require patients to be on bed rest, thereby limiting their mobility and rehabilitation and most importantly preventing them from being discharged to home.

RVAD IMPLANTATION STRATEGY

Continuous-flow pumps can provide excellent right circulatory support via a 50-cm percutaneously placed femoral vein cannula advanced into the right atrium. Blood is easily returned to the main PA. The right pulmonary artery[39] and right pulmonary outflow tract[40] have also been successfully used. In our experience, pulsatile pumps provide the best support when their access cannula are placed directly into the right ventricle beneath the acute margin of the heart. Blood is easily returned through a Dacron graft sewn to the main pulmonary artery. RVADs can almost always be placed without the use of cardiopulmonary bypass, even in the presence of an implanted LVAD. Aside from higher flows, an additional advantage of direct right ventricular drainage is that it minimizes the chances of producing right ventricular stasis thrombosis which can occur when the right heart endocardium is damaged and low right ventricular flow conditions are created due to right atrial drainage.

RVAD EXPLANTATION STRATEGY

The RVAD is removed when right circulatory pumping capacity is adequate to fill the LVAD well enough to allow it to provide sufficient systemic flow and blood pressure with low systemic venous pressure. Since the risk of leaving an RVAD in place is low, relative to leaving an LVAD in place, it is not removed until the patient's systemic organs have recovered enough to indicate that they will continue to recover. RVAD flows are progressively reduced over 24 to 48 hours. Tricuspid valve function is assessed, pulmonary vascular resistance is minimized, and right ventricular contractility is assessed using echo to determine the impact of PCWP and LVAD flow on RV function and LV size. If the pulmonary capillary wedge is high and LV size is large, LVAD apical cannula obstruction should be suspected and corrected if present. Changes in LVAD cannula position can dramatically reduce the performance demands on the right ventricle and

allow prompt RVAD removal. Removal can be accomplished without reopening the sternum if the pulmonary artery return conduit is a graft which has been sewn to the pulmonary artery, and the graft can be accessed through a lower sternotomy. Transection and oversewing portions of the graft and retaining parts of the long return segment do not present a significant liability to the patient provided the graft is not infected.

Despite recent advances in miniaturizing LVAD design, improved outcomes with mechanical circulatory support, and an enhanced ability to predict the occurrence of RV failure, an implantable and durable RVAD has not been approved for long-term support. This area represents an opportunity for future discovery and improved outcomes in a field that is currently experiencing rapid growth.

REFERENCES

1. Dang NC, Topkara VK, Mercando M, et al. Right heart failure after left ventricular assist device implantation in patients with chronic congestive heart failure. *J Heart Lung Transplant.* 2006;25(1):1-6.
2. Patel ND, Weiss ES, Schaffer J, et al. Right heart dysfunction after left ventricular assist device implantation: a comparison of the pulsatile HeartMate I and axial-flow HeartMate II devices. *Ann Thorac Surg.* 2008 Sep;86(3):832-840.
3. Kavarana MN, Pessin-Minsley MS, Urtecho J, et al. Right ventricular dysfunction and organ failure in left ventricular assist device recipients: a continuing problem. *Ann Thorac Surg.* 2002;73(3):745-750.
4. Boyle AJ, Russell SD, Teuteberg JJ, et al. Low thromboembolism and pump thrombosis with the HeartMate II left ventricular assist device: analysis of outpatient anti-coagulation. *J Heart Lung Transplant.* 2009;28(9):881-887.
5. Morgan JA, John R, Lee BJ, Oz MC, Naka Y. Is severe right ventricular failure in left ventricular assist device recipients a risk factor for unsuccessful bridging to transplant and post-transplant mortality. *Ann Thorac Surg.* 2004;77(3):859-863.
6. Eda K. Optimal pulse pressure of pulmonary circulation under biventricular assist after cardiogenic shock. *Ann Thorac Cardiovasc Surg.* 1999 Dec; 5(6):365-369.
7. Faber MJ, Dalinghaus M, Lankhuizen IM, et al. Right and left ventricular function after chronic pulmonary artery banding in rats assessed with biventricular pressure-volume loops. *Am J Physiol Heart Circ Physiol.* 2006 Oct;291(4):H1580-H1586.
8. Klima UP, Lee MY, Guerrero JL, Laraia PJ, Levine RA, Vlahakes GJ. Determinants of maximal right ventricular function: role of septal shift. *J Thorac Cardiovasc Surg.* 2002;123(1):72-80.
9. Santamore WP, Dell'Italia LJ. Ventricular interdependence: significant left ventricular contributions to right ventricular systolic function. *Prog Cardiovasc Dis.* 1998 Jan;40(4):289-308.
10. Santamore WP, Gray L, Jr. Significant left ventricular contributions to right ventricular systolic function. Mechanism and clinical implications. *Chest.* 1995;107(4):1134-1145.
11. Klima U, Guerrero JL, Vlahakes GJ. Contribution of the interventricular septum to maximal right ventricular function. *Eur J Cardiothorac Surg.* 1998 Sep;14(3):250-255.
12. Laver MB, Strauss HW, Pohost GM. Herbert Shubin Memorial Lecture. Right and left ventricular geometry: adjustments during acute respiratory failure. *Crit Care Med.* 1979;7(12):509-519.
13. Taylor RR, Covell JW, Sonnenblick EH, Ross J, Jr. Dependence of ventricular distensibility on filling of the opposite ventricle. *Am J Physiol.* 1967 Sep;213(3):711-718.
14. Moon MR, Castro LJ, DeAnda A, et al. Right ventricular dynamics during left ventricular assistance in closed-chest dogs. *Ann Thorac Surg.* 1993 Jul;56(1):54-66.
15. Santamore WP, Gray LA, Jr. Left ventricular contributions to right ventricular systolic function during LVAD support. *Ann Thorac Surg.* 1996;61(1):350-356.
16. Farrar DJ, Chow E, Compton PG, Foppiano L, Woodard J, Hill JD. Effects of acute right ventricular ischemia on ventricular interactions during prosthetic left ventricular support. *J Thorac Cardiovasc Surg.* 1991 Oct;102(4):588-595.

17. Hendry PJ, Ascah KJ, Rajagopalan K, Calvin JE. Does septal position affect right ventricular function during left ventricular assist in an experimental porcine model? *Circulation.* 1994 Nov;90(5 Pt 2):II353-II358.

18. Moon MR, Castro LJ, DeAnda A, Daughters GT, Ingels NB, Jr, Miller DC. Effects of left ventricular support on right ventricular mechanics during experimental right ventricular ischemia. *Circulation.* 1994 Nov;90(5 Pt 2):II92-II101.

19. Daly RC, Chandrasekaran K, Cavarocchi NC, Tajik AJ, Schaff HV. Ischemia of the interventricular septum. A mechanism of right ventricular failure during mechanical left ventricular assist. *J Thorac Cardiovasc Surg.* 1992; 103(6):1186-1191.

20. Rose EA, Gelijns AC, Moskowitz AJ, et al. Long-term mechanical left ventricular assistance for end-stage heart failure. *N Engl J Med.* 2001 Nov 15;345(20):1435-1443.

21. Slaughter MS, Rogers JG, Milano CA, et al. Advanced heart failure treated with continuous-flow left ventricular assist device. *N Engl J Med.* 2009 Dec 3;361(23):2241-2251.

22. Kormos RL, Teuteberg JJ, Pagani FD, et al. Right ventricular failure in patients with the HeartMate II continuous-flow left ventricular assist device: incidence, risk factors, and effect on outcomes. *J Thorac Cardiovasc Surg.* 2010;139(5):1316-1324.

23. Fitzpatrick JR, III, Frederick JR, Hsu VM, et al. Risk score derived from pre-operative data analysis predicts the need for biventricular mechanical circulatory support. *J Heart Lung Transplant.* 2008;27(12):1286-1292.

24. Ochiai Y, McCarthy PM, Smedira NG, et al. Predictors of severe right ventricular failure after implantable left ventricular assist device insertion: analysis of 245 patients. *Circulation.* 2002 Sep 24;106(12 Suppl 1):I198-I202.

25. Fukamachi K, McCarthy PM, Smedira NG, Vargo RL, Starling RC, Young JB. Preoperative risk factors for right ventricular failure after implantable left ventricular assist device insertion. *Ann Thorac Surg.* 1999 Dec;68(6): 2181-2184.

26. Jaski BE, Lingle RJ, Kim J, et al. Comparison of functional capacity in patients with end-stage heart failure following implantation of a left ventricular assist device versus heart transplantation: results of the experience with left ventricular assist device with exercise trial. *J Heart Lung Transplant.* 1999;18(11):1031-1040.

27. Kucuker SA, Stetson SJ, Becker KA, et al. Evidence of improved right ventricular structure after LVAD support in patients with end-stage cardiomyopathy. *J Heart Lung Transplant.* 2004;23(1):28-35.

28. Taggart P, Sutton P, John R, Lab M, Swanton H. Monophasic action potential recordings during acute changes in ventricular loading induced by the Valsalva manoeuvre. *Br Heart J.* 1992;67(3):221-229.

29. Matthews JC, Koelling TM, Pagani FD, Aaronson KD. The right ventricular failure risk score a pre-operative tool for assessing the risk of right ventricular failure in left ventricular assist device candidates. *J Am Coll Cardiol.* 2008 Jun 3;51(22):2163-72.

30. Jaski BE, Miller D. Ultrafiltration in decompensated heart failure. *Curr Heart Fail Rep.* 2005 Sep;2(3):148-154.

31. Klodell CT, Jr, Morey TE, Lobato EB, et al. Effect of sildenafil on pulmonary artery pressure, systemic pressure, and nitric oxide utilization in patients with left ventricular assist devices. *Ann Thorac Surg.* 2007;83(1):68-71.

32. Trachte AL, Lobato EB, Urdaneta F, et al. Oral sildenafil reduces pulmonary hypertension after cardiac surgery. *Ann Thorac Surg.* 2005;79(1):194-197.

33. Van MC, Jr, Robbins RJ, Ochsner JL. Technique of right heart protection and deairing during heartmate vented electric LVAD implantation. *Ann Thorac Surg.* 1997;63(4):1191-1192.

34. Kaul TK, Kahn DR. Postinfarct refractory right ventricle: right ventricular exclusion. A possible option to mechanical cardiac support, in patients unsuitable for heart transplant. *J Cardiovasc Surg (Torino).* 2000 Jun;41(3): 349-355.

35. Moazami N, Pasque MK, Moon MR, et al. Mechanical support for isolated right ventricular failure in patients after cardiotomy. *J Heart Lung Transplant.* 2004;23(12):1371-1375.

36. Berman M, Tsui S, Vuylsteke A, Klein A, Jenkins DP. Life-threatening right ventricular failure in pulmonary hypertension: RVAD or ECMO? *J Heart Lung Transplant.* 2008;27(10):1188-1189.

37. Adamson RM, Dembitsky WP, Daily PO, Moreno-Cabral R, Copeland J, Smith R. Immediate cardiac allograft failure. ECMO versus total artificial heart support. *ASAIO J.* 1996 Jul;42(4):314-316.

38. Loebe M, Potapov E, Sodian R, Kopitz M, Noon GP. A safe and simple method of preserving right ventricular function during implantation of a left ventricular assist device. *J Thorac Cardiovasc Surg.* 2001 Nov;122(5):1043.

39. Minami K, Bonkohara Y, Arusoglu L, El Banayosy A, Korfer R. New technique for the outflow cannulation of right ventricular assist device. *Ann Thorac Surg.* 1999 Sep;68(3):1092-1093.

40. Dewey TM, Chen JM, Spanier TB, Oz MC. Alternative technique of right-sided outflow cannula insertion for right ventricular support. *Ann Thorac Surg.* 1998 Nov;66(5):1829-1830.

CHAPTER 15

BLEEDING COMPLICATIONS OF CONTINUOUS FLOW

Daniel D. Joyce and Sheri S. Crow

INTRODUCTION

Left ventricular assist devices (LVADs) have become a viable long-term treatment option for end-stage heart failure.[1-3] Continuous-flow LVADs (CF-LVAD) have replaced the earlier pulsatile devices due to their smaller size and increased durability, better functional status, and improved probability of survival.[4] Unfortunately, nonsurgical bleeding in CF-LVAD recipients has become a major concern and detractor from the improved quality of life these patients have come to expect following device placement.[5] The most common source for bleeding complications involves the gastrointestinal (GI) tract and nasal mucosa. Understanding the etiology of these complications will facilitate development of effective treatment strategies for device recipients, ultimately improving the quality and longevity of CF-LVAD recipients. This chapter explores the nature of nonsurgical bleeding among CF-LVAD recipients and proposes strategies for minimizing the impact of these complications.

BLEEDING RISKS ASSOCIATED WITH LVAD SUPPORT

Bleeding is a common adverse event associated with cardiac surgery[6] and occurs in up to 60% of LVAD implants.[7] Bleeding events can be classified into one of two categories: surgical (due to unrecognized bleeding in unligated vessels or leaking anastomotic suture lines) and nonsurgical (bleeding that occurs outside of the immediate postoperative period). While surgical bleeding is a substantial risk in LVAD recipients, the majority of adverse bleeding events are nonsurgical.[2] The exact cause for the development of nonsurgical bleeding is unknown at this time. Recent investigations have highlighted several potential explanations, including alterations in thrombostatic function due to exposure to biomaterials[8] and right heart failure–induced hepatic insufficiency.

The earliest LVAD designs provided pulsatile blood flow. Initial comparisons between the pulsatile and CF-LVADs reported similar surgical and nonsurgical bleeding rates in these recipients.[2] Over the last 3 years, several independent analyses have identified an isolated increase in the rate of GI bleeding in CF-LVAD recipients compared to pulsatile recipients. In fact the CF-LVAD GI bleed rate is nearly 10 times higher than that observed in pulsatile device recipients (Fig. 15–1).[5,9] These findings are surprising when one considers that pulsatile device recipients are more likely to be in poorer health, based on significantly lower albumin and longer bypass times that might increase the propensity for GI bleeding. Improved ease of implantation, prolonged survival, and increased durability have resulted in the CF-LVAD almost completely replacing the earlier pulsatile designs. As a result, understanding the potential causes for the increase in bleeding events has become one of the top priorities for improving outcomes.

POTENTIAL MECHANISMS FOR INCREASED BLEEDING DURING CF-LVAD SUPPORT

Perhaps the most obvious explanation for the observed difference between pulsatile and CF-LVAD bleeding rates is anticoagulation therapy. CF-LVAD recipients are typically anticoagulated with warfarin sodium to a goal international normalized ration (INR) of 1.5 to 2.5, whereas pulsatile recipients are not anticoagulated. Aspirin therapy is currently recommended and utilized for both the pulsatile and CF-LVAD recipient. Despite the difference in anticoagulation strategy, several factors suggest that warfarin therapy alone does not account for the difference in bleeding rates. First, the observed CF-LVAD bleeding rate of 40% in most studies far exceeds the expected rate observed in patients anticoagulated for other reasons.[10] For instance, patients who undergo mechanical valve placement require an INR in the 3.0 to 4.0 range. Despite a much higher-targeted INR, these patients experience bleeding rates of only 2.68 to 4.6 bleeding events per 100 patient years.[11] In comparison, CF-LVAD recipients have reported bleeding rates as high as 63 events per 100 patient years.[5] Furthermore, despite the differences in anticoagulation strategy, Crow et al found no significant differences in the INRs between the pulsatile and nonpulsatile groups at follow-up or during a bleeding event (2.1 vs 2.0).[5] Therefore, it seems likely that the device itself may pose an independent risk.

The isolated increase in GI bleeding observed in CF-LVAD recipients is similar to that seen in patients with severe aortic stenosis. Heyde first described this association between aortic stenosis and GI bleeding in a letter to the *New England Journal of Medicine* in 1958.[12] Heyde's observation would later be attributed to the dysfunction of von Willebrand factor (vWF), now known as acquired von Willebrand syndrome (AvWS).[13-15] vWF is a 250-kDa glycoprotein stored within endothelial cells and is essential to the blood clotting process. Large vWF multimers exceeding 10 dimers, also known as high-molecular-weight multimers (HMWMs), promote platelet adhesion in high shear stress areas (Fig. 15–2). In aortic stenosis, the calcified aortic valve creates an area of high shear stress that causes proteolysis and cleavage of these HMWM.[16] Acquired loss of these vital multimers leads to an inability to bind collagen and platelets in high shear stress areas of the body such as GI arteriovenous malformations. One explanation for why bleeding does not occur throughout the body in individuals with HMWM loss is the consistency of overall vWF in the blood. Only sites dependent on the

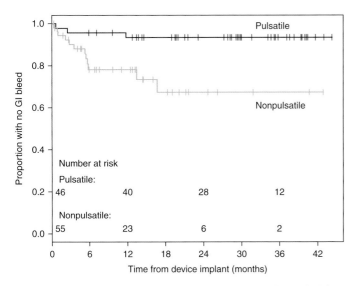

FIGURE 15-1. Bleeding rates after LVAD implantation reveal a much higher-risk profile associated with continuous-flow assist devices. (Reproduced with permission from Crow et al.[5] Copyright © Elsevier.)

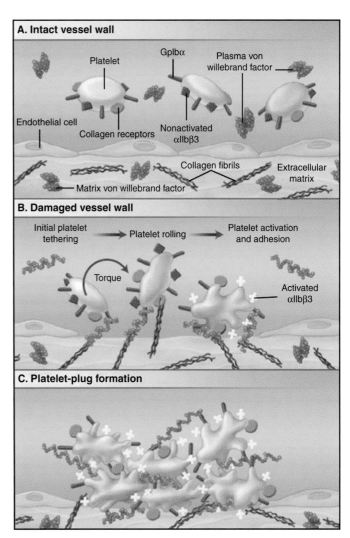

FIGURE 15-2. Mechanism of von Willebrand factor function in platelet-plug formation. (Reproduced with permission from Mannucci PM. Treatment of von Willebrand's disease. *N Engl J Med*. 2004;351:683-694. Copyright © Massachusetts Medical Society. All rights reserved.)

high-molecular-weight version of the protein will be affected. The association between HMWM loss and bleeding was confirmed by the observation that following aortic valve replacement, bleeding stops and HMWM levels return to normal.

Recent studies have observed similar HMWM loss in CF-LVAD patients. This led to the hypothesis that the mechanical design and speed of the impeller system creates an environment of high shear stress similar to that of the calcified aortic valve.[17-19] It is less well understood why only some CF-LVAD patients experience GI bleeds when HMWM loss occurs universally following CF-LVAD placement.[20] The presence or absence of preoperative angiodysplasia is one possible explanation. An alternative explanation is that the nonpulsatile flow of the CF-LVAD induces the formation of GI angiodysplasia. Early studies examining nonpulsatile flow in animal models demonstrated normal end-organ function despite the nonphysiologic circulation.[21] However, follow-up of CF-LVAD recipients is in the early stages. Alterations in recipient vascular systems may only become apparent as the device is in place for prolonged periods of time. As longer-term follow-up of recipients is completed, further details regarding the impact of prolonged nonpulsatile flow on the human body will become available.

Previous studies investigating the hematologic attributes of CF-LVAD recipients with bleeding complications have identified a number of other distinguishing features. There appears to be a significant relationship between blood type and the development of bleeding complications. Patients who bled were more likely to have blood type O. We found that only 6% of VAD recipients who bleed had blood type A, indicating that even distribution of blood types among bleeders does not occur.[22] Further analysis of blood type comparison in continuous-flow recipients is needed to confirm this as a potential contributing factor. vWF antigen (vWF:Ag) levels and factor VIII percentages were significantly higher in CF-LVAD patients who bled. These levels were higher than the normal ranges both pre- and 30 days

post–VAD placement in patients with bleeding. vWF:Ag is an acute-phase reactant, and the higher levels observed in bleeders may suggest that these patients were sicker surrounding their CF-LVAD implantation. Theoretically, sicker patients may have more risk factors for developing bleeding in the postoperative period (unpublished data).

The HMWM loss documented following CF-LVAD implantation certainly hinders platelet adhesion in high shear areas. In addition to this derangement, LVAD support has been shown to have a direct effect on the platelets themselves. Koster et al compared bleeding profiles between six continuous-flow (DeBakey VAD) recipients and six pulsatile (Novacor) recipients. They found that β-thromboglobulin (β-TG), platelet factor 4 (PF4), factor XIIa, thrombin/antithrombin complexes, and D-dimer levels were elevated in both groups. The levels of β-TG, PF4, factor XIIa, and plasmin/α_2-antiplasmin were significantly increased in CF-LVAD recipients.[23] Although both nonpulsatile and pulsatile devices contribute to platelet destruction, the elevated PF4 and β-TG levels suggest a greater degree of platelet damage and α-granule release in the CF-LVAD patients. Steinlechner and colleagues compared 12 outpatient CF-LVAD patients to 12 healthy volunteers utilizing a variety of platelet function tests that included thromboelastography, platelet mapping, thromboelastometry, platelet function analyzer, and a whole blood aggregometer (Multiplate).[24] CF-LVAD patients demonstrated substantial impairment in platelet function that was only partially attributable to the shear stress–mediated decrease in vWf activity.[24] The healthy volunteers demonstrated a threefold higher ristocetin-induced aggregation assay, suggesting additional impairment in platelet function due to the CF-VAD.[24]

CONCLUSION

The implications of the hemostatic perturbations that occur during VAD support remain unclear. The HMWM vWF loss following CF-LVAD implantation is now well recognized. However, the fact that not all CF-LVAD recipients experience bleeding complications suggests that further evaluation is required to identify additional contributing factors. Predictive indices of bleeding risk would facilitate the development of individualized strategies for anticoagulation and antiplatelet management in CF-LVAD recipients. The ability to balance the risk for pump thrombosis with a patient's individualized bleeding risk would greatly improve the ability to minimize hemorrhagic complications. Given the significant morbidity associated with bleeding events, this complication remains an important obstacle to overcome in improving patient outcomes.

REFERENCES

1. Slaughter MS, Rogers JG, Milano CA, et al. Advanced heart failure treated with continuous-flow left ventricular assist device. *N Engl J Med.* 2009; 361(23):2241-2251.
2. Miller LW, Pagani FD, Russell SD, et al. Use of a continuous-flow device in patients awaiting heart transplantation. *N Engl J Med.* 2007;357(9):885-896.
3. Rose EA, Gelijns AC, Moskowitz AJ, et al. Long-term mechanical left ventricular assistance for end-stage heart failure. *N Engl J Med.* 2001;345(20):1435-1443.
4. Fang JC. Rise of the machines—left ventricular assist devices as permanent therapy for advanced heart failure. *N Engl J Med.* 2009;361(23):2282-2285.
5. Crow S, John R, Boyle A, et al. Gastrointestinal bleeding rates in recipients of nonpulsatile and pulsatile left ventricular assist devices. *J Thorac Cardiovasc Surg.* 2009;137(1):208-215.
6. Whitlock R, Crowther MA, Ng HJ. Bleeding in cardiac surgery: its prevention and treatment—an evidence-based review. *Crit Care Clin.* 2005; 21(3):589-610.
7. Goldstein DJ, Beauford RB. Left ventricular assist devices and bleeding: adding insult to injury. *Ann Thorac Surg.* 2003;75(6 Suppl):S42-S47.
8. John R, Lee S. The biological basis of thrombosis and bleeding in patients with ventricular assist devices. *J Cardiovasc Transl Res.* 2009;2(1):63-70.
9. Geisen U, Heilmann C, Beyersdorf F, C et al. Non-surgical bleeding in patients with ventricular assist devices could be explained by acquired von Willebrand disease. *Eur J Cardiothorac Surg.* 2008;33(4):679-684.
10. Stern DR, Kazam J, Edwards P, et al. Increased incidence of gastrointestinal bleeding following implantation of the HeartMate II LVAD. *J Card Surg.* 2010; 25(3):352-356.
11. Cannegieter SC, van der Meer FJ, Briet E, Rosendaal FR. Warfarin and aspirin after heart-valve replacement. *N Engl J Med.* 1994;330(7):507-508.
12. Massyn MW, Khan SA. Heyde syndrome: a common diagnosis in older patients with severe aortic stenosis. *Age Ageing.* 2009;38(3):267-270.
13. Sucker C, Feindt P, Scharf RE. Aortic stenosis, von Willebrand factor, and bleeding. *N Engl J Med.* 2009; 349(18):1773-1774.
14. Love JW, Jahnke EJ, Zacharias D, Davidson WA, Kidder WR, Luan LL. Calcific aortic stenosis and gastrointestinal bleeding. *N Engl J Med.* 2009; 302(17):968.
15. Williams RC, Jr. Aortic stenosis and unexplained gastrointestinal bleeding. *Arch Intern Med.* 2004;164(6):679.
16. Vincentelli A, Susen S, Le Tourneau T, et al. Acquired von Willebrand syndrome in aortic stenosis. *N Engl J Med.* 2003;349(4):343-349.
17. Uriel N, Pak SW, Jorde UP, et al. Acquired von Willebrand syndrome after continuous-flow mechanical device support contributes to a high prevalence of bleeding during long-term support and at the time of transplantation. *J Am Coll Cardiol.* 2010 Oct 5;56(15):1207-1213.
18. Meyer AL, Malehsa D, Bara C, et al. Acquired von Willebrand syndrome in patients with an axial flow left ventricular assist device. *Circ Heart Fail.* 2010 Nov 1;3(6):675-681.
19. Klovaite J, Gustafsson F, Mortensen SA, Sander K, Nielsen LB. Severely impaired von Willebrand factor-dependent platelet aggregation in patients with a continuous-flow left ventricular assist device (HeartMate II). *J Am Coll Cardiol.* 2009;53(23):2162-2167.
20. Crow S, Milano C, Joyce L, et al. Comparative analysis of von Willebrand factor profiles in pulsatile and continuous left ventricular assist device recipients. *ASAIO J.* 2010;56(5):441-445.
21. Saito S, Westaby S, Piggot D, et al. End-organ function during chronic nonpulsatile circulation. *Ann Thorac Surg.* 2002;74(4):1080-1085.
22. Souto JC, Almasy L, Muniz-Diaz E, et al. Functional effects of the ABO locus polymorphism on plasma levels of von Willebrand factor, factor VIII, and activated partial thromboplastin time. *Arterioscler Thromb Vasc Biol.* 2000;20(8):2024-2028.
23. Koster A, Loebe M, Hansen R, et al. Alterations in coagulation after implantation of a pulsatile Novacor LVAD and the axial flow MicroMed DeBakey LVAD. *Ann Thorac Surg.* 2000;70(2):533-537.
24. Steinlechner B, Dworschak M, Birkenberg B, et al. Platelet dysfunction in outpatients with left ventricular assist devices. *Ann Thorac Surg.* 2009; 87(1):131-137.

CHAPTER 16
MECHANICAL CIRCULATORY SUPPORT IN INFANTS AND CHILDREN

Seema Mital

INTRODUCTION

Despite advances and widespread availability in technology for adult ventricular assist devices (VADs), the development and availability of mechanical cardiopulmonary support for children remains poor. The evolution of surgical repair in complex congenital heart defects and the availability of cardiac transplantation as a treatment option in end-stage heart disease have increased the need for mechanical cardiopulmonary support in children. A third of children listed for transplantation die waiting due to progression of disease while awaiting a suitable donor heart. Mechanical circulatory support improves survival to transplant by allowing critically ill patients with end-stage heart disease to be bridged to transplant. In the absence of appropriate-sized VADs, extracorporeal membrane oxygenation (ECMO) is still the most widely used modality for circulatory support in children but has several limitations, including a relatively high risk of complications, limited duration of support, and incomplete decompression of the failing ventricle. Despite these limitations, ECMO does have the advantage of providing oxygenation for the circulating blood which is important in situations where respiratory failure and pulmonary hypertension are important causes of cardiac failure. A recent review of the Extracorporeal Life Support Organization (ELSO) database of 2376 patients younger than 18 who received ECMO support postcardiotomy for congenital heart disease revealed an overall mortality of 37% (unpublished data), thereby highlighting the need for the development of improved methods of cardiopulmonary support, such as VAD therapy. There has been considerable experience with the use of VADs in the pediatric age group in Europe, with somewhat less experience in the United States.

INDICATIONS FOR MECHANICAL CIRCULATORY SUPPORT

The following indications for mechanical circulatory support (VADs) in children are comparable to those in adults:

A. Bridge-to-recovery for potentially reversible myocardial dysfunction
- Postcardiotomy (following palliative or reparative open heart operations) for postoperative low cardiac output or for inability to wean from cardiopulmonary bypass
- Posttransplant for donor heart dysfunction
- Acute allograft rejection
- Acute myocarditis
- Recoverable metabolic cardiac dysfunction
- Resuscitation after cardiac arrest

B. Bridge-to-transplantation (BTT) for end-stage irreversible cardiac dysfunction
- Inoperable congenital heart defects
- End-stage cardiomyopathy
- Intractable malignant arrhythmias

Unlike adults, VADs are not currently used as permanent or destination therapy in pediatric patients with end-stage failure in whom cardiac transplant is contraindicated.

CONTRAINDICATIONS

The contraindications to mechanical circulatory support in children are similar to those in adults. When the indication for a VAD is as a BTT, any contraindication to transplant constitutes a contraindication to use of mechanical support. Several contraindications are listed. However, several of these are relative contraindications and need to be evaluated on an individual patient basis. These include the following:

- Irreversible multiorgan system failure
- Severe coagulopathy
- Intracranial hemorrhage, irreversible neurological insult
- Active systemic infection
- Severe systemic disorder or other severe congenital anomalies
- Eisenmenger syndrome
- Pregnancy
- Very low weight (< 1.5 kg)

■ RELATIVE CONTRAINDICATIONS

The presence of multisystem organ failure is a relative contraindication since mechanical circulatory support may permit sufficient organ recovery to allow bridging to transplant. However, the presence of severe neurologic insult or of irreversible end-organ dysfunction that precludes transplantation remains a contraindication to device support.

While the presence of irreversible pulmonary hypertension is a contraindication to use of an assist device, the presence of pulmonary hypertension alone is not a contraindication but necessitates evaluation of the patient for biventricular rather than left ventricular support alone. Mechanical circulatory support for resuscitation after a cardiac arrest is controversial in light of the uncertain neurologic status following prolonged resuscitation and the uncertainty of return of end-organ function. Temporary support (eg, ECMO) may be used initially while assessing end-organ function postarrest, followed by conversion to a mechanical assist device if feasible and indicated for longer duration of support.

■ SPECIAL CONSIDERATIONS IN CHILDREN WITH CONGENITAL HEART DEFECTS

In the congenital heart disease population, several anatomic issues may make it technically difficult to implant an assist device. This is particularly true of patients with a single ventricle physiology, for example following the total cavopulmonary connection. There are only isolated reports of use of an assist device with this anatomy. Matsuda et al reported implanting a pneumatic VAD for cardiogenic shock in a 10-year-old after a modified Fontan operation.[1] The device was placed between the functional left atrium and ascending aorta, serving as an "artificial single ventricle" with neither pumping chamber nor artificial support on the right side of the heart. The systemic circulation was maintained by keeping a relatively high central venous pressure. The patient remained on support for 5 days but was unable to be weaned from support. The currently available assist devices need to be redesigned to permit implantation into hearts with a single ventricle anatomy. All patients should be evaluated for severe valvar insufficiency prior to device implantation. In patients with severe aortic insufficiency, the aortic valve needs to be oversewn prior to implantation of the device to prevent runoff of the systemic output.[2] Likewise, a systemic-pulmonary shunt including a patent ductus arteriosus, aortopulmonary window or surgical shunt needs to be ligated or divided prior to implantation of the device. In patients with severe mitral insufficiency, the severity of mitral insufficiency often improves after device implantation.[3] However in others, the valve may need to be repaired at the time of device implantation. The presence of a mechanical aortic or mitral valve is not a contraindication but significantly increases the risk of valve thrombosis following device implantation, and these patients require aggressive anticoagulation and monitoring for development of thrombus. Another issue that requires special consideration is the implantation of an assist device into either a systemic right ventricle or a severely hypertrophic ventricle.

There is a risk of inflow cannula occlusion by muscle trabeculations or hypertrophied muscle bundles. A cannula with a flared inflow should be used to reduce the risk of occlusion.

OPTIMAL TIMING FOR MECHANICAL CIRCULATORY SUPPORT

Children requiring mechanical circulatory support as BTT must meet institutional criteria for transplantation prior to implantation of an assist device. It is critical to identify the optimal timing for mechanical circulatory support in patients with advanced heart failure. Elective implantation in the absence of significant impairment of end-organ function has been shown to be a predictor of a positive outcome.[4] The evaluation of the need for mechanical support should begin early in any patient requiring multiple inotropes and/or showing signs of worsening heart failure with early evidence of end-organ dysfunction despite maximal medical support. Since placement of an indwelling pulmonary catheter is not technically feasible in all children for continuous measurement of cardiac hemodynamics caused by their smaller size, these patients need to be monitored closely for clinical signs of worsening heart failure and decompensation. An increase in serum blood urea nitrogen (BUN), creatinine, hepatic enzymes, worsening pulmonary edema, rising serum lactate, and decrease in mixed venous oxygen saturations are all indicators of worsening cardiac output.[5] Continuous hemodynamic monitoring via an indwelling catheter should be attempted in older patients with advanced heart failure awaiting transplant if feasible. The criteria for device implantation in these patients include the following:

Left atrial or pulmonary capillary wedge pressure > 18 mm Hg

Mean arterial pressure < 90 mm Hg

Cardiac index < 2 L/min/m^2

LV ejection fraction < 25%

Incomplete response to intravenous inotropes or pressors

Intraaortic balloon pump support

High risk for sudden cardiac arrest

INFLUENCE OF PATIENT SELECTION ON OUTCOME AFTER MECHANICAL CIRCULATORY SUPPORT

■ FACTORS INFLUENCING THE CHOICE OF TYPE OF CIRCULATORY SUPPORT

Appropriate patient selection is an important factor in patient survival following institution of mechanical circulatory support. ECMO or centrifugal support is often preferred in postcardiotomy patients with failure to wean off cardiopulmonary bypass who have a potential for myocardial recovery. The main advantage of using centrifugal support is that it provides a reduction in preload and wall stress that can lead to a reduction in inotropic requirements which can promote myocardial recovery by decreasing myocardial oxygen consumption, afterload, and arrhythmias. Prior to using circulatory support as a bridge-to-recovery following surgery, it is critical to assess the potential for recovery by excluding the presence of a residual cardiac defect which is the strongest correlate of failure of extracorporeal support. If patients cannot be weaned from bypass despite maximum pharmacologic intervention and adequate surgical repair, right ventricular function and pulmonary function should be evaluated while still on bypass to assess suitability for a mechanical assist device. At full flow, good right ventricular contraction and right atrial pressure less than 12 mm Hg (without pulmonary hypertension or right heart distension) suggest adequate right heart function. Serial blood gases should be done to assess adequacy of pulmonary function. If right ventricular or pulmonary function is inadequate, ECMO is the preferred option. ECMO is the only option if intracardiac shunts persist or respiratory failure is present which would require an oxygenator in the circuit. For patients on an assist device as a bridge-to-recovery, device flow is usually maintained for a minimum of 24 hours before attempting to wean. The flow is reduced to allow left ventricular ejection at left atrial pressures of 8 to 10 mm Hg. Evidence of stable hemodynamics and adequate echocardiographic left ventricular function on minimal safe flow suggests myocardial recovery and attempt should be made to wean off circulatory support.

◼ OUTCOME AFTER MECHANICAL CIRCULATORY SUPPORT BASED ON INDICATION FOR SUPPORT

In several studies reporting experience with pulsatile pneumatic support in children, the primary indication for support was a major factor in outcome with highest survival in patients with cardiomyopathies and myocarditis and lowest in those with congenital heart defects and postcardiotomy patients. This was shown by Reinhartz et al who reported on the outcome of pediatric patients on pulsatile circulatory support, including the Thoratec VAD, Berlin Heart, and Medos VAD. Overall survival rate for patients on Thoratec devices was 68.8% with 65.6% survival to discharge. Overall survival rate in 45 patients supported on the Berlin Heart was 48.9% with 75% survival to discharge. Of 56 patients supported with Medos devices, overall survival rate was 37.5%.[6]

Outcome of Mechanical Assist Devices as Bridge-to-Recovery

Ishino and colleagues reported their experience with the use of pneumatic paracorporeal VAD in 28 infants and children using the Berlin Heart.[7] Indications included BTT in 18, "rescue" after corrective surgery for congenital heart defects in 5, and bridge-to-recovery or transplant for myocarditis in 5. Overall survival was 40%. There were seven long-term survivors in groups I and III but none in group II again highlighting the need to be judicious in patient selection for mechanical assist device as "rescue" therapy. Thuys et al reported their experience related to the use of centrifugal ventricular assist as a bridge-to-recovery in neonates and small children (< 6 kg) requiring ventricular support postcardiopulmonary bypass.[8] This included children who could not be weaned from bypass and for postoperative low

cardiac output unresponsive to maximal medical management. Of the 34 patients requiring ventricular support, the most common defect was hypoplastic left heart syndrome in 12, transposition of great arteries in 8, and complete atrioventricular septal defect in 3. Twenty-five failed to wean from bypass and 10 developed low cardiac output postoperatively (median time from bypass to device implantation was 23.5 hours; median duration of support was 68 hours). Twenty-two were successfully weaned and decannulated; 5 were converted to ECMO. Fourteen of the 22 patients were discharged from hospital of whom 11 were alive 1 year postdischarge. Therefore, survival to discharge was 40% which was equivalent to that reported in patients supported by ECMO in previous studies. The type of cardiac lesion was an important determinant of survival with 5 of 8 patients with transposition of great arteries surviving to discharge while only 3 of 12 patients with hypoplastic left heart syndrome survived to discharge.

Outcome of Mechanical Assist Devices as BTT

Stiller et al reviewed the course of 45 pediatric patients with VADs as BTT.[9] Five patients were successfully weaned from support after recovery of function, 14 died of peripheral circulatory failure within 3 days of device implantation, and 8 died while awaiting donor hearts. Eighteen survived to transplant. Thirteen of 18 required biventricular support and all were on the Berlin Heart assist device. The 5-year survival of the transplant patients on device support was similar to that of patients who were transplanted without mechanical support with no difference in neurologic outcome, acute cardiac rejection, or transplant failure. This study highlighted several important factors related to use of VADs in pediatric patients as BTT. Forty-eight percent patients requiring mechanical assist device as BTT died while awaiting heart transplant with a relatively high early attrition (14 of the 22 patients who died did so within 3 days of device implantation of peripheral circulatory failure). This may reflect poor patient selection criteria with possible implantation of the device after the onset of irreversible peripheral organ failure. While ventricular support allows peripheral organ recovery while awaiting transplant, this may not be achievable once irreversible organ dysfunction has set in. This underscores the importance of close monitoring of patients with heart failure for signs of low cardiac output and implantation of device before multiorgan system failure develops. The ongoing loss of patients awaiting transplant on support indicates the need for improving patient management while on support with particular attention to management of anticoagulation, infection, and optimizing organ recovery. The finding that patients who were transplanted after device support had a similar 5-year survival as medically managed patients suggests that these patients are not at higher risk of posttransplant complications. In a recent study by Brancaccio et al, 10 children weighing less than 10 kg were implanted with the Berlin Heart as a BTT. The median duration of support in this study was 61 days (range: 2-168 days) with four deaths and five patients successfully BTT.[10] In a multi-institutional study from the Pediatric Heart Transplant Study Investigators, outcomes were analyzed in 99 pediatric patients with VAD implantation

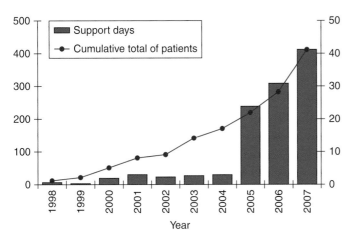

FIGURE 16–1. As experience with LVAD support in the pediatric population expands, the days of mechanical support offered per year is steadily increasing. (Reproduced with permission from Cassidy et al.[12] Copyright © Elsevier.)

as BTT between 1993 and 2003.[11] Mean duration of support was 57 days. Seventy-three percent were supported with a long-term device; 39% required biventricular support. Seventy-seven percent survived to transplant, 5 patients were successfully weaned off support, and 17% died on support. Risk factors for death while awaiting transplant included earlier era of implantation, female gender, and congenital heart disease diagnosis. Overall these are encouraging results. With an increase in waiting times, VAD support is likely to play an increasing role in pediatric transplantation (Fig. 16–1).[12]

CURRENT STATUS OF PEDIATRIC VENTRICULAR ASSIST DEVICES

Most of the experience with the use of VADs in the United States has included small series of patients. The experience with the use of Thoratec HeartMate and Novacor devices in 12 adolescents as a BTT was reported by Helman et al and in younger children with body surface area less than 1.3 m² by Reinhartz et al.[13,14] Ashton et al reviewed their experience with the use of the Abiomed BVS 5000 or the Biomedicus centrifugal pump in nine pediatric patients aged 12 days to 15 years.[15] In contrast, there has been a relatively extensive European experience, some of which was reviewed by Reinhartz et al related to use of the Thoratec, Berlin Heart, and Medos VAD in children.[16] The overall outcome and survival to discharge has been comparable across different device types. Despite attempts to miniaturize adult pumps, there are few pediatric devices available in the United States. A Humanitarian Use Device designation was awarded to the DeBakey VAD *Child*, and a Humanitarian Device Exemption has been granted to allow implant of the DeBakey VAD *Child*—a fully implantable VAD in 5- to 16-year-old, with end-stage heart failure pediatric patients who need mechanical circulatory support as a bridge-to-cardiac transplantation. Berlin Heart, Inc recently announced that its Excor Pediatric VAD was given approval from the US Food and Drug Administration (FDA) for the ongoing Investigational Device Exemption (IDE) in the United States. The National Institutes

of Health recently awarded five contracts over a 5-year period for the development of mechanical circulatory support in children. The objective of this initiative was to develop a range of devices (both intra- and extracorporeal as well as axial and pulsatile flow) that could support patients up to 2 years of age with mixed flow.[17] Examples of these devices are given in Fig. 16–2.

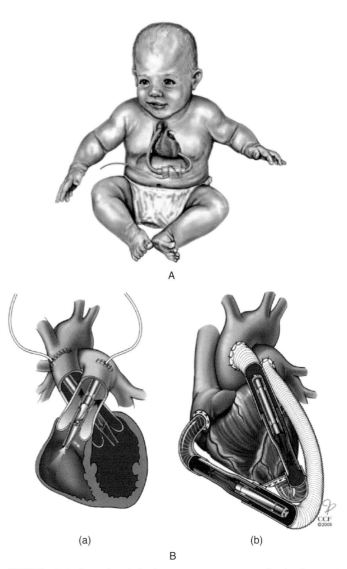

FIGURE 16–2. Examples of circulatory support systems under development for children. **A.** PediaFlow system: a mixed-flow turbodynamic blood pump for patients up to 2 years old. (Reproduced with permission from Baldwin et al.[17] Fig 1.) **B.** (a) Intravascular PediPump: biventricular assist device for patients weighing more than 15 kg; placed across both semilunar valves to provide biventricular support. (b) Extravascular, intracorporeal PediPump deployed as a biventricular assist device for patients weighing less than 15 kg. (Reprinted with permission, Cleveland Clinic Center for Medical Art & Photography © 2005-2010. All Rights Reserved.) (c) The Ension pCAS system. Blue and red arrows demonstrate inflow and outflow, respectively. Gas exchange occurs in the rotor's microporous hollow fibers. This system was designed to improve outcomes in ECMO therapy. (Reproduced with permission from Baldwin et al.[17] Fig 4.) (d) The adult, child, and infant Jarvik-2000 devices. (e) The Penn State PVADs is an extracorporeal pulsatile device designed to produce rotational blood flow patterns within the pump chambers. The 12-mL infant-size VAD is shown. (Reproduced with permission from Baldwin et al.[17] Fig 8.)

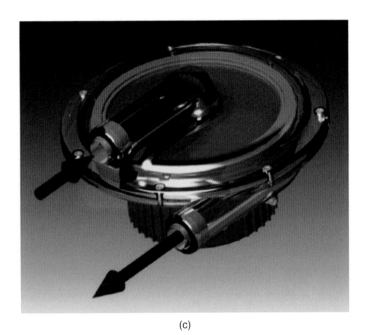

(c)

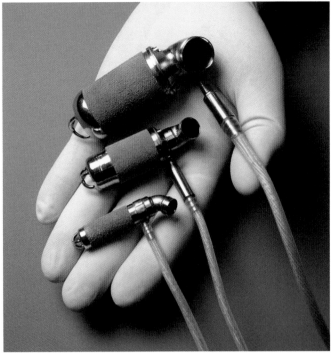

(d)

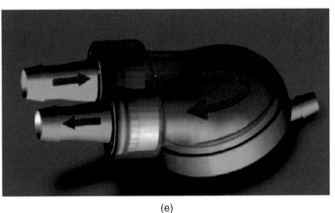

(e)

FIGURE 16–2B. *Continued.*

It is hoped that with these initiatives, there will be better devices and improved availability of these devices for use in infants and children requiring mechanical circulatory support.

REFERENCES

1. Matsuda H TY, Ohkubo N, Ohtani M, et al. Use of a paracorporeal pneumatic ventricular assist device for postoperative cardiogenic shock in two children with complex cardiac lesions. *Artif Organs.* 1988;12:423-430.

2. Park SJ, Liao KK, Segurola R, Madhu KP, Miller LW. Management of aortic insufficiency in patients with left ventricular assist devices: a simple coaptation stitch method (Park's stitch). *J Thorac Cardiovasc Surg.* 2004;127:264-266.

3. Holman WL, Bourge RC, Fan P, Kirklin JK, Pacifico AD, Nanda NC. Influence of longer term left ventricular assist device support on valvular regurgitation. *ASAIO J.* 1994;40:M454-M459.

4. Salzberg S, Lachat M, Zund G, et al. Left ventricular assist device as bridge to heart transplantation—lessons learned with the MicroMed DeBakey axial blood flow pump. *Eur J Cardiothorac Surg.* 2003;24:113-118.

5. Reddy SLC, Hasan A, Hamilton LRJ, et al. Mechanical versus medical bridge to transplantation in children. What is the best timing for mechanical bridge? *Eur J Cardiothorac Surg.* 2004;25:605-609.

6. Reinhartz O, Keith FM, El-Banayosy A, et al. Multicenter experience with the thoratec ventricular assist device in children and adolescents. *J Heart Lung Transplant.* 2001;20:439-448.

7. Ishino K, Loebe M, Uhlemann F, Weng Y, Hennig E, Hetzer R. Circulatory support with paracorporeal pneumatic ventricular assist device (VAD) in infants and children. *Eur J Cardiothorac Surg.* 1997;11:965-972.

8. Thuys CA, Mullaly RJ, Horton SB, et al. Centrifugal ventricular assist in children under 6 kg. *Eur J Cardiothorac Surg.* 1998;13:130-134.

9. Stiller B, Hetzer R, Weng Y, et al. Heart transplantation in children after mechanical circulatory support with pulsatile pneumatic assist device. *J Heart Lung Transplant.* 2003;22:1201-1208.

10. Brancaccio G, Amodeo A, Ricci Z, et al. Mechanical assist device as a bridge to heart transplantation in children less than 10 kilograms. *Ann Thorac Surg.* 2010;90(1):58-62.

11. Blume ED, Naftel DC, Bastardi HJ, et al; Pediatric Heart Transplant Study Investigators. Outcomes of children bridged to heart transplantation with ventricular assist devices: a multi-institutional study. *Circulation.* 2006;113(19):2313-2319.

12. Cassidy J, Haynes S, Kirk R, et al. Changing patterns of bridging to heart transplantation in children. *J Heart Lung Transplant.* 2009;28(3):249-254.

13. Helman DN, Addonizio LJ, Morales DLS, et al. Implantable left ventricular assist devices can successfully bridge adolescent patients to transplant. *J Heart Lung Transplant.* 2000;19:121-126.

14. Reinhartz O, Copeland JG, Farrar DJ. Thoratec ventricular assist devices in children with less than 1.3 m2 of body surface area. *ASAIO J.* 2003;49:727-730.

15. Ashton RC, Jr, Oz MC, Michler RE, et al. Left ventricular assist device options in pediatric patients. *ASAIO J.* 1995;41:M277-M280.

16. Reinhartz O, Stiller B, Eilers R, Farrar DJ. Current clinical status of pulsatile pediatric circulatory support. *ASAIO J.* 2002;48:455-459.

17. Baldwin JT, Borovetz HS, Duncan BW, et al. The National Heart, Lung, and Blood Institute Pediatric Circulatory Support Program. *Circulation.* 2006;113(1):147-155.

CHAPTER 17

PULMONARY HYPERTENSION DURING LVAD SUPPORT

Robert E. Southard and Gerald J. Berry

Congestive heart failure (CHF) is commonly complicated by pulmonary hypertension. The presence of pulmonary hypertension in the setting of CHF can further worsen the prognosis.[1] Pulmonary hypertension is usually defined when one or more of the following criteria are met: systolic pulmonary artery pressure (SPAP) greater than 50 mm Hg, pulmonary vascular resistance (PVR) greater than 4 Wood units, PVR index greater than 6 Wood units, or transpulmonary gradient (TPG) greater than 15 mm Hg (Table 17–1).[2] The World Health Organization (WHO) defines pulmonary hypertension as a sustained elevation of pulmonary arterial pressure to more than 25 mm Hg at rest (or to > 30 mm Hg with exercise) as well as a mean pulmonary wedge pressure and left ventricular end-diastolic pressure less than 15 mm Hg. The pathologic basis for pulmonary hypertension was described by Donald Heath and Jesse Edwards in 1958 as a classification scheme to describe the progressive histologic changes that occur in the pulmonary arteries and arterioles in patients with congenital septal defects.[3] The six pathologic grades are summarized in Table 17–2, and examples are given in Fig. 17–1A-H. In general, Heath-Edwards grade 3 or greater lung lesions are thought to represent irreversible pulmonary hypertension. The scheme does not reflect a morphologic continuum or sequence of developmental changes and therefore has limited clinicopathologic utility. It does, however, illustrate the wide range of lesions that can develop in the setting of clinical pulmonary hypertension.

Right heart failure is more likely to occur following cardiac transplantation in patients whose preoperative TPG is elevated. One study has shown that a TPG greater than 12 mm Hg is associated with 6-month and 1-year mortality rates, five and seven times higher than those of patients with a normal TPG.[4] Furthermore, early transplant mortality (0-2 days) has been shown to be three times higher in patients with TPG greater than or equal to 15 mm Hg.[5] Therefore, many centers consider fixed pulmonary hypertension to be a relative contraindication to heart transplantation.[6,7]

REVERSAL OF PULMONARY HYPERTENSION

The phenomenon of normalization of pulmonary arterial pressures with left ventricular assist device (LVAD) support has been described in several case reports and small series.[8,9] Al Khaldi and colleagues reported a patient who underwent reduction in TPG

from 22 to 6 mm Hg after 11 months of mechanical unloading.[10] Adamson and colleagues reported similar results in a patient who was supported for 10 weeks.[11] Nguyen et al demonstrated a lowering of the TPG in three patients supported with an assist device.[12] In another series of six patients, a reduction in PVR from 5.7 ± 0.7 to 2.0 ± 1.2 Wood units was demonstrated.[13] In this series, all six patients underwent heart transplant with only one mortality 3 months after transplant. A larger series of 54 bridge-to-transplant patients (41% with fixed pulmonary hypertension) suggested that LVAD support removed the negative influence of pulmonary hypertension on posttransplant outcomes.[14]

The study by Martin et al included one patient who underwent a device change to a HeartMate after initially receiving a Jarvik-2000.[15] However, they report that this patient was large and had little residual left ventricular function and so required a device with the ability to generate a large amount of flow. In a study involving only patients with axial-flow devices, Salzberg et al demonstrated a decrease in PVR in six patients who received a DeBakey LVAD.[16] In a comparison between axial-flow and pulsatile devices in patients with pulmonary hypertension, Wieselthaler and colleagues saw no difference between device types.[17] Our series of nine patients (two with pulsatile and seven with axial-flow ventricular assist devices [VADs]) suggested a similar improvement in pulmonary hemodynamics and post-transplant outcome regardless of device type.[18] A larger series of 50 patients demonstrated normalization of pulmonary hemodynamics after axial-flow LVAD support, with preservation of this effect following cardiac transplantation.[19] Despite the marked difference in physiology, this phenomenon also seems to occur in response to axial-flow as well as pulsatile devices. The fact that PVR may be reduced in the setting of both axial-flow and pulsatile devices suggests that reversal of pulmonary hypertension does not require complete unloading of the left ventricle.

Although these studies demonstrate that reversal of fixed pulmonary hypertension may occur in some patients, there has not been a systematic study of a large number of patients with pulmonary hypertension supported by assist devices. The relatively small number of patients who not only receive a device, but also have severe pulmonary hypertension is a major obstacle for such a study to be performed at a single center. Registry data and multicenter trials will likely be necessary to determine the effectiveness of LVADs to reverse pulmonary hypertension at the population level.

APPLICATION OF ASSIST DEVICES IN THE SETTING OF PULMONARY HYPERTENSION

Elevated pulmonary resistance has consequences not only after heart transplantation, but during LVAD support as well. Right heart failure after LVAD implantation is a common problem and multiple risk factors have been identified.[20] Interestingly, low preoperative pulmonary arterial pressures are associated with right heart failure after LVAD implantation, whereas elevated pulmonary pressures were not a risk factor. This is likely because a right ventricle capable of generating supranormal pulmonary arterial pressures is unlikely to fail, but a right ventricle that is

TABLE 17–1. Clinical Parameters Used to Define Pulmonary Hypertension (Where TPG = Mean Pulmonary Artery Pressure–Pulmonary Capillary Wedge Pressure)

Clinical Parameter	Threshold
Systolic pulmonary artery pressure (SPAP)	> 50 mm Hg
Pulmonary vascular resistance (PVR)	> 4 Wood units
PVR index	> 6 Wood units
Transpulmonary gradient (TPG)	> 15 mm Hg

incapable of producing such pressures has a high risk of failure once required to keep up with an increased cardiac output.

Because LVADs may reverse pulmonary hypertension in some patients, some have advocated the use of device support prior to heart transplantation in the subset of patients with pulmonary hypertension.[21] This approach might result in a number of patients becoming eligible for heart transplant as well as a decrease in posttransplant mortality by decreasing pulmonary resistance prior to transplantation. Furthermore, if some of these patients do not experience a significant decrease in pulmonary resistance, the device could be left in place as destination therapy or as bridge-to-recovery when the clinical situation dictates.

PATHOPHYSIOLOGY OF SECONDARY PULMONARY HYPERTENSION

The mechanism by which chronic CHF leads to the development of pulmonary hypertension is poorly understood. Multiple vasoactive drugs can affect pulmonary arterial pressures. Nesiritide is recombinant human B-type natriuretic peptide and is commonly used in the treatment of severe CHF. Nesiritide can decrease PVR in the setting of CHF.[22] The effect of this drug suggests that neurohormones play a role in the development of secondary pulmonary hypertension. Furthermore, nitric oxide is a vasoactive inhalation agent that is normally produced by endothelial cells as a regulator of vascular resistance.[23] Inhaled nitric oxide is often effective in treating pulmonary hypertension in the acute setting. Therefore, a derangement of the regulation of vascular resistance by endothelial cells has also been implicated in the pathogenesis of secondary pulmonary hypertension. However, a subset of patients has fixed pulmonary hypertension that is not responsive to either intravenous drugs or inhaled nitric oxide.[24] These patients may respond to mechanical unloading despite unresponsiveness to pharmacologic therapy. The lack of response to pharmacologic therapy suggests that there may be a structural change induced in the pulmonary vasculature over time in response to elevated left-sided volumes and low-flow states. Presumably, a structural change would only be responsive to chronic unloading such as that seen with LVADs.

BIVENTRICULAR SUPPORT WITH AXIAL-FLOW DEVICES

The high risk of right-sided failure on LVAD support often mandates the use of biventricular support with either two assist devices or a single total artificial heart (TAH). The TAH has successfully supported up to 70% of patients in whom it is placed.[25] However, one of the serious problems with biventricular support is the need to accurately match left- and right-sided cardiac outputs. This problem is especially difficult to overcome in patients with elevated PVR. The use of biventricular support with axial-flow devices can deal with this problem. Using biventricular Jarvik-2000 support, Kindo and colleagues supported a calf with varying degrees of PVR.[26] Because axial-flow devices are more sensitive to preload pressures than pulsatile devices, relatively small increases in right-sided output were compensated for by increases in left-sided output without adjusting the speed setting on the device itself.

TABLE 17–2. Heath-Edwards Pathologic Classification for Pulmonary Hypertension

Grade	Pathologic Findings
1	Medial hypertrophy in arteries and arterioles; minimal to no intimal changes
2	Medial hypertrophy; cellular intimal proliferation
3	Medial hypertrophy; intimal fibrosis; early generalized vascular dilatation in severe instances
4	Progressive generalized vascular dilatation and occlusion by intimal fibrosis and fibroelastosis
5	Appearance of the other "dilatation lesions," including vein-like branches of hypertrophied muscular arteries, cavernous lesions, and angiomatoid lesions; highly vascular lung due to vein-like arterial branches; pulmonary hemosiderosis
6	Necrotizing arteritis

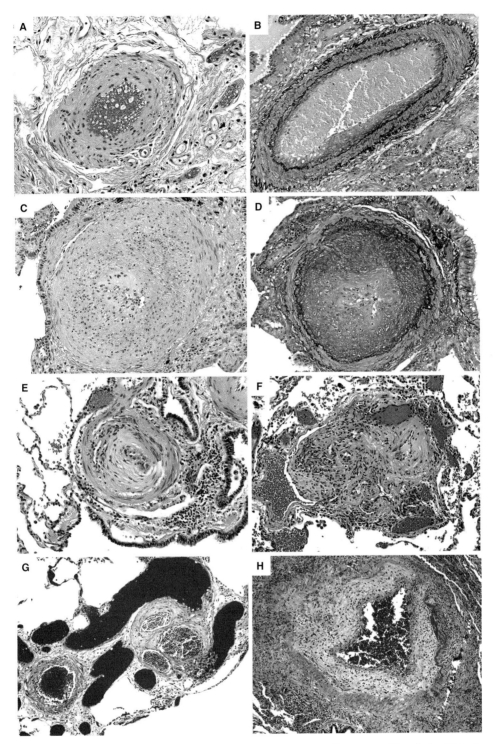

FIGURE 17–1. A. Grade I. Muscular hypertrophy of muscular arteries. The small muscular arteries and arterioles display thickening of the medial layer by smooth muscle cells. **B.** The elastic van Gieson stain (EVG) demonstrates the internal and external elastic layers. In this case of grade I hypertrophy, there is little or no intimal thickening but medial expansion. **C.** Grade II. Intimal proliferation of muscular arteries. The muscular arteries exhibit marked luminal narrowing, often with slit-like or pinpoint lumens. **D.** The EVG stain shows a mild degree of medial layer thickening but profound concentric intimal thickening. The intimal proliferation is composed of both cellular elements and connective tissue stroma. **E.** Grade III. Concentric laminar fibrosis of muscular arteries. The muscular arteries show concentric intimal expansion by a predominantly fibrous matrix admixed with some cellular elements. This produces a whorled or lamellated arrangement of the intimal layer. **F.** Grade IV. Plexiform lesion. The left-sided portion of the muscular artery displays a proliferation of slit-like, thick-walled vascular channels lined by endothelial cells. These appear to arise in an eccentric fashion from the muscular artery. In this example the residual part of the artery on the right shows intimal and medial thickening. **G.** Dilatation lesion. The muscular artery displays an increase in thin-walled, dilated, blood-filled vascular spaces around a plexiform lesion. **H.** Necrotizing arteritis with fibrinoid necrosis. This uncommon pattern of pulmonary hypertension is characterized by eosinophilic fibrinoid accumulations in the wall of the arteries, usually at the intimamedial layer interface. (All Images reproduced with permission from Gerald J. Berry, MD.)

In the setting of fixed pulmonary hypertension secondary to chronic heart failure, VADs have the potential to become a mainstay of therapy. Reversal of pulmonary hypertension with LVAD support prior to heart transplantation may soon become a common indication for device implantation. Also, in patients with severely elevated PVR and a failing right ventricle, newer-generation continuous-flow devices offer the unique ability to match left- and right-sided flows spontaneously.

REFERENCES

1. Cappola TP, Felker GM, Kao WH, Hare JM, Baughman KL, Kasper EK. Pulmonary hypertension and risk of death in cardiomyopathy: patients with myocarditis are at higher risk. *Circulation.* 2002;105(14):1663-1668.

2. Ross H, Hendry P, Dipchand A, et al. 2001 Canadian Cardiovascular Society Consensus Conference on cardiac transplantation. *Can J Cardiol.* 2003;19(6):620-654.

3. Heath D, Edwards JE. The pathology of hypertensive pulmonary vascular disease: a description of six grades of structural changes in the pulmonary arteries with special reference to congenital cardiac septal defects. *Circulation.* 1958;18(4 Part 1):533-547.

4. Erickson KW, Costanzo-Nordin MR, O'Sullivan EJ, et al. Influence of preoperative transpulmonary gradient on late mortality after orthotopic heart transplantation. *J Heart Transplant.* 1990;9(5):526-537.

5. Murali S, Kormos RL, Uretsky BF, et al. Preoperative pulmonary hemodynamics and early mortality after orthotopic cardiac transplantation: the Pittsburgh experience. *Am Heart J.* 1993;126(4):896-904.

6. Kirklin JK, Naftel DC, Kirklin JW, Blackstone EH, White-Williams C, Bourge RC. Pulmonary vascular resistance and the risk of heart transplantation. *J Heart Transplant.* 1988; 7(5):331-336.

7. Costard-Jackle A, Fowler MB. Influence of preoperative pulmonary artery pressure on mortality after heart transplantation: testing of potential reversibility of pulmonary hypertension with nitroprusside is useful in defining a high risk group. *J Am Coll Cardiol.* 1992;19(1):48-54.

8. Gallagher RC, Kormos RL, Gasior T, Murali S, Griffith BP, Hardesty RL. Univentricular support results in reduction of pulmonary resistance and improved right ventricular function. *ASAIO Trans.* 1991;37(3):M287-M288.

9. Bhat G, Costea A. Reversibility of medically unresponsive pulmonary hypertension with nesiritide in a cardiac transplant recipient. *ASAIO J.* 2003;49(5):608-610.

10. Al Khaldi A, Ergina P, DeVarennes B, Lachappelle K, Cecere R. Left ventricular unloading in a patient with end-stage cardiomyopathy and medically unresponsive pulmonary hypertension. *Artif Organs.* 2004;28(2):158-160.

11. Adamson RM, Dembitsky WP, Jaski BE, et al. Left ventricular assist device support of medically unresponsive pulmonary hypertension and aortic insufficiency. *ASAIO J.* 1997;43(4):365-369.

12. Nguyen DQ, Ormaza S, Miller LW, et al. Left ventricular assist device support for medically unresponsive pulmonary hypertension from left ventricular failure. *J Heart Lung Transplant.* 2001;20(2):190.

13. Martin J, Siegenthaler MP, Friesewinkel O, et al. Implantable left ventricular assist device for treatment of pulmonary hypertension in candidates for orthotopic heart transplantation-a preliminary study. *Eur J Cardiothorac Surg.* 2004;25(6):971-977.

14. Alba AC, Rao V, Ross HJ, et al. Impact of fixed pulmonary hypertension on post-heart transplant outcomes in bridge-to-transplant patients. *J Heart Lung Transplant.* 2010;29(11):1253-1258.

15. Martin J, Siegenthaler MP, Friesewinkel O, et al. Implantable left ventricular assist device for treatment of pulmonary hypertension in candidates for orthotopic heart transplantation—a preliminary study. *Eur J Cardiothorac Surg.* 2004;25(6):971-977.

16. Salzberg SP, Lachat ML, von Harbou K, Zund G, Turina MI. Normalization of high pulmonary vascular resistance with LVAD support in heart transplantation candidates. *Eur J Cardiothorac Surg.* 2005;27(2):222-225.

17. Wieselthaler GM, Roethy WK, Schima H, et al. Treatment of fixed pulmonary hypertension in end-stage heart failure patients with LVAD therapy as bridge to transplantation: comparison of pulsatile vs. non-pulsatile pumps [Abstract]. Second EACTS/ESTS Joint Meeting, Vienna [October 12-15]. 2003. Ref Type: Generic.

18. Torre-Amione G, Southard RE, Loebe MM, et al. Reversal of secondary pulmonary hypertension by axial and pulsatile mechanical circulatory support. *J Heart Lung Transplant.* 2010;29(2):195-200.

19. John R, Liao K, Kamdar F, Eckman P, Boyle A, Colvin-adams M. Effects on pre- and posttransplant pulmonary hemodynamics in patients with continuous-flow left ventricular assist devices. *J Thorac Cardiovasc Surg.* 2010;140(2):447-452.

20. Ochiai Y, McCarthy PM, Smedira NG, et al. Predictors of severe right ventricular failure after implantable left ventricular assist device insertion: analysis of 245 patients. *Circulation.* 2002;106(12 Suppl 1):I198-I202.

21. Martin J, Siegenthaler MP, Friesewinkel O, et al. Implantable left ventricular assist device for treatment of pulmonary hypertension in candidates for orthotopic heart transplantation—a preliminary study. *Eur J Cardiothorac Surg.* 2004;25(6):971-977.

22. Bhat G, Costea A. Reversibility of medically unresponsive pulmonary hypertension with nesiritide in a cardiac transplant recipient. *ASAIO J.* 2003;49(5):608-610.

23. Moraes DL, Colucci WS, Givertz MM. Secondary pulmonary hypertension in chronic heart failure: the role of the endothelium in pathophysiology and management. *Circulation.* 2000;102(14):1718-1723.

24. Martin J, Siegenthaler MP, Friesewinkel O, et al. Implantable left ventricular assist device for treatment of pulmonary hypertension in candidates for orthotopic heart transplantation—a preliminary study. *Eur J Cardiothorac Surg.* 2004;25(6):971-977.

25. Copeland JG, Smith RG, Arabia FA, et al. Cardiac replacement with a total artificial heart as a bridge to transplantation. *N Engl J Med.* 2004;351(9):859-867.

26. Kindo M, Radovancevic B, Gregoric ID, et al. Biventricular support with the Jarvik 2000 ventricular assist device in a calf model of pulmonary hypertension. *ASAIO J.* 2004;50(5):444-450.

CHAPTER 18

PHYSIOLOGY OF CONTINUOUS BLOOD FLOW

Wilfried Roethy, Georg M. Wieselthaler, Heinrich Schima and Ernst Wolner

BACKGROUND

The majority of the current generation of ventricular assist devices (VADs) rely on application of continuous flow for providing mechanical circulatory support. However, prior to the first long-term clinical application of axial-flow VADs in 1998, the compatibility of different human end-organ systems to pulseless blood flow patterns was unknown. In fact, only a number of experiments performed in animal models revealed promising initial results. With the introduction of roller pumps for cardiopulmonary bypass in the early 1950s, it was demonstrated for the first time that the human organism could tolerate nonpulsatile blood flow for at least a limited time of support. Today, long-term follow-up in patients with continuous-flow devices has shown that end-organ function is well maintained during VAD support, and doubts about the feasibility of long-term low-pulsatile circulation have nearly disappeared.

INTRODUCTION

Although it was demonstrated more than 50 years ago with the use of roller pumps in cardiopulmonary bypass that the human body could tolerate nonpulsatile blood flow at least for a short time, most early work in the field of mechanical circulatory support focused on pulsatile volume-displacement pumps. Nevertheless, scientists were intrigued by the idea of a technically simple, low-cost continuous-flow pump with the potential of miniaturization, maximum freedom of movement, superior quality of life, and lower cost than comparable pulsatile systems. Despite this optimism, however, even after promising initial results in short-term animal models, there were concerns about whether or not nonpulsatile flow would be compatible with human life over a longer period of time. The effect on end-organ function remained a concern.

In the early 1950s, the first clinically applicable continuous-flow pumps were developed by DeBakey and Gibbon.[1] These heart/lung machines were based on a roller pump that was previously introduced by Michael E. DeBakey in 1934 for use in blood transfusion.[2] The physiologic compatibility of short-term nonpulsatile perfusion was demonstrated in 1955 by Adam

Weslowski.[3] Despite these early promising results, concerns persisted in subsequent decades about the possible negative effects of low-pulsatile blood flow on the physiologic function on different organ systems, such as the brain, kidneys, splanchnic organs as well as the hormonal response of endocrine organs. As a result, only pulsatile cardiac assist devices were the main focus of development until 20 years ago.

As a next step to further investigate the acceptance of continuous-flow, chronic animal studies were designed which allowed an easy switchover from pulsatile to nonpulsatile support. Consistent data were derived from these experiments that provided further insight into possible disturbances of physiologic reactions in single organs as well as more complex organ systems. A number of different continuous-flow pumps were developed for short-, medium-, and long-term support. In 1998, with the MicroMed DeBakey VAD, developed by Michael DeBakey, George Noon, and the National Aeronautics and Space Administration (NASA), the first fully implantable continuous-flow left ventricular assist device (LVAD) became available for long-term clinical testing. Important new data were derived about the compatibility of nonpulsatile blood flow with human life in areas such as hemostasis, end-organ function, flow adjustment (autoregulation) during physical exercise, immunologic response, and the patient's mental status during chronic support. Furthermore, because of the excellent early outcomes of these systems, it was possible to discharge patients to their homes while bridging them for cardiac transplantation for more than 400 days. The positive results derived from these early patients led to the development of a variety of other continuous-flow pumps, which today dominate the field among patients requiring solitary left ventricular support. This chapter discusses the historical context of the current push toward continuous-flow physiology with additional discussion on the effects of nonpulsatile flow regarding cardiac function, cerebral blood flow, neurocognitive function, neuroendocrine function, end-organ perfusion, pulmonary hypertension, and humoral sensitization. The hematologic ramifications of continuous flow and their impact on bleeding rates are discussed in Chapter 15.

HISTORICAL BACKGROUND

In 1958, T. Akutsu and W.J. Kolff summarized their first experience with permanent pulsatile substitutes for the heart, revealing results of animal experiments that even go back to the early 1930s.[4] They successfully implanted a hydraulic, polyvinyl chloride total artificial heart in a dog, keeping the animal alive for 90 minutes. Compatibility of nonpulsatile perfusion of the pulmonary circulation using a roller pump was later published in 1953, by Weslowski and coworkers.[5] In 1960, Saxton and Andrews demonstrated the application of centrifugal blood pumps for assistance of the failing heart[6] and even added their thoughts about the potential benefits compared to pulsatile systems. In 1976, Johnston and coworkers[7,8] described their animal studies using a centrifugal pump for pulsatile and nonpulsatile bypass of the left ventricle. Four out of nine animals survived until the preset endpoint of 14 days without any complications.

In 1979, T. Murakami from Yukihiko Nosé's group at the Cleveland Clinic Foundation published the first manuscript on nonpulsatile biventricular bypass using two rotary blood pumps.[9] In 1980, Golding et al from the same group added their findings on chronic nonpulsatile blood flow in a conscious animal that survived for 34 days.[10] For these studies two Blackshear-Medtronic centrifugal blood pumps were implanted paracorporeally, mounted on the back of calves, and started up after ventricular fibrillation was induced. That pump, developed by Blackshear and coworkers in the late 1960s, was a centrifugal pump with a small impeller with a shaft inside the pump head that was rotated by a relatively small DC motor.[11] This pump performed well for 2 weeks without blood clot formation. Five animals were kept alive for up to 99 days in experiments with totally nonpulsatile blood flow, although it was essential to keep blood flow 20% above the physiologic pulsatile perfusion rate. However, after 6 weeks this increased blood flow was no longer necessary and returned to normal values. At the same time an arterial pressure pulsation, the so-called *ideoperipheral pulsation*, at a rate of 40 beats/min was observed.[12,13] Interestingly, the physiology of these supported animals was not significantly different from that of animals undergoing implantation of pulsatile total artificial hearts (TAH),[9,12,14] at no time was there any evidence of neurologic damage, subcutaneous edema, or ascites. The animals did well with good oral intake and were even intermittently exercised in treadmill tests.[10]

In 1990, Taenaka et al repeated the experiments in conscious animals and investigated the physiologic response to an immediate switch between pulsatile and nonpulsatile blood flow.[15] In this study, they tried to eliminate as much as possible the potential adverse effects caused by anesthesia and/or the surgical procedure by choosing a different time point for the switchover to nonpulsatile flow. Using this modified protocol, they no longer observed relevant changes in hemodynamics, oxygen consumption, or blood catecholamines and proved the ability of mammals to immediately adapt to systemic nonpulsatile circulation.

However, these very promising results failed to convince most scientists, and the majority favored a pulsatile strategy in their blood pumps for clinical application. A growing number of investigators started to develop a variety of rotary blood pumps. Systems with different kinds of bearings and later magnetically levitated rotors were presented at specific workshops on rotary blood pumps in smaller meetings which were first held in Austria in 1988 and 1991.[16,17] These international meetings evolved into the International Society for Rotary Blood Pumps (ISRBP), established in 1992 in Houston, Texas, to further support the development of continuous-flow blood pumps. In November 1998, the first clinical application of the first implantable, miniaturized continuous axial-flow blood pump, the MicroMed DeBakey VAD, was performed almost at the very same time in Berlin and Vienna. After a period of 73 days following the implantation in Vienna, carried out by Drs G. Noon, E. Wolner, and G. Wieselthaler, a donor heart became available and this first patient with long-term support of a continuous-flow pump was successfully transplanted. Later, other axial-flow pumps like the Jarvik-2000 pump, the HeartMate II, and the Berlin Heart INOCOR system were introduced for clinical

investigation. These were in turn followed by an entire third generation of continuous-flow VADs that represent the current strategy under investigation.

■ PHYSIOLOGIC IMPLICATIONS OF CONTINUOUS FLOW

Return of Low-Pulsatile Blood Flow

It was long believed, that nonpulsatile blood flow would lead to dysfunction of different organ systems. However, in vivo, pulsatile flow is only present in the aorta, large and small arteries, and arterioles, and diminishes in capillaries, venules, and smaller vasculature of the circulatory system. Therefore, in normal individuals pulsatile flow is not present at the end-organ level. The safety of continuous flow at the end-organ level was also borne out in early animal experiments with biventricular continuous-flow assistance, where low pulsatility in the arterial pressure was observed during fibrillation to avoid any natural pulsatility.[10,18] In other studies, rhythmic idioperipheral pulsations of 40 beats/min were observed during chronic nonpulsatile perfusion.[12,13,19,20] It was speculated that this phenomenon was triggered by peripheral vasoconstriction, with the vasomotor center as the origin of this effect. In 1994, Fukamachi from L.A. Golding's group demonstrated in calves supported with nonpulsatile biventricular bypass that such effects can also be caused by respiration.[21]

In any case, it is only during the very early postoperative period that complete nonpulsatile arterial pressure curves can be detected. After the initial period of complete nonpulsatile flow, low pulsatility of blood flow reoccurs with recovery of the native left heart function.[22,23] Because of the low amplitude of oscillating pressure signals, in many patients measurement of the systemic arterial pressure with the conventional Riva-Rocci cuff method is impossible and requires invasive blood pressure monitoring or a new, more sophisticated ultrasonic Doppler-based method (Fig. 18–1).[24]

Hemodynamic Consequences of Continuous Unloading

Although some pulsatility returns in the early postoperative period after placement of a continuous-flow pump, flatline flow patterns can be provoked by increasing the speed of the pump. In contrast to pulsatile assist devices, excessive continuous unloading of the left ventricle can cause the complete collapse of the left ventricle and suction is detected. Furthermore, a concomitant shift of the interventricular septum can lead to severe incompetence of the tricuspid valve and subsequent right heart failure with low pump-flow conditions.[25] In this scenario, only speed reduction immediately resolves the problem and restores normal hemodynamic conditions.

Therefore, control circuits with suction detection and automatic adjustment of the pump speed to physiologic requirements have been developed to provide further enhancement of pump performance and adaptation to exercise.[26]

Effects on Cerebral Metabolism

Before the first clinical application of a nonpulsatile assist device in humans, there was much concern about its possible

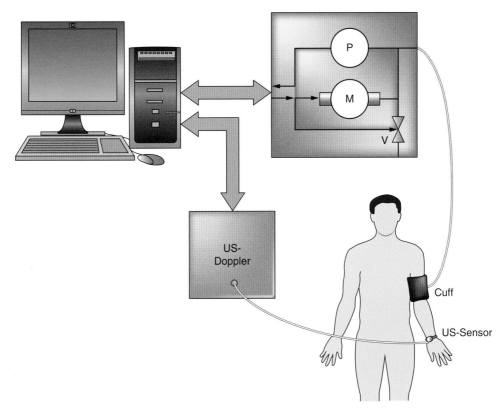

FIGURE 18–1. Patients supported on continuous-flow devices require either invasive pressure monitoring or newer ultrasound Doppler techniques as shown. This system incorporates a PC-controlled electropneumatic board with a motor compressor (M) for inflating the cuff in the upper arm, a pressure sensor (P), a deflation valve (V), and an ultrasound Doppler system with a wristwatch sensor. (Reproduced with permission from Schima et al.[24] Copyright © John Wiley & Sons.)

consequences on cerebral metabolism, neurologic function, and subsequent changes in physical examination or mental status. Previous studies from various groups, either with an acute setup or short-term clinical studies, demonstrated varying data on the potential negative effects of nonpulsatility on cerebral blood flow, autoregulation, and metabolism.[27-35] However, these varying results are most likely caused by the inconsistency of the experimental conditions. A more recent chronic animal study in goats performed by Nishinaka et al investigated the effects of reduced pulse pressure on the cerebral metabolism during prolonged nonpulsatile left heart bypass.[36] These experiments failed to demonstrate any significant changes in cerebral metabolism during long-term nonpulsatile perfusion, supporting early clinical findings in which no adverse effects on cerebral function or any kind of neurologic or behavioral disorders were reported.

Effects on Ocular Microcirculation and Cerebral Blood Flow

In Vienna, we enrolled patients implanted with one continuous-flow device in a pilot study in which repeated ocular examination was performed to further investigate possible alterations in ocular microcirculation. Since this test is considered specific as a "window to the brain," it sheds light on general cerebral perfusion. The circulation in arterioles and capillaries was noninvasively assessed in the chorioidea by laser Doppler and interferometric fundus pulsation diagnostics. These investigations were performed during VAD support at various speeds

of support and later repeated 2 years after cardiac transplant. Careful analysis of the data revealed that fundus pulse amplitude strongly correlated with the percentage of support and therefore pulsatility, whereas blood flow in the choroidal microvasculature did not show any relevant changes.[37] After transplant, fundus pulse amplitude and choroidal blood flow only changed by 3.2% and 3.6%, respectively.

Effects on Neurocognitive Function

Previous studies in patients who underwent open-heart surgery with cardiopulmonary bypass have shown that postoperative neurocognitive function, evaluated with the P300 test, can be significantly impaired. To evaluate the effect of long-term continuous-blood flow on neurocognitive capabilities, Zimpfer et al compared P300 auditory–evoked potentials from patients supported by pulsatile VADs (Novacor LVAS and Thoratec pVAD) with data generated from patients bridged with the MicroMed DeBakey VAD before operation, at intensive care unit (ICU) discharge, and at 8 and 12 weeks follow-ups.[38] Careful evaluation of these data revealed that implanting a cardiac assist improves neurocognitive function irrespective of device type (Fig. 18–2, pulsatile vs continuous flow).

Effects on Neuroendocrine Function

In 2000, a manuscript was published by Nishinaka et al describing the influence of pulsatile and nonpulsatile left heart bypass

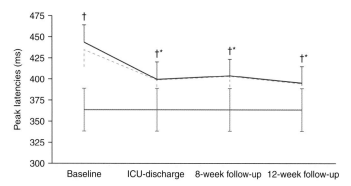

FIGURE 18–2. Neurocognitive function as measured by P300-evoked potentials. The black line represents patients with continuous-flow VADs, while the dotted line represents patients with pulsatile VADs. The gray line represents controls ($P < .05$). (Reproduced with permission from Zimpfer D, Wieselthaler G, Czerny M, et al. Neurocognitive function in patients with ventricular assist devices: a comparison of pulsatile and continuous blood flow devices. *ASAIO J.* 2006;52(1). Copyright © Wolters Kluwer Health.)

on the hormonal circadian rhythm in goats.[39] Although a change from pulsatile to nonpulsatile flow did not alter melatonin concentrations, measurements of cortisol and renin activity demonstrated more variability: both cortisol and renin followed a circadian rhythm, but the acrophase revealed abnormal variations. Additional stress on the animals during bypass or a masking effect caused by altered hemodynamic conditions could possibly explain these observations.

In our institution, Wieselthaler et al investigated the effect of long-term continuous assist on the neuroendocrine axis in patients supported with the MicroMed DeBakey VAD.[40] Six to 8 weeks after VAD implantation, total anterior pituitary function was screened by defining basal hormone concentrations followed by evaluation of the response to a bolus of hypothalamic releasing hormones (corticotropin-releasing hormone [CRH], thyrotropin-releasing hormone [TRH], growth hormone–releasing hormone [GHRH], luteinizing hormone–releasing hormone [LHRH]). Blood samples were then drawn at multiple time points. An adequate, prompt increase in serum concentrations of ACTH, TSH, GH, FSH, and LH was noted, suggesting a normal response to this stimulus. In addition, the cortisol response to ACTH release and basal concentrations of thyroid hormones, testosterone, aldosterone, and catecholamines in plasma and urine as well as renin activity were not different compared to healthy, sex- and age-matched individuals, demonstrating a normal physiologic regulation of the neuroendocrine axis.

Effects on Regional Organ Perfusion and End-Organ Function

In 1982, Losert et al from the Ludwig Boltzmann Institute for Cardiac Research in Vienna investigated the regional myocardial blood flow during nonpulsatile left ventricular bypass in calves.[21] Using radioactively labeled microspheres, they could provide evidence that the resistance in cardiac microcirculation was increased while myocardial oxygen consumption was

significantly reduced during total left ventricular unloading. Later, scientists further examined organ perfusion and microcirculation during continuous-flow circulatory support and did not experience adverse effects in histologic studies performed in hearts and kidneys after long-term support.[41] Others focused on hematologic effects, hemolysis, and biochemical aspects of hepatic and renal function after long-term support,[42] which remained within normal ranges.

However, other groups have identified negative effects on the microcirculation of splanchnic organs, such as the stomach, kidneys, and liver, after periods of nonpulsatile support following experimental acute myocardial infarction.[43-45] Structural pathologic changes have been noted in the kidneys and liver under these conditions, combined with alterations in regional organ perfusion. These data suggest an improved response to pulsatile blood flow during recovery of splanchnic organs after cardiogenic shock. One key difference between these studies and other similar studies was that these data were derived from animals in cardiogenic shock that subsequently developed impaired organ function.

In contrast to these findings, a clinical study published in 2003 by Letsou et al investigated renal and hepatic function in 10 patients who received the Jarvik-2000 continuous axial-flow VAD as a bridge-to-cardiac transplantation.[46] Pump support was maintained for up to 6 months and blood parameters were monitored at least weekly. At the time of heart transplant, all renal and hepatic parameters were within the normal physiologic range. In addition to these findings, other laboratory values such as hematologic variables, coagulation parameters, and electrolytes were seen to normalize during VAD support. Other parameters related to pulmonary and neurologic function also normalized on device support when measured at the time of heart transplant. In the HeartMate II experience, and even larger group of patients were followed to monitor changes in renal and hepatic function under VAD support. In this group of 309 patients, mean blood urea nitrogen and serum creatinine decreased significantly 37 ± 14 to 23 ± 10 mg/dL ($P < .0001$) and from 1.8 ± 0.4 to 1.4 ± 0.8 mg/dL ($P < .01$), respectively among patients with impaired baseline function.[47] Meanwhile, aspartate transaminase and alanine transaminase dropped from 121 ± 206 and 171 ± 348 to 36 ± 19 and 31 ± 22 IU ($P < .001$), respectively while total bilirubin decreased from 2.1 ± 0.9 mg/dL at baseline to 0.9 ± 0.5 mg/dL by 6 months ($P < .0001$) among patients with impaired hepatic function (Fig. 18–3).[47] Patients with normal preop renal and liver values remained normal during support in this study. These studies provides clear evidence that an implantable continuous-flow device can improve or maintain good renal and hepatic function despite reduced pulsatility and correspond well with clinical data derived from patients on continuous-flow support in Vienna.

Effects on Pulmonary Arterial Pressure and Pulmonary Vascular Resistance

Many end-stage heart failure patients waiting for cardiac transplant suffer from concomitant secondary fixed pulmonary hypertension due to chronic elevation of the left atrial

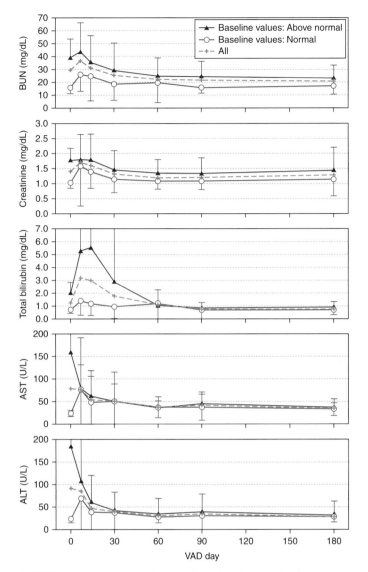

FIGURE 18–3. Improvement/preservation of end-organ function is seen after supporting the circulation with continuous flow (in this case due to HeartMate II implantation). (Reproduced with permission from Russell et al.[47] Copyright © Wolters Kluwer Health.)

pressure. Over time, this elevation of pulmonary artery pressures becomes medically unresponsive and represents a contraindication for orthotopic heart transplantation. However, continuous unloading of the failing left ventricle has been shown to reduce the amount of fixed pulmonary hypertension and elevated pulmonary vascular resistance (PVR) in these individuals.[48] Wieselthaler and coworkers demonstrated that preoperative elevation in PVR up to 10 Wood Units starts to decline after 3 to 4 days postoperatively and further decreases to normal values below 2.5 Wood Units in all patients within 6 weeks. This reduction in PVR was shown to be stable during the time of device support as well as after cardiac transplant. These data suggest that continuous nonpulsatile blood flow is therapeutically effective in unloading the pulmonary circulation

and allows patients with otherwise increased risk for orthotopic heart transplantation to be considered for a two-staged therapy.

Immunologic Response and Development of Panel Reactive Antibodies

Antibodies to major histocompatibility (HLA) class I or II antigens are developed in approximately 60% of patients following implantation of a pulsatile LVAD.[49-51] In the 1990s, it was shown by two different groups that patients with elevated panel reactive antibody (PRA) levels less than 20% demonstrate a significantly higher incidence of allograft rejection, and survival is adversely affected.[52,53] No standardized therapy for elimination of those antibodies has been clinically proven. In a recent review of the International Society for Heart and Lung Transplant (ISHLT) registry, LVAD support was found to increase the rate of humoral sensitization with no significant difference among different pulsatile device types. However, the rate of rejection and mortality among patients in the registry did not show a clinically significant difference between patients who were supported on a device and those who were not.[54] We evaluated the incidence of antibody development to HLA class I or II antigens by PRA screening following implantation of the MicroMed DeBakey VAD to investigate the possible relationship between axial-flow support and subsequent posttransplantation rejection and mortality. The incidence of development of HLA class I or II antibodies (PRA) in these patients remained extremely low and was significantly lower than previously reported with other VADs. In addition to these findings, the incidence of allograft rejection was quite low after successful cardiac transplant.[55]

SUMMARY

Since the first implantation of a MicroMed DeBakey VAD axial-flow pump in 1998, continuous flow has become the standard of therapy among patients on mechanical circulatory support. Although experimental animal data on the impact of continuous flow began to emerge in the 1950s, inconsistent results raised questions about the compatibility of continuous flow with normal organ function. Recent clinical studies have proven that even long-term support with continuous-flow blood pumps is well tolerated by the human body. Not only is there no significant difference in laboratory tests derived from various organs when compared to data from normal individuals, but a physiologic hormonal response can be observed as well as normal cerebral function, mental status, and behavior in continuous-flow VAD recipients.

Continuous-flow pumps have demonstrated excellent clinical outcomes during long-term or even permanent support despite the differences in blood distribution compared to normal physiology. Recent clinical data suggest that pulseless blood flow is well tolerated, but these results are derived from early studies and a limited number of patients. Animal studies have been plagued by both design flaws and the limited applicability to the clinical realm. As surgical therapy of chronic heart failure with small, implantable, continuous-flow blood pumps gains more experience, the impact of nonpulsatile blood flow on the human physiology will become more clearly elucidated. However, recent clinical trials have shown that these assist devices are well tolerated and have an excellent potential to recover patients from this multiorgan disease combined with good quality of life. Future examinations will provide more insight about optimization of rotary blood pumps to further enhance compatibility with human physiology.

REFERENCES

1. Gibbon J. Application of a mechanical heart and lung apparatus to cardiac surgery. *Minn Med.* 1954:171-180.
2. DeBakey M. A simple continuous flow blood transfusion instrument. *New Orleans M&S J.* 1934;87:386.
3. Weslowski S. The role of the pulse in maintenance of the systemic circulation during heart-lung bypass. *Trans Am Soc Artif Intern Organs.* 1956;1:84-86.
4. Akutsu T, Kolff W. Permanent substitutes for valves and hearts. *Trans Am Soc Artif Intern Organs.* 1958;4:230-235.
5. Weslowski S, Fisher J, Welch C. Perfusion of the pulmonary circulation by non-pulsatile flow. *Surgery.* 1953;33:370.
6. Saxton GA, Jr, Andrews CB. An ideal heart pump with hydrodynamic characteristics analogous to the mammalian heart. *Trans Am Soc Artif Intern Organs.* 1960;6:288-291.
7. Johnston GG, Hammill F, Marzec U, et al. Prolonged pulseless perfusion in unanesthetized calves. *Arch Surg.* 1976;111:1225-1230.
8. Johnston GG, Hammill FS, Johansen KH, et al. Prolonged pulsatile and nonpulsatile LV bypass with a centrifugal pump. *Trans Am Soc Artif Intern Organs.* 1976;22:323-231.
9. Murakami T, Golding L, Jacobs G, et al. Nonpulsatile biventricular bypass using centrifugal blood pumps. *Jap Soc Artif Organs.* 1979;8:636-639.
10. Golding LR, Jacobs G, Murakami T, et al. Chronic nonpulsatile blood flow in an alive, awake animal 34-day survival. *Trans Am Soc Artif Intern Organs.* 1980;26:251-255.
11. Dorman F, Bernstein EF, Blackshear PL, Sovilj R, Scott DR. Progress in the design of a centrifugal cardiac assist pump with trans-cutaneous energy transmission by magnetic coupling. *Trans Am Soc Artif Intern Organs.* 1969;15:441-448.
12. Tsutsui T, Nose Y. Arterial pressure pulsation during nonpulsatile biventricular bypass experiments: possible idioperipheral pulsation. *Artif Organs.* 1986;10:153-155.
13. DeVries WC, Joyce LD. The artificial heart. *Clin Symp.* 1983;35:1-32.
14. Valdes F, Takatani S, Jacobs GB, et al. Comparison of hemodynamic changes in a chronic nonpulsatile biventricular bypass (BVB) and total artificial heart (TAH). *Trans Am Soc Artif Intern Organs.* 1980;26:455-460.
15. Taenaka Y, Tatsumi E, Nakamura H, et al. Physiologic reactions of awake animals to an immediate switch from a pulsatile to nonpulsatile systemic circulation. *ASAIO Trans.* 1990;36:M541-M544.
16. Thoma H, Schima H. Proceedings of the International Workshop 1988 on Rotary Blood Pumps. In: Thoma H, Schima H, eds. *International Workshop on Rotary Blood Pumps.* Vienna: Austria, ISBN 3-900928-00-2 1988; 1988.
17. Schima H, Wieselthaler G, Thoma H, Wolner E. Proceedings of the International Workshop 1991 on Rotary Blood Pumps. In: Schima H, Wieselthaler G, Thoma H, Wolner E, eds. Vienna-Austria, ISBN 3-900928-00-2, 1991; 1991.
18. Losert U, Glogar D, Mayr H, et al. Regional myocardial blood flow during nonpulsatile left ventricular bypass in calves. *Trans Am Soc Artif Intern Organs.* 1982;28:86-92.
19. Tsutsui T, Sutton C, Harasaki H, Jacobs G, Golding L, Nose Y. Idioperipheral pulsation during nonpulsatile biventricular bypass experiments. *ASAIO Trans.* 1986;32:263-268.
20. Nose Y. Is it possible to have pulse during nonpulsatile perfusion with a continuous flow pump? Idioperipheral pulsation? *Artif Organs.* 1994;18:187.
21. Fukamachi K, Tominaga R, Harasaki H, Smith WA, Golding LA. Effect of respiration on the arterial pressure wave in calves with nonpulsatile biventricular bypass. *ASAIO J.* 1994;40:981-985.
22. Wieselthaler GM, Schima H, Lassnigg AM, et al. Lessons learned from the first clinical implants of the DeBakey ventricular assist device axial pump: a single center report. *Ann Thorac Surg.* 2001;71:S139-43; discussion S144-S146.
23. Potapov EV, Loebe M, Nasseri BA, et al. Pulsatile flow in patients with a novel nonpulsatile implantable ventricular assist device. *Circulation.* 2000;102:III183-III187.
24. Schima H, Boehm H, Huber L, et al. Automatic system for noninvasive blood pressure determination in rotary pump recipients. *Artif Organs.* 2004;28:451-457.
25. Wieselthaler G, Schima H, Deckert Z, Röthy W, Wolner E. Excessive unloading of the left ventricle can severely impair right ventricular function. In: *10th Congress of the Int Soc Rot Blood Pumps: A1, 2002*; 2002.
26. Vollkron M, Schima H, Huber L, Benkowski R, Morello G, Wieselthaler G. Development of a suction detection system for axial blood pumps. *Artif Organs.* 2004;28:709-716.
27. Tominaga R, Smith WA, Massiello A, Harasaki H, Golding LA. Chronic nonpulsatile blood flow. I. Cerebral autoregulation in chronic nonpulsatile biventricular bypass: carotid blood flow response to hypercapnia. *J Thorac Cardiovasc Surg.* 1994;108:907-912.
28. Kashiwazaki S. Effects of artificial circulation by pulsatile and non-pulsatile flow on brain tissues. *Ann Thorac Cardiovasc Surg.* 2000;6:389-396.
29. Murkin JM, Farrar JK, Tweed WA, McKenzie FN, Guiraudon G. Cerebral autoregulation and flow/metabolism coupling during cardiopulmonary bypass: the influence of PaCO2. *Anesth Analg.* 1987;66:825-832.
30. Hindman B. Cerebral physiology during cardiopulmonary bypass: pulsatile versus nonpulsatile flow. *Adv Pharmacol.* 1994;31:607-616.
31. Onoe M, Mori A, Watarida S, et al. The effect of pulsatile perfusion on cerebral blood flow during profound hypothermia with total circulatory arrest. *J Thorac Cardiovasc Surg.* 1994;108:119-125.
32. Geha AS, Salaymeh MT, Abe T, Baue AE. Effect of pulsatile cardiopulmonary bypass on cerebral metabolism. *J Surg Res.* 1972;12:381-387.
33. Watanabe T, Orita H, Kobayashi M, Washio M. Brain tissue pH, oxygen tension, and carbon dioxide tension in profoundly hypothermic cardiopulmonary bypass. Comparative study of circulatory arrest, nonpulsatile low-flow perfusion, and pulsatile low-flow perfusion. *J Thorac Cardiovasc Surg.* 1989;97:396-401.
34. Henze T, Stephan H, Sonntag H. Cerebral dysfunction following extracorporeal circulation for aortocoronary bypass surgery: no differences in neuropsychological outcome after pulsatile versus nonpulsatile flow. *Thorac Cardiovasc Surg.* 1990;38:65-68.
35. Anstadt MP, Tedder M, Hegde SS, et al. Pulsatile versus nonpulsatile reperfusion improves cerebral blood flow after cardiac arrest. *Ann Thorac Surg.* 1993;56:453-461.
36. Nishinaka T, Tatsumi E, Nishimura T, et al. Effects of reduced pulse pressure to the cerebral metabolism during prolonged nonpulsatile left heart bypass. *Artif Organs.* 2000;24:676-679.
37. Schmetterer L, Polska E, Wieselthaler G, Schima H. Ocular microcirculation in patients with rotary cardiac assist devices [Abstract, 2001]. *Int J Artif Organs.* 2001;24:545.
38. Zimpfer D, Wieselthaler G, Czerny M, et al. Neurocognitive function in patients with ventricular assist devices a comparison of pulsatile and continuous blood flow devices. *ASAIO J.* 2006 Jan-Feb;52(1):24-7.
39. Nishinaka T, Tatsumi E, Taenaka Y, Takano H, Koyanagi H. Influence of pulsatile and nonpulsatile left heart bypass on the hormonal circadian rhythm. *ASAIO J.* 2000;46:582-586.
40. Wieselthaler G, Riedl M, Schima H, et al. Endocrine function is not impaired in patients with a continuous MicroMed-DeBakey axial flow pump. *J Thorac Cardiovasc Surg.* 2004;133(1):2-6.
41. Parnis SM, Macris MP, Jarvik R, et al. Five month survival in a calf supported with an intraventricular axial flow blood pump. *ASAIO J.* 1995;41:M333-M336.
42. Saito S, Westaby S, Piggott D, et al. Reliable long-term non-pulsatile circulatory support without anticoagulation. *Eur J Cardiothorac Surg.* 2001;19:678-683.
43. Sezai A, Shiono M, Orime Y, et al. Comparison studies of major organ microcirculations under pulsatile- and nonpulsatile-assisted circulations. *Artif Organs.* 1996;20:139-142.
44. Orime Y, Shiono M, Nakata K, et al. The role of pulsatility in end-organ microcirculation after cardiogenic shock. *ASAIO J.* 1996;42:M724-M729.
45. Nakata K, Shiono M, Orime Y, et al. Effect of pulsatile and nonpulsatile assist on heart and kidney microcirculation with cardiogenic shock. *Artif Organs.* 1996;20:681-684.
46. Letsou GV, Myers TJ, Gregoric ID, et al. Continuous axial-flow left ventricular assist device (Jarvik 2000) maintains kidney and liver perfusion for up to 6 months. *Ann Thorac Surg.* 2003;76:1167-1170.

47. Russell SD, Rogers JG, Milano CA, et al. Renal and hepatic function improve in advanced heart failure patients during continuous-flow support with the HeartMate II left ventricular assist device. *Circulation.* 2009;120(23):2352-2357.

48. Wieselthaler G, Schima H, Czerny M, et al. Decrease of medically unresponsive elevated pulmonary vascular resistance with LVAD [Abstract, 2001]. *Artif Organs.* 2001;25:813.

49. Itescu S, Tung TC, Burke EM, et al. Preformed IgG antibodies against major histocompatibility complex class II antigens are major risk factors for high-grade cellular rejection in recipients of heart transplantation. *Circulation.* 1998;98:786-793.

50. Moazami N, Itescu S, Williams MR, Argenziano M, Weinberg A, Oz MC. Platelet transfusions are associated with the development of anti-major histocompatibility complex class I antibodies in patients with left ventricular assist support. *J Heart Lung Transplant.* 1998;17:876-880.

51. Massad MG, Cook DJ, Schmitt SK, et al. Factors influencing HLA sensitization in implantable LVAD recipients. *Ann Thorac Surg.* 1997;64:1120-1125.

52. Lavee J, Kormos RL, Duquesnoy RJ, et al. Influence of panel-reactive antibody and lymphocytotoxic crossmatch on survival after heart transplantation. *J Heart Lung Transplant.* 1991;10:921-929; discussion 929-930.

53. Kobashigawa JA, Sabad A, Drinkwater D, et al. Pretransplant panel reactive-antibody screens. Are they truly a marker for poor outcome after cardiac transplantation? *Circulation.* 1996;94:II294-II297.

54. Joyce DL, Southard RE, Torre-Amione G, Noon GP, Land GA, Loebe M. Impact of left ventricular assist device (LVAD)-mediated humoral sensitization on post-transplant outcomes. *J Heart Lung Transplant.* 2005;24(12):2054-2059.

55. Roethy W, Oezpeker C, Schima H, Grimm M, Wolner E. Development of panel reactive antibodies following continuous flow MicroMed-DeBakey VAD implantation and subsequent effects on allograft rejection [Abstract]. *J Heart Lung Transplant.* 2004;23:S109.

CHAPTER 19

CEREBRAL BLOOD FLOW IN LEFT VENTRICULAR ASSIST DEVICE SUPPORT

Evgenij V. Potapov and Roland Hetzer

BACKGROUND

Debate concerning the effect of short-term nonpulsatile flow on organ function is extensive and has been under way since cardiopulmonary bypass (CPB) became routine.[1-5] However, the pathophysiology of long-term nonpulsatile flow is poorly understood. The benefit of pulsatile perfusion for the peripheral organs is probably mediated by its effect on systemic vascular resistance and on the microcirculation[6] as a result of less damage to the endothelium[7] and normalization of NO release.[8] Pulsatile flow improves splanchnic perfusion[9] and plays a fundamental role in the movement of lymph into and out of the intestine, thereby preventing edema and maintaining capillary patency by preventing sludging. The brain microcirculation and liquor movements are reported to be improved by pulsatility.[10] Pulsation also improves aerobic tissue metabolism.[4] The influence of nonpulsatile flow on the renin-angiotensin system and catecholamine release remains controversial.[5,11]

Compared to the pulsatile left ventricular assist devices (LVADs) which dominated early experience with mechanical circulatory support, continuous-flow ventricular assist devices (VADs) have the advantages of small size, low energy consumption, easier implantation, and the absence of valves.[12] These advantages have resulted in pulsatile VADs being largely replaced by miniaturized continuous-flow pumps for long-term support.[13-16] The continuous-flow VAD produces a nonpulsatile blood flow during the first weeks after implantation; after some time the blood flow becomes pulsatile.[17] However, the nonpulsatile blood flow during the early postoperative period may have some disadvantages.[3,5,6,8,18] Impairment of the microcirculation and of cerebrospinal fluid movement in the brain has been reported.[10,19]

The impact on cerebral blood flow after implantation of a continuous-flow LVAD may be investigated in various ways. The most direct way is to compare pre- and postoperative cerebral function. However, the valid and reliable evaluation of preoperative cerebral function in critically ill patients requiring LVAD implantation and assessment of these patients during prolonged recovery periods with a complex battery of psychological tests are difficult.[20,21]

An indirect strategy involves comparing pre- and postoperative cerebral blood flow using transcranial Doppler (TCD) sonography. This method allows quantitative analysis of the cerebral blood flow, but its correlation with cerebral function is not well-established. A third possibility is to measure serum protein S-100B (S100B) and neuron-specific enolase (NSE) as markers of brain damage and therefore indirect markers of the impact of continuous blood flow on brain function.

Our experience in monitoring changes in cerebral perfusion due to continuous flow is based on early data collected from the DeBakey VAD™ (MicroMed Technology, MicroMed Inc, Houston, TX). Data presented in this discussion are from implants in 39 patients with end-stage heart failure at the Deutsches Herzzentrum Berlin. The mean age of the patients (34 men and 5 women) was 55.4 years. The mean time on the system was over 3 months, with the longest period being 1.5 years. In 20 patients who had had previous heart surgery, a lateral thoracotomy approach was used and the device was connected to the descending aorta.[22]

ANESTHESIA AND CARDIOPULMONARY BYPASS

Anesthesia was performed using propofol and sufentanil, and patients were paralyzed with pancuronium. Mannitol (100 mL of 20% solution) was given during the first hour of operation. Standard, nonpulsatile cardiopulmonary bypass (CPB) with uncoated lines, roller pumps, and membrane oxygenator (Medtronic, Parker, CO) and a 40-μm arterial filter (Pall, Dreieich, Germany) was used in all patients. The CPB was primed with 1.6 L of crystalloid solution and then prefiltered using a 0.2-μm filter (Pall, Dreieich, Germany) for 10 minutes with a flow of 4 L/min. Perfusion was performed in mild hypothermia with a body temperature of 32°C and a systemic flow rate of 2.8 to 3 L × min^{-1} × m^{-2} employing an α-stat acid-base management. Preoperative anticoagulation was performed with unfractionated heparin to an activated thromboplastin time of 40 to 60 seconds. The anticoagulation during CPB was accomplished with unfractionated heparin according to the Hepcon HMS regimen (Medtronic, Parker, CO). In all patients during CPB, aprotinin was given as an IV bolus of 2 ×10^6 kIU, 2 ×10^6 kIU in the priming solution, and 0.5 × 10^6 kIU × h^{-1} as a continuous infusion during and for 4 to 6 hours after CPB. In all patients cardiotomy suction was used during CPB. Before and after CPB the cell-saving device CATS® (Fresenius GmbH, Bad Homburg, Germany), which allows continuous washing and retransfusion of the suctioned blood, was used to minimize blood transfusion. Postoperative anticoagulation was performed according to the protocol established in our institution.[23] In patients with heparin-induced thrombocytopenia, type II heparin and tirofiban were used during CPB followed by r-hirudin infusion for 4 to 6 hours after CPB.[24]

CEREBRAL BLOOD FLOW

To study the effects of the long-term continuous flow produced by the MicroMed DeBakey VAD on the blood flow in the cerebral vessels, we performed TCD sonographic measurements of flow parameters in the middle cerebral arteries (MCAs) in patients after implantation of the VAD.[17] Both MCAs were isolated through the temporal window. We used a low gain for spectra display and a low acoustic intensity (33 mW/cm²). The 5-mm pulsed wave sample volume was placed on the first segment of the vessel, ranging from 47 to 63 mm deep (deeper volume). A 64-point fast Fourier transform with length of 2 milliseconds and an overlap of 60% was set. These parameters were kept constant throughout the study. A total of 60 studies were performed in four mobilized patients for up to 12 weeks after device implantation. In each session blood velocity (V) was measured and the Gosling pulsation index ($[V_{max} - V_{min}]/V_{mean}$, PI) was calculated for both MCAs. The study showed that the PI in both MCAs continually increased in all patients after VAD implantation (median 0.21 vs 0.37; $P = .022$). The course of mean PI after implantation is shown in Fig. 19–1. No correlation was found between PI and the mean arterial blood pressure in any patient. The V_{mean} slightly decreased in all patients after 6 weeks of support (median 0.71 vs 0.48 m/s, $P = .07$). During long-term support the continuous-flow DeBakey VAD produces, after a short period of nonpulsatility, increased pulsatility due to pulsatile preload of the pump. This is produced by contractions of the unloaded and, with time, partially recovered left ventricle. In some patients opening of the aortic valve was seen and caused some degree of pulsatility. The typical TCD signal immediately after implantation is shown in Fig. 19–2. We found that the flow pulsatility in the peripheral vessels continually increased after VAD implantation in all patients (Fig. 19–3) while simultaneous echocardiography during some TCD studies demonstrated that the aortic valve did not move. The pulsatility of blood flow continually increased in patients due to improving left ventricular function and was seen in the PI as values of between 0.3 and 0.5 after some weeks of support and in some patients at times up to 0.6 to 0.7. An almost normal relationship between systolic and diastolic blood flow acceleration was seen in some patients as soon as 4 weeks after the commencement of support.

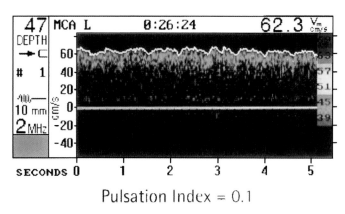

Pulsation Index = 0.1

FIGURE 19–2. Transcranial Doppler signal from the middle coronary artery on the second postoperative day. (Reprinted with permission from Potapov et al.[17])

The question then arises as to what can be the origin of this pulsation. The continuous-flow VADs are pressure-dependent. This means that the output of the pump is dependent on the pressure difference (Δp) between the inflow (p_{in}) and outflow cannulas (p_{out}) during the cardiac cycle. The constant Δp during the cardiac cycle leads to nonpulsatile flow through the pump. After unloading by the MicroMed DeBakey VAD and recovery to some extent of the left ventricle (not lasting recovery but an increase in contractility of the unloaded ventricle), the contractions of the left ventricle cause pressure changes at the inflow cannula (ie, different Δp between the inlet and the outlet of the pump during one cardiac cycle) and the flow becomes pulsatile with high flow during the systole and low flow during the diastole. The pulsatility is independent of the afterload of the pump.

A brief example of the development of pulsatility: immediately after implantation of a continuous-flow VAD the end-diastolic and end-systolic pressures in the badly damaged and poorly contracting left ventricle are nearly identical, for example 10 mm Hg.

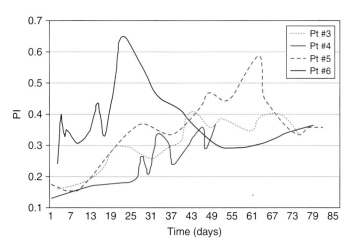

FIGURE 19–1. The course of the pulsation indices after DeBakey VAD implantation. (Reprinted with permission from Potapov et al.[17])

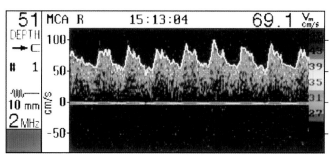

Pulsation Index = 0.63

FIGURE 19–3. Transcranial Doppler signal from the left middle coronary artery in patient no. 5 after 4 weeks of support with a nearly normal relationship between systolic and diastolic blood acceleration. (Reprinted with permission from Potapov et al.[17])

Given that the mean arterial pressure (MAP) is 70 mm Hg, the Δp between the pump's inlet and outlet is 60 mm Hg during a whole cardiac cycle and the pump flow and subsequent blood pressure are nonpulsatile. After a period of unloading (in some patients this takes some weeks) the almost empty left ventricle begins to contract. With constant rpm (revolutions per minute) the end-diastolic pressure in the left ventricle remains 10 mm Hg ($\Delta p = 60$ mm Hg), but the end-systolic pressure in the recovered and now contracting left ventricle rises to up to 40 mm Hg. This pressure is not sufficient to open the aortic valve (MAP 70 mm Hg), but the Δp at the end of the systole is $70 - 40 = 30$ mm Hg. Because the VAD is a pressure-dependent pump and the rpm remain unchanged, the pump delivers more blood at the end of the systole due to lower Δp and the flow becomes pulsatile. This hypothesis has been proven in a mock circulation with a pneumatically driven pulsatile pump and with pulsatile and nonpulsatile Δp with large numbers of fluids, hydrodynamic conditions, and pumping parameters.[25] In vitro, on the basis of the flow characteristic chart ($F = f(\Delta p)$, rpm) with given rpm, p_{in} and p_{out}, and their curvature, the flow pulsatility can be calculated and is comparable to that of clinical findings. The continuous-flow VAD acts as a pressure amplifier for a low ventricular pulsatile pressure. Figure 19–4 explains the pulsatility in vitro as a pressure amplification by pulsatile Δp and shows the pulsatile flow produced by the continuous-flow VAD.

During the early period after implantation, continuous-flow VADs produce a slightly pulsatile blood flow. The pulsatility rises with recovery of the left ventricle and almost reaches physiological levels in some patients. In some patients contraction of the left ventricle leads to opening of the aortic valve and blood flow through the aortic valve with pulsatility. These findings accordingly preclude the use of the term "nonpulsatile pump" in connection with the axial- and centrifugal-flow VADs. In our opinion, the term "continuous-flow pump" better reflects the flow form produced by the device.

The possibility of myocardial recovery in patients with dilated cardiomyopathy during support with a continuous-flow VAD has been proven, as we have seen this in some patients and have explanted the continuous-flow pump in more than 10 patients with sustained good cardiac function. However, the level of pulsatility is dependent on pump flow. During high pump flow, the empty left ventricle does not produce pulsatility. If the speed of the pump is further increased, the typical "suction" phenomenon with flow cessation caused by collapse of the left ventricle without flow increase occurs. In patients with some degree of myocardial recovery, lowering of the pump speed leads to increased filling of the left ventricle with an increase in contractility and consequently in pulsatility.

MICROEMBOLIC SIGNALS IN PATIENTS WITH THE MICROMED DEBAKEY VAD

The pattern of the blood flow during long-term LVAD support may also influence thromboembolic complications. The rate of such complications in the postoperative course has been reported to be as high as 19.8% in patients with pulsatile LVAD support.[26] The complication rate is predominantly device specific, related to the characteristics of the surfaces in contact with the blood and the configuration of the device.[27] The decrease in thromboembolic complications after modification of the inflow graft and valve of the Novacor® (Edwards Lifesciences, Oakland, CA) is well known. The preimplantation status of the patients[28] and the genotype[29] are also important.

The dependence of microembolism on the mode and intensity of anticoagulation has been discussed.[30,31] However, microemboli have a predictive value for stroke,[32] can provide crucial prognostic information on the individual embolic risk,[31] and may be used to evaluate the efficacy of the anticoagulation regimen. In order to determine the effect of the continuous flow and high-speed revolutions on the generation of microthrombi or bubbles from cavitation, we measured the microembolic signals (MESs) with TCD sonography in patients after implantation of the MicroMed DeBakey VAD.[33] No MES or thromboembolic events were noted in four out of seven patients. In one patient the MESs were detected both before and after VAD implantation. The preoperative incidence of MES in this patient was 0.22 per minute. The postoperative incidence in the same patient did not significantly change and was 0.2 per minute; the prevalence of MES was 50%. Two transient ischemic attacks (TIAs) were noted in this patient during the study period of 55 days. In this patient the average V_{mean} was significantly higher ($P = .00002$) for the left MCA at 0.66 ± 0.16 m/s (range 0.46-0.9 m/s) than for the right MCA at 0.33 ± 0.11 m/s (range 0.22-0.6 m/s). The average V_{mean} in other patients was similar for both sides and is given in Table 19–1.

The prevalence of MES in patients with prosthetic heart valves is high,[34,35] and in patients with the TCI HeartMate® (Thoratec Corporation, Pleasanton, CA) or the Novacor® N100 LVAD it ranges from 18% to 84%.[30,31,36,37] However, Wilhelm et al showed no significant relationship between coagulation, fibrinolysis, and cellular activation and MES in patients supported by assist systems with artificial valves.[30] These data suggest that the type of assist device and the presence of artificial valves, but not the hemostatic parameters, caused MES. The MES could be

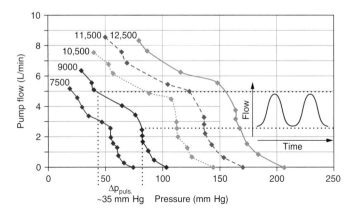

FIGURE 19–4. In vitro exemplification (mock circulation) of pressure amplification by pulsatile Δp, resulting in pulsatility of the flow produced by the MicroMed DeBakey VAD. (Reprinted with permission from Potapov et al.[25])

TABLE 19–1. Results of TCD Measurements and VAD Performance in Patients With the DeBakey VAD

Patient No	Sex	Age (y)	Diagnosis	MES preoperatively	MES postoperatively Prevalence (%)	Average V_{mean} left or right MCA (m/s)	Mean speed (1000 × rpm)	Mean pump flow (L/min)	Mean power consumption (W)	Comments
3	m	37	CMP	No	No	0.54/0.53	10.1 ± 0.6	4.0 ± 0.3	11.6 ± 1.6	SR
4	m	62	CHD	Yes	50	0.66ª/0.33	9.4 ± 0.3	3.0 ± 0.4	9.4 ± 1	AF, ICA stenosis
5	f	46	CHD	No	No	0.66/0.62	9.5 ± 0.2	4.3 ± 0.6	9.1 ± 1.1	SR
6	f	33	CMP	No	No	0.51/0.46	9.8 ± 0.2	4.6 ± 0.5	8.7 ± 0.6	SR
7	m	43	CMP	No	No	0.53/0.52	9.3 ± 0.2	5.6 ± 0.4	9.8 ± 1.2	SR

ª$P < .05$.

AF, atrial fibrillation; CHD, coronary heart disease; CMP, cardiomyopathy; ICA, internal carotid artery; MES, microembolic signal; SR, sinus rhythm.

related to the solid particles or to microbubbles appearing from the cavitation effect.[34,38-42] The identification of platelet microthrombi related to CPB in an experiment has been reported.[43] The differentiation between microbubbles and solid microemboli by using TCD in clinical practice is a matter of controversial discussion in the literature. The device and software used in the present study did not allow definitive differentiation between microbubbles and solid particles. However, they both may cause microembolization and are clinically relevant.

The impeller is the only moving element in the axial-flow VAD and produces a continuous flow. The blood flow through the impeller fluctuates but at any time during the cardiac cycle it is present, which means that the inlet pressure is positive all the time. If the inlet pressure became negative, it would lead to a cessation of blood flow. However, an increase in rpm leads to ventricular collapse and negative inlet pressure. The absence of MES in four patients without preoperatively detected MES in our study could be based on the smaller blood contact surface, the continuous flow through the inflow cannula, impeller and outflow graft, and the absence of artificial valves. These data suggest that the MicroMed DeBakey VAD does not produce microemboli or microbubbles due to the cavitation effect. However, the microbubbles may be too small to be detected with our equipment.[44] The bigger bubbles possibly produced by the impeller cannot be detected in the MCA due to the large distance between the impeller and the probes. The absence of any thromboembolic events in four patients during the study period correlates with that of MES. However, the imbalance between thrombin generation and additional platelet trauma,[23] as well as partial stimulation of the inflammatory system,[45] found in patients with the MicroMed DeBakey VAD may increase the risk of thromboembolism.

In patient no. 4 who had atrial fibrillation, carotid artery stenosis, and a history of stroke events, the MESs were detected preoperatively. The patient suffered two TIAs during the study period. The left lateral TIAs were related to thrombus formation in the right internal carotid artery (ICA) detected by Doppler sonography. The V_{mean} in the right MCA in patient no. 4 before the TIAs was approximately 50% of the V_{mean} in the left MCA because of thrombosis formation or due to stenosis of the distal part of the right ICA/MCA. After the TIAs, the V_{mean} in the right MCA rose for a short time to about 75% of the V_{mean} in the left MCA. The incidence of MES did not significantly change after VAD implantation. No changes in anticoagulation (target international normalized ratio [INR] 2.5-3.5) were introduced during the study period in this patient. The unchanged incidence of MES in patient no. 4 and the absence of MES or thromboembolic events in the other four patients suggest that the DeBakey VAD does not produce microemboli. TCD is a time-consuming procedure: The study time is as long as 1 hour or even longer in patients with a VAD. Also, performance of the procedure on a daily basis is not possible in outpatients. In our opinion, the use of TCD as a method for monitoring the anticoagulation status of these patients should be further investigated in larger studies. However, for patients with neurological events during VAD support, the method may be used additionally to control and adjust the anticoagulation.[40]

RELEASE OF PROTEIN S100B AND NSE IN PATIENTS WITH A CONTINUOUS-FLOW VAD

Injured brain cells release protein S100B into the cerebral spinal fluid, but S100B will only appear in serum if there is a concomitant increase in blood-brain barrier permeability.[46,47] Its concentration in serum has been shown to increase after stroke[48] and other cerebral lesions.[47,49] NSE occurs mainly in the nerve cells and in the neuroectodermal cells. As an enzyme from the cellular cytoplasm, NSE is set free in connection with cell destruction. Several studies have shown the utility of NSE as a specific marker for brain damage.[49-53] The serum concentrations of S100B and NSE have been used to identify cerebral injuries after cardiac surgery.[21,54-60] These studies suggested that transient elevations of S100B and NSE levels may reflect subclinical cerebral deterioration in the absence of frank neurological signs.[21,54-58,60] In order to compare the impact of the pattern of cerebral blood flow on the release of these markers, we performed a prospective study comparing serum concentrations of S100B and NSE in patients treated with the MicroMed DeBakey VAD and the pulsatile flow Novacor N100 LVAD. Additionally, patients' neurological status was examined preoperatively and on the 3rd and 14th days after LVAD implantation.[61] The study showed no correlation between age and preoperative values of S100B and NSE in either group (r = 0.12, r = 0.34, respectively). The analysis of variance with repeated measurements of S100B and NSE showed significant time effects (P = .004, P = .009, respectively) but no group effects (P = .06, P = .26) and no interaction between groups and time (P = .12, P = .48, respectively). The mean preoperative value of S100B was significantly elevated in the DeBakey VAD group (P = .03). The mean preoperative values of NSE were similar in both groups (P = .68). Four hours after the end of CPB, the mean values of S100B had significantly increased sixfold in both groups (DeBakey VAD group: P = .006; Novacor group: P = .001). The mean values of NSE were also increased twofold 4 hours after termination of CPB (DeBakey VAD group: P = .01; Novacor group P = .019). The elevation of S100B was significantly higher in the DeBakey VAD group (P = .031). No difference was found in NSE values 4 hours after terminating CPB between the groups (P = .9). The values returned to preoperative levels in the DeBakey VAD group on day 1 after implantation (S100B: P = .069, NSE: P = .093) and in the Novacor group S100B on day 3 (P = .05) and NSE on day 1 (P = .46). Postoperative mean values of S100B and NSE were significantly elevated in the DeBakey VAD group compared with those of the Novacor group only on the third postoperative day (POD) (P = .005, P = .023, respectively). The release patterns of S100B and NSE in both groups are shown in Figs. 19–5 and 19–6, respectively. There were no differences between

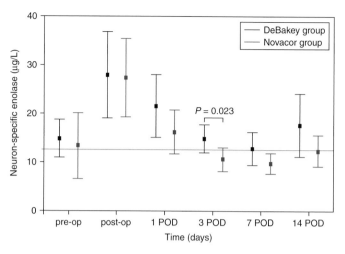

FIGURE 19–6. Time courses of mean neuron-specific enolase (NSE) values in the groups. The vertical bars show 95% confidence intervals and the horizontal line the upper reference limit for the test. POD, postoperative day. (Reprinted by permission from Potapov et al.[61] Copyright © Elsevier.)

groups regarding pre- and postoperative platelet counts. Four patients in the DeBakey VAD group required intraoperative transfusion of platelet concentrates (mean 1.3 ± 1.6 concentrates per patient), while no patients in the Novacor group required transfusions of platelet concentrates. In the postoperative period no platelet concentrates were transfused in either group.

The neurological examinations, which were performed on the 3rd and 14th POD, revealed no neurological deficits in patients in the DeBakey VAD group, while two patients in the Novacor group presented neurological deficits: one patient had late awakening, attaining conscious awareness on the 5th POD; during this period no focal neurological deficits occurred. The preoperative S100B value (0.054 μg/L) was normal and the NSE value slightly elevated (14.46 μg/L). The postoperative values of both markers were within standard deviations of mean values in the Novacor group. Another Novacor patient suffered a cerebral infarction on the 13th POD followed by global aphasia. This patient showed abnormal elevation of both S100B and NSE values on the 14th POD compared with the 7th POD (0.373 vs 0.088 μg/L and 17.2 vs 9.6 μg/L, respectively). This study showed no impact of the continuous-flow DeBakey VAD on serum concentrations of S100B and NSE in the early postoperative period. During the first 2 weeks no significant pulsatility of the blood flow occurred in the DeBakey VAD group. This was confirmed by examining signals from the invasive arterial pressure measurements and TCD studies. The aortic valve remained closed during the study period.[17] However, later on the pulsatility significantly increased due to recovery of the unloaded left ventricle. Elevated NSE values before LVAD implantation were observed in both groups. The significantly higher preoperative S100B serum level in the DeBakey VAD group in the absence of frank neurological deficits and the significantly higher level immediately postoperatively may be explained by the significantly higher preoperative serum creatinine in the DeBakey

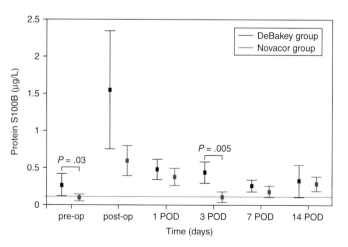

FIGURE 19–5. Time courses of mean S100B values in the groups. The vertical bars show 95% confidence intervals and the horizontal line the upper reference limit for the test. POD, postoperative day. (Reprinted with permission from Potapov et al.[61] Copyright © Elsevier.)

VAD group and by two critically ill patients with preoperative low cardiac output who were dependent on a ventilator and intra-aortic balloon pump. The preoperative low cardiac output in patients with end-stage heart failure may lead to impairment of brain perfusion and to brain injury with subsequent elevation of S100B and NSE concentrations in serum. Improvement of the hemodynamic situation after LVAD implantation should lead to an improvement of brain perfusion and a subsequent decrease in concentrations of both markers. However, prospective neuropsychological evaluation may reveal some impairment of brain function in patients with progressed heart failure.[55] The preoperative elevated NSE values decrease to the normal level in both groups after LVAD implantation (see Fig. 19–6). S100B values returned to the preoperative level in both groups on days 1 and 3. However, two patients with preoperative S100B values elevated above 0.5 μg/L (0.544 and 0.541 μg/L, both from the DeBakey VAD group) revealed a marked decrease on day 7 (0.217 and 0.095 μg/L, respectively). The present study allowed comparison of the impact of different types of blood flow after LVAD implantation on the release of S100B and NSE in serum, while other factors known to significantly affect the release of S100B and NSE, such as operation trauma, CPB, hemolysis, and cardiotomy suction, were similar in the two groups. However, as previously demonstrated in our patients, the DeBakey VAD influences the system of contact activation and fibrinolysis more than the Novacor LVAD and leads to platelet damage.[23] Nevertheless, no platelet concentrates were transfused postoperatively in either group. Despite the increased intraoperative use of platelet concentrates in the DeBakey VAD group, which may contribute to increased NSE serum levels,[56,62] no significant differences were found between the groups regarding the course of NSE levels. The particular influence of the inflammatory response with increased interleukin-6 and C5a levels[45] in the study patients may also increase the permeability of the blood-brain barrier without injury to the brain itself. However, none of the patients in whom the DeBakey VAD had been implanted showed neurological complications during the study period, while two patients in the Novacor group presented neurological abnormalities, in one case caused by a thromboembolism on the 13th POD. Our recently published study[33] confirmed the absence of thromboembolic events in the DeBakey VAD group by the absence of MESs related to the DeBakey VAD, as shown by the use of TCD examination of the MCA. This study suggests that the risk of thromboembolic events may be minimal when using valveless continuous-flow pumps. The release patterns of both markers found in our study were comparable to the values reported after cardiac surgery using CPB.[55,56,63-69] The significantly higher preoperative values of S100B in the DeBakey VAD group may explain the significantly higher values of S100B 4 hours after the end of CPB and on the 3rd POD in the DeBakey VAD group.[59] This may suggest that preoperative deterioration of astroglial and Schwann cells results in increased risk for intraoperative injury with subsequent release of S100B. The fact that analysis of variance showed no group effects and no interaction between groups and time for either marker of brain injury suggests that the continuous flow produced by the DeBakey VAD in the early postoperative period[17] and the influence on

hemostasis and inflammatory response systems found in the same patients[23,45] did not lead to brain injury. In conclusion, the study shows that implantation of continuous-flow LVADs does not lead to injury of the brain or the blood-brain barrier. The measurements of S100B and NSE are applicable for diagnosis of brain injury in patients after LVAD implantation. However, the preoperative and serial postoperative blood samples provide more comprehensive information.

CLINICAL FINDINGS

Our clinical experience showed no significant differences with regard to neurological or mental status of patients in the early and late postoperative period after implantation of continuous-flow VADs in comparison to pulsatile pumps. In some patients no significant myocardial recovery occurs and they remain "pulseless" for a long time. This status may excite publications in medical journals, but it is of little consequence to the patients themselves. Because of the low noise profile of continuous-flow VADs, they are able to return to normal social activities, including cinema and theater visits; some patients report sexual activity. Additionally, a significant number of patients return to their previous work. In conclusion, the continuous, "less pulsatile" blood flow in cerebral vessels does not markedly impact cerebral function.

ACKNOWLEDGMENT

The authors thank Anne Gale for editorial assistance.

REFERENCES

1. Finlayson D. Con: Nonpulsatile flow is preferable to pulsatile flow during cardiopulmonary bypass. *J Cardiothorac Anesthesia*. 1987;1(2):169-170.
2. Shevde K, DeBois WJ. Pro: pulsatile flow is preferable to nonpulsatile flow during cardiopulmonary bypass. *J Cardiothorac Anesth*. 1987;1(2):165-168.
3. Taylor K, Bain W, Davidson K, Turner M. Comparative clinical study of pulsatile and non-pulsatile perfusion in 350 consecutive patients. *Thorax*. 1982;37:324-330.
4. Mori F, Ivey T, Itoh T, Thomas R, Breazeale D, Misbach G. Effect of pulsatile reperfusion on postischemic recovery of myocardial function after global hypothermic cardiac arrest. *J Thorac Cardiovasc Surg*. 1987;93:719-727.
5. Canivet J, Larbusson R, Damas P, et al. Plasma renin activity and urine b2-microglobulin during and after cardiopulmonary bypass: pulsatile vs non-pulsatile perfusion. *Eur Heart J*. 1990;11:1079-1082.
6. Fukae K, Tominaga R, Tokunaga S, Kawachi Y, Imaizumi T, Yasui H. The effects of pulsatile and nonpulsatile systemic perfusion on renal sympathetic nerve activity in anesthetized dogs. *J Thorac Cardiovasc Surg*. 1996;111(2):478-484.
7. Waaben J, Wulf H, Wettermark G, Andersen K, Husum B. ATP-content in muscular interstitial fluid during pulsatile and non-pulsatile cardiopulmonary bypass in pigs. *Biomed Biochem Acat*. 1985;44(7/8):1113-1118.
8. Busse R, Fleming I. Pulsatile stretch and shear stress: physical stimuli determining the production of endothelium-derived relaxing factors. *J Vasc Res*. 1998;35(2):73-84.
9. Gaer J, Shaw A, Wild R, et al. Effect of cardiopulmonary bypass on gastrointestinal perfusion and function. *Ann Thorac Surg*. 1994;57:371-375.
10. Vainshtein G, Moskalenko Y. The significance of pulsation factor for functioning of the cerebral circulation system. *Fisiol Zh Im I M Sechenova*. 1995;81(6):54-58.
11. Taenaka Y, Tatsumi E, Nakamura H, et al. Physiologic reactions of awake animals to an immediate switch from a pulsatile to nonpulsatile systemic circulation. *ASAIO Trans*. 1990;36(3):M541-M544.

12. Noon G, Morley D, Irwin S, DeBakey M. The DeBakey Ventricular Assist Device. In: Goldstein D, Oz M, editors. Cardiac Assist Devices. New York: Futura Publishing Company; 2000. p. 375-386.

13. Hon JK, Yacoub MH. Bridge to recovery with the use of left ventricular assist device and clenbuterol. *Ann Thorac Surg.* 2003;75(6 Suppl):S36-S41.

14. Frazier OH, Shah NA, Myers TJ, Robertson KD, Gregoric ID, Delgado R. Use of the Flowmaker (Jarvik 2000) left ventricular assist device for destination therapy and bridging to transplantation. *Cardiology.* 2004;101(1-3): 111-116.

15. Goldstein DJ. Worldwide experience with the MicroMed DeBakey ventricular assist device as a bridge to transplantation. *Circulation.* 2003;108 Suppl 1: II272-II277.

16. Griffith BP, Kormos RL, Borovetz HS, et al. HeartMate II left ventricular assist system: from concept to first clinical use. *Ann Thorac Surg.* 2001;71 (3 Suppl):S116-S120; discussion S114-S116.

17. Potapov EV, Loebe M, Nasseri BA, et al. Pulsatile flow in patients with a novel nonpulsatile implantable ventricular assist device. *Circulation.* 2000;102(19 Suppl 3):III183-III187.

18. Toda K, Tatsumi E, Taenaka Y, Masuzawa T, Takano H. Impact of systemic depulsation on tissue perfusion and sympathetic nerve activity. *Ann Thoracic Surg.* 1996;62(6):1737-1742.

19. Tranmer B, Gross C, Kindt G, Adey G. Pulsatile versus nonpulsatile blood flow in the treatment of acute cerebral ischemia. *Neurosurgery.* 1986;19(5):724-731.

20. Balestroni G, Bosimini E, Corra U, Giannuzzi P, Zotti AM. The usefulness of the clinical interview in the psychological evaluation of the patient with heart failure. *Giornale Italiano di Cardiologia.* 1998;28(6):653-660.

21. Wimmer-Greinecker G, Matheis G, Brieden M, et al. Neuropsychological changes after cardiopulmonary bypass for coronary artery bypass grafting. *Thorac Cardiovasc Surg.* 1998;46(4):207-212.

22. Hetzer R, Potapov EV, Weng Y, et al. Implantation of MicroMed DeBakey VAD through left thoracotomy after previous median sternotomy operations. *Ann Thorac Surg.* 2004;77(1):347-350.

23. Koster A, Loebe M, Hansen R, et al. Alterations in coagulation after implantation of a pulsatile Novacor LVAD and the axial flow MicroMed DeBakey LVAD. *Ann Thorac Surg.* 2000;70(2):533-537.

24. Koster A, Kukucka M, Bach F, et al. Anticoagulation during cardiopulmonary bypass in patients with heparin-induced thrombocytopenia type II and renal impairment using heparin and the platelet glycoprotein IIb-IIIa antagonist tirofiban. *Anesthesiology.* 2001;94(2):245-251.

25. Potapov EV, Koster A, Loebe M, et al. The MicroMed DeBakey VAD—part I: the pump and the blood flow. *J Extra Corpor Technol.* 2003;35(4):274-283.

26. Mehta SM, Aufiero TX, Pae WE, Jr, Miller CA, Pierce WS. Combined Registry for the Clinical Use of Mechanical Ventricular Assist Pumps and the Total Artificial Heart in conjunction with heart transplantation: sixth official report—994. *J Heart Lung Transplant.* 1995;14(3):585-593.

27. Livingston ER, Fisher CA, Bibidakis EJ, et al. Increased activation of the coagulation and fibrinolytic systems leads to hemorrhagic complications during left ventricular assist implantation. *Circulation.* 1996;94 (9 Suppl):II227-II234.

28. Himmelreich G, Ullmann H, Riess H, et al. Pathophysiologic role of contact activation in bleeding followed by thromboembolic complications after implantation of a ventricular assist device. *ASAIO J.* 1995;41(3): M790-M794.

29. Potapov EV, Ignatenko S, Nasseri BA, et al. Clinical significance of PlA polymorphism of platelet GP IIb/IIIa receptors during long-term VAD support. *Ann Thorac Surg.* 2004;77(3):869-874; discussion 874.

30. Wilhelm CR, Ristich J, Knepper LE, et al. Measurement of hemostatic indexes in conjunction with transcranial Doppler sonography in patients with ventricular assist devices. *Stroke.* 1999;30(12):2554-2561.

31. Nabavi DG, Georgiadis D, Mumme T, et al. Clinical relevance of intracranial microembolic signals in patients with left ventricular assist devices. A prospective study. *Stroke.* 1996;27(5):891-896.

32. Siebler M, Nachtmann A, Sitzer M, et al. Cerebral microembolism and the risk of ischemia in asymptomatic high-grade internal carotid artery stenosis. *Stroke.* 1995;26(11):2184-2186.

33. Potapov EV, Nasseri BA, Loebe M, et al. Transcranial detection of microembolic signals in patients with a novel nonpulsatile implantable LVAD. *ASAIO J.* 2001;47(3):249-253.

34. Deklunder G, Roussel M, Lecroart JL, Prat A, Gautier C. Microemboli in cerebral circulation and alteration of cognitive abilities in patients with mechanical prosthetic heart valves. *Stroke.* 1998;29(9):1821-1826.

35. Dauzat M, Deklunder C, Aldis A, Rabinovitch M, Burte F, Bret P. Gas bubble emboli detected by transcranial Doppler sonography in patients with prosthetic heart valves. *J Ultrasound Med.* 1994;13:129-135.

36. Schmid C, Wilhelm M, Rothenburger M, et al. Effect of high dose platelet inhibitor treatment on thromboembolism in Novacor patients. *Eur J Cardiothorac Surg.* 2000;17(3):331-335.

37. Moazami N, Roberts K, Argenziano M, et al. Asymptomatic microembolism in patients with long-term ventricular assist support. *ASAIO J.* 1997;43(3):177-180.

38. Raco L, Belcher PR, Sim I, McGarrity A, Bernacca GM, Wheatley DJ. Platelet aggregation and high-intensity transient signals (HITS) in a sheep model of mitral valve replacement. *J Heart Valve Dis.* 1999;8(5):476-480; discussion 481.

39. Lagos R, Cabezas FM. Microemboli in cerebral circulation and alteration of cognitive abilities in patients with mechanical prosthetic heart valves. *Stroke.* 1999;30(5):1150.

40. Goertler M, Baeumer M, Kross R, et al. Rapid decline of cerebral microemboli of arterial origin after intravenous acetylsalicylic acid. *Stroke.* 1999;30:66-69.

41. Dauzat M, Deklunder C, Aldis A, Rabinovitch M, Burte F, Bret P. Gas bubble emboli detected by transcranial Doppler sonography in patients with prosthetic heart valves. *J Ultrasound Med.* 1994;13:129-135.

42. Deklunder G, Lecroart JL, Savoye C, Coquet B, Houdas Y. Transcranial high-intensity Doppler signals in patients with mechanical heart valve prostheses: their relationship with abnormal intracavitary echoes. *J Heart Valve Dis.* 1996;5(6):662-667.

43. Dewanjee MK, Zhai P, Hsu LC, Twardock AR. A new method for quantitation of platelet microthrombi and microemboli from cardiopulmonary bypass in organs using 111In labeled platelets. *ASAIO J.* 1997;43(5):M701-M705.

44. Ries F, Tiemann K, Pohl C, Bauer C, Mundo M, Becher H. High-resolution emboli detection and differentiation by characteristic postembolic spectral patterns. *Stroke.* 1998;29(3):668-672.

45. Loebe M, Koster A, Sanger S, et al. Inflammatory response after implantation of a left ventricular assist device: comparison between the axial flow MicroMed DeBakey VAD and the pulsatile Novacor device. *ASAIO J.* 2001;47(3):272-274.

46. Aberg T. Signs of brain cell injury during open heart operations: past and present. *Ann Thorac Surg.* 1995;59(5):1312-1315.

47. Persson L, Hardemark HG, Gustafsson J, et al. S-100 protein and neuron-specific enolase in cerebrospinal fluid and serum: markers of cell damage in human central nervous system. *Stroke.* 1987;18(5):911-918.

48. Fassbender K, Schmidt R, Schreiner A, et al. Leakage of brain-originated proteins in peripheral blood: temporal profile and diagnostic value in early ischemic stroke. *J Neurol Sci.* 1997;148(1):101-105.

49. Hardemark HG, Ericsson N, Kotwica Z, et al. S-100 protein and neuron-specific enolase in CSF after experimental traumatic or focal ischemic brain damage. *J Neurosurg.* 1989;71(5 Pt 1):727-731.

50. Usui A, Kato K, Murase M, et al. Neural tissue-related proteins (NSE, G0 alpha, 28-kDa calbindin-D, S100b and CK-BB) in serum and cerebrospinal fluid after cardiac arrest. *J Neurol Sci.* 1994;123(1-2):134-139.

51. Hay E, Royds JA, Davies-Jones GA, Lewtas NA, Timperley WR, Taylor CB. Cerebrospinal fluid enolase in stroke. *J Neurol Neurosurg Psychiatry.* 1984;47(7):724-729.

52. Dauberschmidt R, Zinsmeyer J, Mrochen H, Meyer M. Changes of neuron-specific enolase concentration in plasma after cardiac arrest and resuscitation. *Mol Chem Neuropathol.* 1991;14(3):237-245.

53. Schaarschmidt H, Prange HW, Reiber H. Neuron-specific enolase concentrations in blood as a prognostic parameter in cerebrovascular diseases. *Stroke.* 1994;25(3):558-565.

54. Johnsson P, Lundqvist C, Lindgren A, Ferencz I, Alling C, Stahl E. Cerebral complications after cardiac surgery assessed by S-100 and NSE levels in blood. *J Cardiothorac Vasc Anesth.* 1995;9(6):694-699.

55. Herrmann M, Ebert AD, Galazky I, Wunderlich MT, Kunz WS, Huth C. Neurobehavioral outcome prediction after cardiac surgery: role of neurobiochemical markers of damage to neuronal and glial brain tissue. *Stroke.* 2000;31(3):645-650.

56. Johnsson P, Blomquist S, Luhrs C, et al. Neuron-specific enolase increases in plasma during and immediately after extracorporeal circulation. *Ann Thorac Surg.* 2000;69(3):750-754.

57. Schmitt B, Bauersfeld U, Schmid ER, et al. Serum and CSF levels of neuron-specific enolase (NSE) in cardiac surgery with cardiopulmonary bypass: a marker of brain injury? *Brain Dev.* 1998;20(7):536-539.

58. Westaby S, Johnsson P, Parry AJ, et al. Serum S100 protein: a potential marker for cerebral events during cardiopulmonary bypass. *Ann Thorac Surg.* 1996;61(1):88-92.

59. Westaby S, Saatvedt K, White S, et al. Is there a relationship between serum S-100beta protein and neuropsychologic dysfunction after cardiopulmonary bypass? *J Thorac Cardiovasc Surg.* 2000;119(1):132-137.

60. Blomquist S, Johnsson P, Luhrs C, et al. The appearance of S-100 protein in serum during and immediately after cardiopulmonary bypass surgery: a possible marker for cerebral injury. *J Cardiothorac Vasc Anesth.* 1997;11(6):699-703.

61. Potapov EV, Loebe M, Abdul-Khaliq H, et al. Postoperative course of S-100B protein and neuron-specific enolase in patients after implantation of continuous and pulsatile flow LVADs. *J Heart Lung Transplant.* 2001;20(12):1310-1316.

62. Gao F, Harris DN, Sapsed-Byrne S, Sharp S. Neurone-specific enolase and Sangtec 100 assays during cardiac surgery: part III—Dose haemolysis affect their accuracy? *Perfusion.* 1997;12(3):171-177.

63. Kilminster S, Treasure T, McMillan T, Holt DW. Neuropsychological change and S-100 protein release in 130 unselected patients undergoing cardiac surgery. *Stroke.* 1999;30(9):1869-1874.

64. Jonsson H, Johnsson P, Alling C, Backstrom M, Bergh C, Blomquist S. S100beta after coronary artery surgery: release pattern, source of contamination, and relation to neuropsychological outcome. *Ann Thorac Surg.* 1999;68(6):2202-2208.

65. Rasmussen LS, Christiansen M, Hansen PB, Moller JT. Do blood levels of neuron-specific enolase and S-100 protein reflect cognitive dysfunction after coronary artery bypass? *Acta Anaesthesiol Scand.* 1999;43(5):495-500.

66. Isgro F, Schmidt C, Pohl P, Saggau W. A predictive parameter in patients with brain related complications after cardiac surgery? *Eur J Cardiothorac Surg.* 1997;11(4):640-644.

67. Gao F, Harris DN, Sapsed-Byrne S. Time course of neurone-specific enolase and S-100 protein release during and after coronary artery bypass grafting. *Br J Anaesth.* 1999;82(2):266-267.

68. Anderson RE, Hansson LO, Vaage J. Release of S100B during coronary artery bypass grafting is reduced by off-pump surgery. *Ann Thorac Surg.* 1999;67(6):1721-1725.

69. Anderson RE, Hansson LO, Liska J, Settergren G, Vaage J. The effect of cardiotomy suction on the brain injury marker S100beta after cardiopulmonary bypass. *Ann Thorac Surg.* 2000;69(3):847-850.

CHAPTER 20

REVERSE REMODELING OF THE MYOCARDIUM AFTER LVAD SUPPORT

Keith A. Youker

The concept of reverse remodeling of failing myocardium is not a new concept but is still poorly understood. In early device studies it was demonstrated that functional recovery could occur and in some cases to the point of device explantation.[1] With the advent of newer more dependable devices, increased experience with implantation, improved postimplant management, and increased length of support, reverse remodeling is beginning to receive more interest. Reverse remodeling and a possible bridge-to-recovery is becoming more widely accepted, but it should also be stated that not all recovery will be significantly beneficial to improve cardiac output and allow device removal. In fact, it is likely that most patients supported by LVAD will still ultimately require cardiac transplantation or permanent support.[2] Reverse remodeling, however, is still an important issue in understanding the improved physiology seen with LVAD support and also to understand the initial remodeling process and suggest alternative ways to reverse the process. Until recent studies, it was unrealized for instance that the reduction in cardiac load (LVAD implantation) could result in decreases in interstitial fibrosis which had been previously thought to be irreversible.[3] This chapter will explore some of the identified changes that occur with cardiac unloading.

NEUROHORMONAL ALTERATIONS

Activation of the sympathetic and renin-angiotensin-aldosterone systems (RAAS) has been shown to play a central role in heart failure progression, and patients with congestive heart failure (CHF) manifest increased levels of many circulating neurohormones.[4] In particular, consistently increased levels have been found in norepinephrine, natriuretic peptides (atrial natriuretic peptide [ANP] and brain natriuretic peptide [BNP]), aldosterone, plasma renin, and endothelin-1 (ET-1).[5,6] The Val-HeFT study randomized 4300 patients and measured baseline neurohormones and compared these values with outcomes which demonstrated that all of these neurohormones were found to be significant markers of outcome.[7] Of these, BNP was the most powerful indicator of poor outcome and is released by myocytes in response to excessive volumetric expansion and pressure overload and possesses compensatory diuretic, natriuretic, and vasodilatory properties.[8]

In our laboratory we looked at BNP and ET-1 levels in 19 CHF patients supported with LVAD using serial serum collections during support. The mean age was 55.2 years old and the average length of LVAD support was 54 days with all devices. Echocardiographic indices were also measured. As shown in Fig. 20–1, LVAD support significantly improved ejection fraction (EF%: 21 ± 3.8% vs 28 ± 3.57%, $P < .04$) and left ventricular end-diastolic diameter (LVEDD) (6.68 ± 0.92 cm vs 4.79 ± 1.54 cm, $P < .0001$). Both BNP and ET-1 levels decreased in these patients postoperatively while on LVAD support with BNP decreasing from a mean of 754.1 ± 261.1 to 221.1 ± 124.2 pg/mL ($P < .0001$) and ET-1 serum levels decreasing from 13.66 ± 11.98 to 3.47 ± 2.96 pg/mL ($P < .001$).

As demonstrated in this small group, decreases were seen in both measured neurohormones while increases in cardiac function occurred. Other laboratories have also demonstrated decreases in BNP and ANP mRNA (messenger RNA)[9] and immunoreactivity[10] as well as increased cardiac function parameters sufficient to allow device explantation[11] When separated by device type in our study, pulsatile devices (Novacor VAD, n = 8; TCI HeartMate, n = 3; Thoratec VAD, n = 3) showed the most significant changes in all measured parameters; however the nonpulsatile devices (MicroMed/DeBakey VAD, n = 6) showed trends in the same direction in all parameters although statistical significance was not reached. This is likely due to the low numbers and the fact that the pulsatile devices were used for a longer period of support than the axial-flow pumps (average days of support: pulsatile = 72 days, axial flow = 27 days). Others have shown that the use of an axial-flow device can reduce plasma BNP levels, New York Heart Association (NYHA) classification and increase exercise tolerance.[12]

EXTRACELLULAR MATRIX

The extracellular matrix composition including collagen content has been implicated in creating myocardial stiffness that contributes to CHF. The idea that fibrosis affects myocardial function is still controversial; however, most agree that increased fibrosis is detrimental to cardiac function. When discussing myocardial fibrosis, it must be kept in mind that there are two types of fibrosis: interstitial and replacement. Replacement fibrosis is matrix which has been deposited to replace contractile myocardial cells which have died due to infarction or apoptosis. This type of fibrosis is rarely remodeled since there are no replacement cells. The interstitial fibrosis, however, surrounds functional myocytes and has been shown to be capable of remodeling. While the quantity of the matrix can certainly impede contraction, the quality of the matrix (ie, cross-linking and protein types) is likely just as important but has received little study. Several studies have now shown decreases in the quantity of fibrosis in response to LVAD implantation although the exact mechanism is still under investigation and not all patients demonstrate significant decreases.[3,13]

Total interstitial collagen was measured in patient heart samples taken at the time of LVAD implantation and again

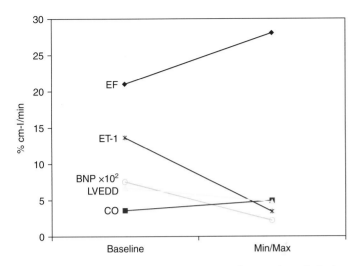

FIGURE 20–1. Baseline versus minimum or maximum values of ejection fraction (EF, %); endothelin-1 levels (ET-1, pg/mL); brain natriuretic peptide (BNP, pg/mL); left ventricular end-diastolic diameter (LVEDD, cm); and cardiac output (CO, L/min) averaged from 19 patients supported by LVAD. (Reproduced with permission from Thompson LO, Skrabal CA, Loebe M, et al. Plasma neurohormone levels correlate with left ventricular functional and morphological improvement in LVAD patients. *J Surg Res.* 2005;123(1):25-32. Copyright © Elsevier.)

MYOCARDIAL CELL CHANGES

A number of changes have been documented to occur to the cardiac myocyte found in heart failure patients. They include changes in genes and proteins such as myosin isotype reversion to the fetal form; changes in metabolic proteins involved energy metabolism, increased cytokine expression, and increased myocardial cell size. The hypertrophy of the cardiac cell is one of the hallmarks used in heart failure along with the increased fibrosis. A few, not all, of the changes seen in the progression to heart failure have been studied in LVAD-supported recovery.

Myocardial cell size is increased in heart failure, and studies now show that along with a decrease in gross ventricular dimensions decreases in myocyte size also occurs. In the same group of

following transplantation of the same patient. These two samples represent a paired pre-LVAD sample and a post-LVAD sample from the same patient allowing for the determination of differences that occur over time with LVAD unloading. To date, we have analyzed the interstitial collagen using area of stain quantitation with Sirius Red staining on 36 pre-LVAD and post-LVAD paired samples (22 dilated cardiomyopathies, 14 ischemic cardiomyopathies). This technique does not differentiate density of collagen-only area versus total cellular area. Of these, 28 showed reduction in interstitial collagen following LVAD support. Seven of the remaining eight patients who remained unchanged or demonstrated an increase in fibrosis were from ischemic cardiomyopathy while only one was from a dilated cardiomyopathy. Figure 20–2 shows the percent of total area of collagen staining from all measured paired samples. While the decrease overall is significant, it was not universal to all patients.

Of the samples where collagen was measured, 6 were from MicroMed/DeBakey VADs and 30 came from pulsatile devices. The decrease in collagen staining was seen in both groups; however, it was greater in the pulsatile group (26% vs 32% decrease). It is likely that this difference is due to the length of support which was greater in the pulsatile group; however, the degree of ventricular unloading may also play a role in the degree of remodeling. The axial-flow pumps are true cardiac assist devices because they do not have valves and cannot completely unload the ventricle and therefore always maintain some ventricular stretch and pressure unlike the pulsatile systems which can completely empty the ventricle.

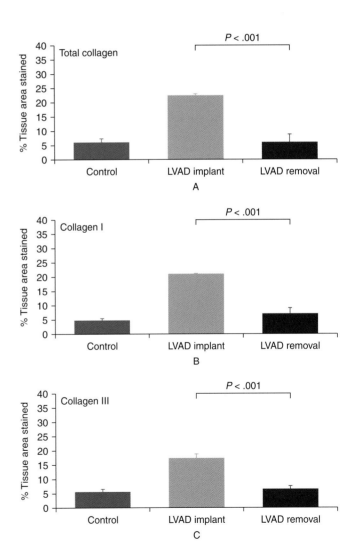

FIGURE 20–2. Change in total collagen in patients supported by LVAD using semiquantitative area of stain using Sirius Red. (Reproduced with permission from Bruckner BA, Stetson SJ, Perez-Verdia A, et al. Regression of fibrosis and hypertrophy in failing myocardium following mechanical circulatory support . *J Heart Lung Transplant.* 2001;20(4):457-464. Copyright © Elsevier.)

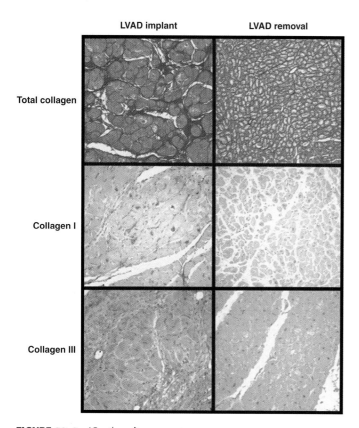

LVAD implant   LVAD removal

Total collagen

Collagen I

Collagen III

FIGURE 20–2. (*Continued*)

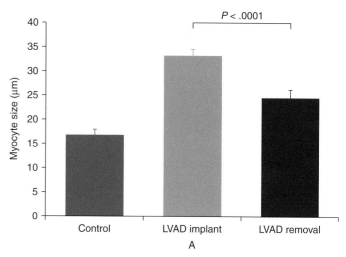

A

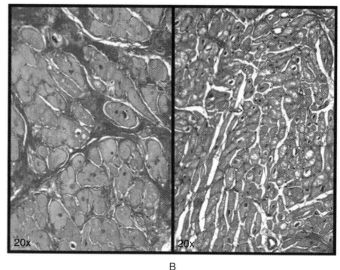

B

patients where collagen was measured, we measured myocardial cell diameters at the level of the nucleus as an indicator of cell size. Of the 36 LVAD supported patients, 34 showed a decrease in myocyte diameters as shown in Fig. 20–3. While this does not demonstrate individual protein changes, it is an indicator of the plasticity of the myocyte and a return toward normal morphology following ventricular unloading. The change in myocyte size was similar in tissues obtained from both pulsatile and axial-flow pumps (25% and 26% decrease, respectively).

It is currently unknown which changes are most important in normalizing function following assist device support. A number of laboratories are studying many aspects of the changes. However, the evidence to date is anecdotal. Most importantly, parallel changes in functional improvement and architectural normalization occur and appear regardless of device type. Whether a particular type of patient, heart failure, or device is best suited for a bridge-to-recovery remains to be determined.

FIGURE 20–3. Myocyte diameters measured in paired myocardial tissue samples taken from LVAD supported patients. (Reproduced with permission from Bruckner BA, Stetson SJ, Perez-Verdia A, et al. Regression of fibrosis and hypertrophy in failing myocardium following mechanical circulatory support. *J Heart Lung Transplant*. 2001;20(4):457-464. Copyright © Elsevier.)

REFERENCES

1. Schiessler A, Warnecke H, Friedel N, Hennig E, Hetzer R. Clinical use of the Berlin Biventricular Assist Device as a bridge to transplantation. *ASAIO Trans*. 1990;36(3):M706-708.
2. Mancini DM, Beniaminovitz A, Levin H, et al. Low incidence of myocardial recovery after left ventricular assist device implantation in patients with chronic heart failure [see comments]. *Circulation*. 1998;98(22):2383-2389.
3. Bruckner BA, Stetson SJ, Farmer JA, et al. The implications for cardiac recovery of left ventricular assist device support on myocardial collagen content. *Am J Surg*. 2000;180(6):498-501.

4. Schrier RW, Abraham WT. Hormones and hemodynamics in heart failure. *N Engl J Med.* 1999;341(8):577-585.
5. Levine TB, Francis GS, Goldsmith SR, Simon AB, Cohn JN. Activity of the sympathetic nervous system and renin-angiotensin system assessed by plasma hormone levels and their relation to hemodynamic abnormalities in congestive heart failure. *Am J Cardiol.* 1982;49(7):1659-1666.
6. Mukoyama M, Nakao K, Hosoda K, et al. Brain natriuretic peptide as a novel cardiac hormone in humans. Evidence for an exquisite dual natriuretic peptide system, atrial natriuretic peptide and brain natriuretic peptide. *J Clin Invest.* 1991;87(4):1402-1412.
7. Latini R, Masson S, Anand I, et al. The comparative prognostic value of plasma neurohormones at baseline in patients with heart failure enrolled in Val-HeFT. *Eur Heart J.* 2004;25(4):292-299.
8. Levin ER, Gardner DG, Samson WK. Natriuretic peptides. *N Engl J Med.* 1998;339(5):321-328.
9. Kuhn M, Voss M, Mitko D, et al. Left ventricular assist device support reverses altered cardiac expression and function of natriuretic peptides and receptors in end-stage heart failure. *Cardiovasc Res.* 2004;64(2):308-314.
10. Altemose GT, Gritsus V, Jeevanandam V, Goldman B, Margulies KB. Altered myocardial phenotype after mechanical support in human beings with advanced cardiomyopathy. *J Heart Lung Transplant.* 1997;16(7):765-773.
11. Farrar DJ, Holman WR, McBride LR, et al. Long-term follow-up of Thoratec ventricular assist device bridge-to-recovery patients successfully removed from support after recovery of ventricular function. *J Heart Lung Transplant.* 2002;21(5):516-521.
12. Salzberg S, Lachat M, Zund G, et al. Left ventricular assist device as bridge to heart transplantation—lessons learned with the MicroMed DeBakey axial blood flow pump. *Eur J Cardiothorac Surg.* 2003;24(1):113-118.
13. Khan T, Delgado RM, Radovancevic B, et al. Dobutamine stress echocardiography predicts myocardial improvement in patients supported by left ventricular assist devices (LVADs): hemodynamic and histologic evidence of improvement before LVAD explantation. *J Heart Lung Transplant.* 2003;22(2):137-146.

CHAPTER 21

PSYCHOSOCIAL ASSESSMENT AND DISCHARGE PLANNING

Importance of the Social Worker in the LVAD Multidisciplinary Team

Monica R. Freeman

INTRODUCTION

The initiation of a left ventricular assist device (LVAD) program requires the formulation of a dedicated and interactive multidisciplinary team. This team approach improves outcomes and survival with ventricular assist device (VAD) therapy.[1] A detailed evaluation of a patient for LVAD placement involves health care professionals from multiple disciplines to ensure that the patient's quality of life can be improved from both the medical and psychosocial perspectives with LVAD implantation. Each member of the multidisciplinary team has a very important role when it comes to patient selection and pre- and postoperative management. Mechanical circulatory support device programs should be organized as an advanced heart failure center, incorporating the following members[2]:

- Cardiothoracic surgeon
- Heart failure cardiologist
- LVAD coordinator(s)
- Pharmacist
- Social worker
- Palliative care (PC) physician
- VAD technicians
- Nurses
- Other medical subspecialties trained in LVAD therapy

For the purposes of the topic of this chapter, the focus is on the importance of the role of a designated social worker within the LVAD team. The designated social worker provides a comprehensive psychosocial assessment specific to LVAD therapy. The primary objective of a pre-LVAD psychosocial assessment is to identify risk factors for difficulty adjusting post-LVAD, as well as behaviors and life situation issues that may place the patient at risk for compromised long-term LVAD care and potential for serious adverse outcome events.

THE PSYCHOSOCIAL ASSESSMENT

For years the psychosocial assessment has been an important part of the pretransplant evaluation of multiple factors affecting a patient's suitability as heart transplant candidate. Currently, patients undergoing LVAD as bridge-to-transplant (BTT) are often assessed by a heart transplant social worker. There is little experience reported in the literature currently available to guide physicians and their medical support staff in the selection of appropriate candidates for LVAD destination therapy (LVAD-DT). An LVAD-DT–specific psychosocial assessment mirrors that of heart transplant but with unique additional issues specific for LVAD-DT patients. Just as with the pre–heart transplant evaluation, a face-to-face interview is conducted between a social worker and the prospective LVAD recipient and his or her family/caregiver. The purpose of the assessment is to learn about the LVAD candidate in a comprehensive fashion. The assessment should be done by a trained social worker and should include

1. Assessment of patient knowledge and motivation for LVAD

2. Presence or absence of family and social support. As part of an informed consent process pre-LVAD, it is important that family members understand the level of commitment required. Education and informed consent are vital in this very important piece of the pre-LVAD assessment. A brief psychosocial assessment can also be conducted with the caregiver. DT patients tend to be older than 65. Commonly, the caregiver of this patient is the spouse who is typically near the same age. An assessment of physical, mental health and level of commitment of the caregiver is vital, regardless of age. A social worker is key in helping the family to develop a short- and long-term caregiving plan. A supportive, committed caregiver can definitely improve patient's long-term outcome and quality of life.

3. Assessment of the mental health and substance abuse history of patient. Administration of mental health screening tools can be useful, such as the Patient Health Questionnaire 9 (PHQ9), mini–mental health examination, or Beck depression inventory.

4. Assessment of level of education, literacy, cognitive issues are crucial. Neurocognitive functioning is an important consideration. When patients in end-stage heart failure are assessed, often times these patients suffer cognitive impairment due to poor cardiac output and/or the sequelae of associated cerebrovascular ischemic events. This necessitates the presence of family and caregivers during psychosocial evaluation. If necessary, psychometric testing can be conducted by a trained neurocognitive psychologist, psychiatrist, or neurologist.

5. Coping. The period of end-stage heart failure leading to LVAD implantation is highly stressful for both patient and

their family. This necessitates a strong commitment from social workers to ensure best possible outcomes in terms of the patient's well-being and coping mechanisms.[3]

6. Past history of treatment compliance. Does the patient consistently take medications as prescribed? Has the patient been able to consistently return for follow-up appointments?

7. Does the patient have financial resources needed to cover the cost of the monthly dressing change supplies, transportation, and potential lodging and meals and time off work required for caregiving and follow-up visits? What are the Medicare or other third-party insurance options available to support the costs related to LVAD?

8. What is the quality of family's communication and working relationship with the heart failure team?

9. Home environment. Does the patient's home have grounded three prong outlets; is it free of clutter and can it be navigated by a patient with an LVAD? How reliable is the electric supply to the patient's home? Is there a bathroom near the master bedroom? It must be remembered that the patient is tethered to the power support cord which is 20 ft long at night.

10. Assistance with the completion of advance directives (AD) pre-op. This topic will be elaborated further.

Repeat psychosocial assessments can also be considered. Social work intervention offers a unique opportunity for preparing patients and families for LVAD.

CASE STUDIES IN PSYCHOSOCIAL ASSESSMENT PRIOR TO LVAD

■ CASE 1

Following is the assessment of a patient who was found to be an appropriate candidate from a psychosocial assessment for LVAD therapy.

Referral

Social services referred as part of program support for LVAD program.

Mr L is being considered for LVAD as BTT versus DT. He was referred to our center by his local physician.

Roles and Relationships

Mr L is a pleasant 61-year-old married gentleman of Indonesian decent. He resides 8 hours from the medical center. Mr L was born in Indonesia, but moved to the Netherlands at age 7 and later moved to the United States at age 11. He speaks fluent Dutch. He is a retired Air Force veteran.

Mr L last worked in December of 2005. He has a master's degree in sociology and a bachelor's degree in higher education. He retired for disability from his career in student services for his local university 5 years ago. He has been married to his wife

for 38 years. His wife reports good health and currently works full time for the local university. She is currently on family medical leave act (FMLA). She reports that she has 12 weeks of FMLA and has 92 days of paid time off, if needed. She does, however, report some anxiety about the work that will be "piled up" for her at her job upon her eventual return.

From their union, they have two adult daughters who are supportive. Their youngest (age 28) lives 45 minutes from their home. This daughter works full time and is married with no children. She plans to come to the center for LVAD training and support in a few weeks. Their oldest daughter, age 32, is married with children and lives in another nearby state. She is Mr L's alternate power of attorney (POA) for health care.

Since retiring for disability, Mr L has been an active volunteer in his community. He had been helping with Special Olympics in his hometown and numerous other activities. Mr L is an active member of a Methodist church in his hometown. As far as chemical use, Mr L does not drink alcohol or use illicit drugs, and denies any history of prescription medication abuse. He denies a history of smoking cigarettes.

Reactions

Mr L admits to feelings of depression and anxiety related to his failing health. He reports that the past 5 years have been difficult for him emotionally due to his failing health, the death of his parents, and the passing away of his youngest brother to cancer. Currently, he is taking Cymbalta, which he reports has helped with his symptoms of depression. Currently, he is also taking a small dose of Xanax to help with anxiety. He describes himself as a "deep thinker" and gets down when he feels like a burden to his family and thinks of his loss of independence. Faith is a source of strength for him. He has been to counseling in the past, which he has found helpful. Overall, he seems to be coping as well as can be expected under the circumstances and seems to have the ability to seek out appropriate help when needed.

Resources

The patient has private insurance from his wife's employer, Medicare A and B, and Tricare (military benefit). He receives social security disability insurance (SSDI), veteran's disability benefit, and a pension. A home safety evaluation was completed today. Mr L resides in a split level home with a three-step entrance. He has a six-step entrance to living room and another seven steps to his bedroom. His home is reported to be free of clutter and loose carpets. His home was built in 1991 and is electrically safe, with grounded three-prong outlets in each room. He has a walker, wheel chair, shower bench, toilet seat riser, and grab bars. His master bed is within 20 ft of his bathroom. He has a home telephone in the event of an emergency at home.

His wife is staying at hotel near the center. Mr L does have an AD which he has placed in his medical records. Mr L was encouraged to have an open and honest conversation with his family before surgery about his wishes so that both his daughters and wife be in agreement regarding the goals, potential outcomes, and long-term commitment involved.

Recommendations

Overall, from a psychosocial perspective, Mr L appears to be a good candidate for LVAD. His wife reports good health and has the ability to take 12 weeks off work to be his primary caregiver. His youngest daughter plans to come to the center in about 9 days for LVAD training as a backup caregiver. I have encouraged his wife to get adequate sleep and practice good self-care so that she is able to be a caregiver for her husband. She does have normal worries about being able to manage caregiving and work, but is not unreasonable. Mr L has lived in his community for 13 years and has several supportive friends. His daughter can also be a backup caregiver if needed, hence lessening the risk of family member caregiver burnout. He has spoken to his family about specific LVAD-related directives in his AD, which is now established in his medical records. The patient and his wife and family have been invited to attend LVAD support group. Social services will continue to follow.

The social worker followed this patient throughout hospitalization to provide continued education, supportive counseling, and assistance with his eventual hospital discharge.

This patient has subsequently done very well following LVAD-DT. He has been completely compliant with LVAD outpatient management recommendations and follow-up. He has also had excellent family support from his wife and his daughter. Mr L has become actively involved with the LVAD-DT support group and enjoys a meaningful and productive quality of life. In addition, he is the author of a new LVAD newsletter for patients at the center.

■ CASE 2

This patient was not suitable for LVAD-DT from a psychosocial perspective. Following is the assessment:

Referral

Referred as part of program support for LVAD program. Interviewed patient and his ex-wife in hospital room this morning. Patient is being evaluated for possible LVAD-DT.

Roles and Relationships

Mr S is a 68-year-old twice divorced Caucasian man from a very rural community in a town of 200 people. The nearest larger town (population 10,000) is 7 miles from his home. Mr S is a retired truck driver with a 10-grade education. Mr S has been married to his ex-wife for 12 years. The couple divorced in 1971 and later both remarried and subsequently both divorced their second spouses. Their current relationship is amicable, but unpredictable. From their union they had four children (three living). Their three living adult sons range in age from 42 to 48. Mr S has been living with his ex-wife and 42-year-old son for the past 4 months. Prior to this living arrangement Mr S lived with his aunt until her death.

Mr S's ex-wife generously took him in, as there are no alternate living arrangements available for patient at this time. His ex-wife is minimally supportive, as she suffers from schizoaffective disorder for which she experiences hallucinations, severe anxiety, and depression. She also reports that she is easily overwhelmed with excessive responsibility and not mechanically inclined. She has had five prior inpatient mental health hospitalizations. Her longest job was as a home health aid for a local home health agency which she held for 7 years. She is a 1 pack per day (PPD) cigarette smoker and smokes in her home. Mr. S's sons are minimally available to provide support. His 42-year-old son works as a painter when he is not laid off. It is doubtful this son would be able to provide support or be educated about the LVAD device. Mr S has a sister who is supportive, but detached as she lives in another state and takes care of her son who is mentally ill. As far as chemical use, patient denies current use of alcohol or illicit drugs. He is a previous 3 PPD cigarette smoker and quit in 1989.

Resources

Medicare A, B, and D; local state medical assistance (non-transferable). Mr S has a medical assistance (MA) arrangement whereby he must spend $550 of his own money before his MA starts. He receives $925/mo social security (SS)—most of which is used for medications and other health care expenses. Mr S has completed an AD. He is currently staying on the second floor of his ex-wife's home (10 steps up). He has utilized home health (HH) in the past.

Reactions

Mr S is having difficulty coping with his illness. He reports "moodiness and irritability" and his ex-wife feels that he is depressed. He recently completed an AD in which he states to have specifically indicated that he does not want nursing home placement at any time. Additionally, his ex-wife reports that she is not able to participate in LVAD training, nor offer hands on caregiver support due to her mental illness.

Recommendations

Overall, Mr S is a 68-year twice divorced Caucasian man from a rural state. From a psychosocial perspective this patient is not a good candidate to receive an LVAD-DT due to the following issues:

1. Lack of reliable home caregiver support.
2. Likely continued instability of current living situation.
3. Distance from his home to adequate health care informed about LVAD-DT.

Additionally, his ex-wife is not comfortable driving outside of her local community and all financial resources are very limiting. On the other hand, Mr S does describe himself as mechanically inclined and does not feel intimated by the LVAD systems controller. His son potentially has a more stable mental health condition than his mother, but is unlikely to assume the role of primary caregiver necessary for his father.

The multidisciplinary team met as a group and discussed Mr S's case in detail; particularly his lack of reliable family support structure needed for long-term care at home, which itself also appeared to be an uncertainty. He was not deemed an appropriate candidate for LVAD-DT therapy.

ADVANCE DIRECTIVES AND ETHICS

All pre-LVAD patients should be encouraged to complete an advance directive (AD). Like any life-supporting device (eg, ventilator, dialysis), there will be a point in time with every LVAD patient where the device will have to be deactivated. This may be due to debilitating stroke, traumatic brain injury, poor postoperative outcome, end-organ failure, or failure to thrive. As more and more LVADs are implanted into an aging population of advanced heart failure patients, it is inevitable that the issue of "deactivation" will have to be addressed by institutions.

A study conducted at the Mayo Clinic concluded that only a minority of patients with LVADs had ADs, and of those who did none mentioned directives regarding the LVAD device in their AD. Physicians should encourage these patients to complete ADs and address LVAD management specifically in the ADs. Not doing so may result in ethical dilemmas (eg, uncertainty following a requested for LVAD deactivation).[4] Clearly, encouraging all pre-LVAD patients to complete an LVAD-specific AD helps ensure good outcomes and is important in order to avoid reaching an ethically complex endpoint, sometimes referred to as "destination nowhere."[5] The Patient Self-Determination Act protects a patient's right to withhold or withdraw medical therapy so that a natural death may occur.[6] An ethical analysis of withdrawing an LVAD concluded that carrying out a request to withdraw VAD support is permissible in accordance with the principles that apply to withdrawing other life-sustaining treatments.[7]

Rizzieri and colleagues emphasize the importance of informed consent and recommend that it should include a detailed discussion and evaluation of particular elements before surgical implantation of the device. A balanced discussion weighing the options of medical management, palliation, hospice care, as well as the surgical procedure itself is encouraged.[8] Clear communication with each patient about goals of care pre- and postoperatively is highly encouraged.

PALLIATIVE CARE

The World Health Organization (WHO) does encourage, as part of a team approach, the use of palliative care (PC) in older persons with serious chronic progressive diseases such as end-stage heart failure.[9] WHO also recommends that PC should be offered as needs develop before they become unmanageable.[8] LVAD-DT has been referred to as "permanent palliation" for advanced heart failure patients.[10] For these reason, a PC physician has proved to be very useful at our center as a member of the multidisciplinary LVAD team. A PC consult is done on every new LVAD-DT patient preoperatively. A PC physician meets the potential candidate in an effort to build an initial relationship with the LVAD-DT patient. The PC physician also speaks to the patient about goals of care and helps elaborate the AD in an effort to create a "preparedness plan" (Fig. 21–1).[11] The involvement of PC will help the patient and medical team devise a precise plan of care for anticipated device-related complications in an effort to avoid ethical dilemmas. Postoperatively,

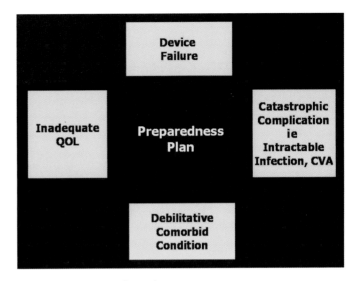

FIGURE 21–1. Preparedness plan.

the PC physician will follow the LVAD-DT patient throughout hospitalization. The PC physician is also useful during hospital readmissions in situations where the patient is medically compromised and facing end-of-life decisions. The PC physician works very closely with the patient and family when a choice is made to deactivate the LVAD.

EDUCATING THE LOCAL COMMUNITY

It is important that local communities be prepared to receive an LVAD patient. LVAD literature must be sent out to the patient's local hospital and emergency room, ambulances, emergency response teams (fire and police departments), local cardiologist, and local primary care physician. Patients should be encouraged to visit with those listed earlier in an effort to advocate for themselves and familiarize themselves with important community contacts. Some patients have even elected to contact local media in an effort to increase their visibility in the community. This is also an important means for educating heart failure patients who may be LVAD candidates.

SUPPORT GROUP FOR LVAD PATIENTS

Transplant support groups have been around for decades and have been a useful connection tool either for patients waiting for an organ or those who have received an organ and wish to identify with others in the same situation. Hildingh describes in an article entitled, "Social support in self-help groups, as experienced by persons having coronary artery disease and their next of kin" that the concept of a support group includes confirmation, trust, sharing, affinity, faith, and empowerment. A support group works best when conducted according to the following tenets: understanding produces humility, a feeling of affinity improves quality of life, and sharing a burden brings relief.[12] Developing an LVAD support group is a positive step in providing pre- and post-LVAD patients with the social support and improving their quality of life. Support groups facilitated by a social worker provide LVAD recipients with a feeling of solidarity and fellowship and encourage members to share their experiences. This in turn enhances their well-being and quality of life. Prior to implantation, LVAD recipients characteristically face a grim prognosis, whereas after therapy they are faced with adjusting to a new lease on life. Patients feel a new sense of optimism and help each other adapt to a new life and in turn live with hope. Social workers and PC physicians help patients through this transition.[13]

The LVAD support group is an excellent venue for patients to feel less isolated, develop a sense of commonality, and help each other learn "tools of the trade." Patients share stories on such things as showering with an LVAD and how to best wear the batteries and system controllers, etc. They talk about their experiences living with an LVAD and how it relates to issues such as perception by others, body image, and traveling. In addition, the LVAD support group is an ideal opportunity for patients considering LVAD therapy to meet patients currently living with a device. It is important for these patients to hear the stories of others in order to guide their own personal decision about LVAD implantation. It is also helpful as an educational venue for hospital personnel who want to know more about living with an LVAD. Caregivers also attend and appreciate being with others who share the same role. This helps to alleviate some of the stress and burden of being a caregiver for an LVAD patient.

DISCHARGE PLANNING OPTIONS FOR PATIENTS WITH LVAD

Discharging the LVAD patient home requires a great deal of preparation. In the era of DT, some LVAD recipients will function quite well in their home environment. However, many will require alternative discharge arrangements. Preparation for discharging LVAD patients to rehabilitation centers, nursing homes (NHs), assisted living centers, or dialysis centers is a paradigm that is likely to become increasingly prevalent in the years ahead.[14] Fortunately, at our center the majority of immediate post-op LVAD patients are referred to our own inpatient acute rehabilitation, where they continue physical and occupational therapy until they are strong enough to return home. At the beginning of the development of our center's LVAD program, this relationship was developed with our acute inpatient program.

Outpatient challenges have been observed in two separate scenarios:

1. Patients who require unanticipated chronic renal dialysis postoperatively.
2. Patients with failure to thrive at home or those who are admitted with other medical conditions such as stroke, traumatic brain injury, loss of caregiver, or other medical comorbities which prohibit them from returning to their home environments.

■ DIALYSIS

In general, dialysis centers are unfamiliar with LVAD therapy. The unique element in dialyzing a patient with an LVAD is measuring of the blood pressure. A patient's heart rate must be measured with a Doppler device as it is not otherwise reliably assessed on clinical examination. Many dialysis centers must obtain a Doppler prior to accepting an LVAD patient for dialysis. Additionally, there must be an accepting nephrologist who will be required to be educated on LVAD therapy. Many dialysis centers are understaffed by nursing and may not have the staff to mangage both the LVAD and dialysis. Some centers have required that caregivers be present during dialysis to manage the device.

Given the potential for renal failure following LVAD insertion, caregivers must understand that dialysis is a potential further commitment they are likely to undertake. Caregivers must commit to sitting with an LVAD patient during dialysis three times a week 4 hours at a time. This can be a tremendous burden, especially if the caregiver must maintain employment. These discussions should occur pre-op as part of the informed consent process.

■ NURSING HOME/REHAB PLACEMENT

Historically, just as placing a ventilator-dependent patient to a nursing home (NH) was difficult, placing an LVAD patient in a NH was noted to be challenging. First, NHs are generally completely unfamiliar with LVAD and therefore often intimidated.

These institutions are appropriately fearful to accept the liability associated with complications due to the LVAD. Maintaining nursing competencies is frequently a problem. If the NH is only being referred one LVAD patient per year, for example, how will the staff maintain their competencies? The discharge planning social worker plays an important role when it comes to complex NH placements. Methods that have proven to be useful are encouraging NHs to accept patients who reside in their own local community and at the same time mailing out of LVAD literature to the potential receiving NH. Additionally, it is important for a center to have resource nursing educators who are able to travel to sites if necessary for LVAD training. Another helpful tool is to refer any NH who is willing to take a look at accepting an LVAD patient to speak with another NH who has previously accepted an LVAD patient. This will help reassure a NH that this strategy is feasible based on the experience of other NHs. Reminding the NH that the hospital LVAD coordinator is available 24 h/d for any LVAD-related concern is another effective strategy in discharging a patient to a NH. It is also often helpful to remind the NH that previously this LVAD patient was living at home and managed well by, often times, an elderly caregiver. It is likely that this caregiver will be at the NH with the patient often and is very familiar with device managing and dress changing protocols. Furthermore, the NH physician may not have had experience caring for an LVAD patient. This physician may benefit from a phone call from the LVAD coordinator and/or heart failure physician for education and reassurance purposes. These forms of empowering are important tools when discharging patients to NHs or rehab centers.

In our experience it has been much easier referring an LVAD patient to a NH when the patient is DNR (Do Not Resuscitate) or hospice appropriate. This again needs to be preordained as directed by the patient's AD. As more LVAD patients age, NHs will need further education on managing end-of-life issues and device deactivation. PC physicians are an excellent resource to NHs in these situations. During these complex placements and situations many questions arise.

- Does the LVAD patient want to be placed in the NH?
- Is the LVAD doing for this patient what he/she had originally intended?
- Is the patient happy with his/her overall quality of life?

These questions should be asked while the patient is hospitalized during the process of discharge planning. Social workers and PC physicians can play an important role in these discussions which will likely be required to occur with all LVAD-DT patients at some point of time. It is also important that any LVAD center begin to nuture relationships and or develop contracts with neighboring rehab centers, NHs, assisted living centers, home health agencies, and dialysis centers. This will avoid unnecessary long-term hospitalizations and expedite hospital discharge. Coordination and communication between LVAD team and local care providers will ensure LVAD patients receive the care they need in a safe and efficient manner.[15] The issue of lack of resources and discharge obstacles should also be presented to patients and caregivers as part of the informed consent process preimplantation so that there are no surprises later down the road.

SUMMARY

Therapy with an LVAD presents a unique set of psychosocial challenges for both patients considered for such intervention and their families. A designated social worker working in conjunction with the LVAD multidisciplinary team plays a pivotal role in the preoperative evaluation of patient's candidacy for LVAD. A comprehensive psychosocial assessment is necessary, as important issues in this regard may escape the purview of the medical and surgical evaluations. Lack of recognition of serious psychosocial issues could have major adverse impact on patient outcomes as well as set the stage for very complicated ethical dilemmas in subsequent management. Social workers are instrumental in aiding the LVAD patients and their families as they develop long-term comprehensive caregiving plans and facilitate integration of such patients into their local medical communities.

REFERENCES

1. Osaki S, Edwards NM, Velez M, et al. Improved survival in patients with ventricular assist device therapy: the U of Wisconsin experience. *Eur J Cardiothorac Surg.*;2008 Aug; 34(2).
2. Cadeiras M, von Bayern M, Deng MC. Managing drugs and devices in patients with permanent ventricular assist devices. *Curr Treat Options Cardiovasc Med.* 2007 Aug;9(4);318-31.
3. Helman DN, Oz MC. Developing a comprehensive mechanical support program. *J Card Surg.* 2001;16:203-208.
4. Swetz K, Mueller P, Ottenberg A, et al. The prevalence and use of advance directives among patients with left ventricular assist devices. *J Card Failure.* 2010 Aug;16(8S).
5. Bramsted KA. Destination nowhere: a potential dilemma with ventricular assist devices. *ASAIO J.* 2008;54:1-2.
6. Dudzinski DM. Ethics guidelines for destination therapy. *Ann Thorac Surg.* 2006;81;1185-1188.
7. Mueller P, Swetz K, Freeman M, et al. Ethical analysis of withdrawing ventricular assist device support. *Mayo Clin Proc.* 2010 Sep;85(39):791-797.
8. Rizzieri AG, Verheijde JL, Rady MY, McGregor JL. Ethical challenges with the left ventricular assist device as a destination therapy. *Pilos Ethics Humanit Med.* 2008;3:20.
9. Swetz K, Freeman M, Carter K, et al. Palliative medicine consultation for preparedness planning and life enhancement in patients receiving left ventricular assist devices as destination therapy. Manuscript in preparation.
10. Davies E, Higginson IJ, eds. Better palliative care for older people. World Health Organization Europe. http://www.euro.who.int/document/E829933.pdg
11. Banning A, Houghton P. Post hospital care of the permanent LVAD patient. *ASAIO J.* 2005;51(6).
12. Swetz K, et al Characterization of patient attitudes toward living with left ventricular assist devices as destination therapy (LVAD-DT)—exploring the natural history of living and dying with LVAD-DT. Manuscript in preparation.
13. Hildingh C, Fridlund B, Segesten K. Social support in self-help groups, as experienced by persons having coronary heart disease and their next of kin. *Int J Nurs Stud.* 1995;32(3):224-232.
14. Maciver J, Ross HJ, Delgado DH, et al. Community support of patients with a left ventricular assist device: the Toronto General Hospital experience. *Can J Cardiol.* 2009;25(11).
15. Freeman M, Swetz K, Mueller P, Ottenberg A, Park S. Coping with a new lease on life after LVAD-DT implantation: value of social work and palliative care in the pre-LVAD assessment and post-implantation. *J Card Failure.* 2010;10(8S).

SECTION II

Device Specific Considerations

CHAPTER 22

DEVICE SELECTION FOR MECHANICAL CIRCULATORY SUPPORT

Matthew D. Forrester, Katherine B. Harrington, and Hari R. Mallidi

INTRODUCTION

Since DeBakey's report of the first successful implant of a ventricular assist device (VAD) in 1966,[1] there has been a remarkable evolution of mechanical circulatory support (MCS) technology. Devices now exist ranging from short-term percutaneous VADs to long-term permanently implantable VADs and total artificial hearts (TAHs). As current devices continue to evolve and new iterations are developed, there is an increasing range of clinical scenarios in which a failing heart can be mechanically supported. With appropriate device selection, treatment can be tailored to the specific needs of each patient. In the broadest terms, MCS can be divided into short- and long-term therapy.

SHORT-TERM CIRCULATORY SUPPORT

Short-term MCS is intended to support a patient with acute decompensated heart failure until the patient recovers sufficient cardiac function or until further long-term therapy is indicated based on recovery of end-organ function. Length of support can be a few hours or several days but is generally limited to fewer than 2 weeks. Most commonly, short-term devices are implanted for patients in acute refractory cardiogenic shock. Common indications for short-term MCS are listed in Table 22–1. This group of patients historically included those who failed to wean from cardiopulmonary bypass (CPB) support or those with early postoperative ventricular failure. More recently, MCS is often implemented for patients with acute cardiogenic shock after myocardial infarction[2] or fulminant myocarditis.[3] There are also a number of emerging roles for short-term MCS, such as during high-risk percutaneous coronary and valvular interventions[4-6] and even during certain cardiac surgical procedures.[7]

ACUTE CARDIOGENIC SHOCK

Acute cardiogenic shock is often a result of either acute myocarditis or myocardial infarction, but can also be seen during periods of rejection after cardiac transplantation. Cardiogenic shock occurs in 2.4% to 12% of patients who suffer an acute myocardial infarction and carries a mortality rate of up to 75%.[8] Despite advancements in percutaneous coronary intervention, improved efficiency in getting patients to the catheterization laboratory, and implementation of intra-aortic balloon counterpulsation, some of these critically ill patients remain unstable and may benefit from more aggressive MCS.

Acute viral myocarditis has been described as "unclear pathophysiology and etiology, uncertain diagnosis, and variable presentation."[3] Nearly 10% of patients with recent onset cardiomyopathy are found to have lymphocytic myocarditis on endomyocardial biopsy.[9] Although cardiomyopathy related to myocarditis is somewhat variable in presentation, patients with acute, fulminant myocarditis often do poorly without mechanical unloading.

MCS allows for restoration of adequate hemodynamics and end-organ perfusion by unloading the ventricle, thereby decreasing myocardial oxygen consumption. Patients may even be stabilized with MCS at a smaller peripheral facility and then be transferred to larger tertiary-care centers for further management. After initial hemodynamic stabilization, a decision can be made regarding further treatment. Some patients recover sufficient cardiac function for explantation of their VAD, while others may require longer ventricular support.[2] These patients can then be transitioned to a long-term VAD either as a bridge-to-transplant (BTT) or as destination therapy (DT).

Several devices are now available for short-term circulatory support and can provide left, right, or biventricular support (Table 22–2). The specific device used is based on the clinical scenario, patient characteristics, goals of support, and device availability. These devices are generally approved by the US FDA (Food and Drug Administration) for up to 6 hours of support; however, they potentially can support a patient for up to 2 weeks. First-generation short-term VADs are implanted surgically as extracorporeal pumps. The Levitronix CentriMag has FDA approval for 30-day support. However, newer-generation devices such as the TandemHeart pVAD (CardiacAssist, Inc, Pittsburgh, PA) and the Impella (Abiomed Inc, Danvers, MA) have become available which can be implanted percutaneously via peripheral cannulation in the catheterization laboratory.

POSTCARDIOTOMY CARDIOGENIC SHOCK

Initial efforts in MCS were often directed toward supporting a failing heart after cardiac surgery.[1,10] While the range of options for treating this condition have expanded dramatically in the years since those early implants, the need for MCS following CPB remains an important indication either after failing to wean from CPB or in cases of early postoperative ventricular failure. Postcardiotomy MCS may be needed for left or right ventricular failure or both. If sufficient ventricular function returns, the VAD can be explanted. Otherwise, the patient must be evaluated as a candidate for either DT or BTT. Unlike cases of myocarditis or acute cardiogenic shock, the exposure available in the setting of postcardiotomy shock permits easy access for any of the available short-term devices.

TABLE 22–1. Common Indications for Short-Term Mechanical Circulatory Support

Indication	Type of Support
Acute cardiogenic shock	LVAD, RVAD, or BiVAD
Postcardiotomy shock	LVAD, RVAD, or BiVAD
Cardiopulmonary failure	ECMO
High-risk percutaneous interventions	LVAD

BiVAD, biventricular assist device; ECMO, extracorporeal membrane oxygenation; LVAD, left ventricular assist device; RVAD, right ventricular assist device.

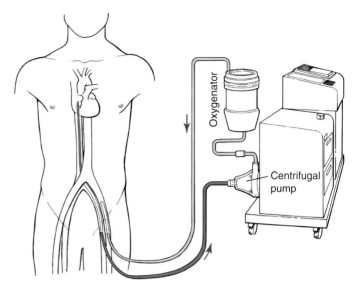

FIGURE 22–1. Percutaneous extracorporeal membrane oxygenation (ECMO) support is attained via femoral vessel access. Right atrial blood is drained via a catheter inserted into the femoral vein and advanced into the right atrium. Oxygenated blood is perfused retrograde via the femoral artery. Distal femoral artery perfusion is not illustrated. (Reproduced with permission from Cohn LH, ed. *Cardiac Surgery in the Adult*, 3rd ed. McGraw-Hill, Inc; 2008:516. Fig. 18–4.)

CARDIOPULMONARY FAILURE

In addition to acute cardiac failure, short-term support can also be instituted for cardiopulmonary failure with extracorporeal membrane oxygenation (ECMO). The principal components of the ECMO circuit are similar to those of CPB machines. The circuit consists of a centrifugal pump, a membrane oxygenator, a heat exchanger, and a heparin-bonded circuit (Fig. 22–1). ECMO can be used for management of life-threatening cardiac or pulmonary failure or both. By providing short-term support, ECMO can be used while awaiting return of cardiopulmonary function or as a bridge to further treatment. Support can be initiated via peripheral or central venoarterial cannulation for cardiac or full cardiopulmonary support or venovenous cannulation for oxygenation when cardiac function is preserved, but the lungs are unable to maintain sufficient gas exchange. Unlike CPB, which is used for several hours during cardiac surgery, ECMO can support a patient for several days.[11]

SHORT-TERM SUPPORT DURING HIGH-RISK INTERVENTIONS

Although VADs are most commonly indicated for heart failure, short-term devices have also been used to support patients undergoing high-risk percutaneous interventions in order to

safeguard against intervention-induced cardiac collapse.[4-6] Frazier recently reported the use of the Impella Recover 5.0 (Abiomed Inc, Danvers, MA) for support during a high-risk off-pump coronary artery bypass grafting procedure.[7] Though these are not yet common applications, they illustrate the increasing utility of ventricular support devices. There will undoubtedly continue to be further clinical roles for short-term devices in the future as technology and clinic experience grow.

LONG-TERM MECHANICAL CIRCULATORY SUPPORT

Although cardiac transplantation remains the gold standard for end-stage heart failure, its application is limited by the persistent shortage of donor organs and increasing heart failure population. Moreover, the requirement of immune suppression

TABLE 22–2. Summary of the Current Short-Term Devices in Use (as of October 1, 2010)

Abiomed AB5000	Abiomed	First generation (pulsatile)	Extracorporeal	Short term	Biventricular
Abiomed BVS 5000	Abiomed	First generation (pulsatile)	Extracorporeal	Short term	Biventricular
Impella	Abiomed	Second generation (axial flow)	Extracorporeal	Short term	Left ventricular
TandemHeart	CardiacAssistInc	Third generation (centrifugal flow)	Extracorporeal	Short term	Biventricular
CentriMag	Levitronix/ Thoratec	Third generation (centrifugal flow)	Extracorporeal	Short term	Biventricular

exposes the patient to a variety of morbid sequelae. Long-term MCS devices are an exciting potential solution to the increasing heart failure population and paucity of donor organs.

Though VADs and TAH devices have been under development since the 1960s,[10] their long-term use has been limited by complications of thromboembolism, infection, and device failure. With continued improvement in both management and design of VADs, their clinical use is rapidly growing. In 1994, the HeartMate Implantable Pneumatic left ventricular assist system (HeartMate IP LVAS, Thoratec Corp, Pleasanton, CA) was approved by the FDA for use as BTT therapy. Iterations of the HeartMate IP LVAS along with other devices of similar concept have since been approved for BTT therapy. The REMATCH (Randomized Evaluation of Mechanical Assistance for the Treatment of Congestive Heart Failure) trial demonstrated a significant survival benefit in patients with VADs as compared to medical therapy alone in patients with decompensated chronic heart failure who were not transplant candidates, which not only supported the concept of BTT but ultimately laid the foundation for DT.[12] Currently, two VADs (HeartMate XVE LVAS and HeartMate II LVAS [Thoratec Corp, Pleasanton, CA]) are approved by the FDA for both BTT and DT. Determining whether a patient is a candidate for BTT versus DT is a complex decision and requires careful consideration by an experienced heart failure team. At present, indications for long-term MCS are based on the REMATCH trial, although these criteria are conservative and many patients who do not meet these criteria may benefit from MCS.[12,13] Continued definition of appropriate patients will undoubtedly clarify the role of long-term MCS in the future.

BRIDGE-TO-TRANSPLANT

Mechanical ventricular assistance in chronic heart failure is directed largely by the defined goals of treatment for each patient. Regardless of the etiology of heart failure, patients with chronic decompensated heart failure can be placed into two categories: those who are transplant candidates and those who are not. Transplant candidates, who are unlikely to receive a donor heart in a timely fashion and are continuing to decompensate despite optimal medical management, may be appropriate candidates for BTT therapy with a VAD. Mechanical ventricular support not only provides improved mortality over medical management alone, but can allow patients an opportunity for transplant who otherwise might die while waiting for a donor organ. For those who are successfully bridged to transplant (BTT), their posttransplant mortality may decrease as compared with patients who were not bridged with a VAD.[13]

Currently available devices for BTT are outlined in Table 22-3. This list is rapidly expanding and several devices are under investigation. Once a patient has been deemed to be a transplant candidate and appropriate for MCS, several patient-related factors help to determine which device is appropriate. Now that several types of devices are available, it is important to carefully choose a specific device for each patient. Some patients may require biventricular mechanical support while others will only require univentricular support. Patient size, anatomy, and ability to tolerate anticoagulation and severity of heart failure are also significant factors in choosing a device. Optimal timing of implantation is also a critical factor in patient selection as outcomes may be dependent on the temporal length of support.[14] Patients with permanent end-organ damage are not likely to have a good outcome despite MCS. As MCS devices improve and morbidities are minimized, there is likely to be a general trend toward earlier device implantation.

Once a patient is determined to be a candidate for a VAD as a BTT, careful consideration must be given to the type of device implanted. Assist devices have characteristically been described based on the stage of development during the evolution of this field. Accordingly, pulsatile, volume displacement pumps are referred to as "first-generation" technology, whereas axial-flow, impeller-driven pumps are described as "second-generation" devices, with centrifugal flow comprising the "third generation." The initial FDA-approved devices generate pulsatile blood flow from a pneumatically or electrically driven pusher-plate or diaphragm mechanisms and can often provide full cardiac support. In general, these devices are fairly large and require an appropriate body habitus for preperitoneal or intraperitoneal implantation of the pump itself. Other devices, such as the Thoratec Paracorporeal Ventricular Assist Device (PVAD) system (Thoratec Corp, Pleasanton, CA) are implanted with an extracorporeal pump and tunneled cannulae. Newer, second-generation, axial-flow, impeller-driven devices generate continuous, nonpulsatile blood flow and are much smaller allowing implantation in patients with a smaller body habitus, including children. Some of these devices can often only provide partial support and are indeed true "assist" devices with the native ventricle generating a portion of the cardiac output. Most recently, third-generation centrifugal pumps have been introduced which also provide continuous nonpulsatile flow and are currently under FDA investigation for long-term support. These pumps are driven by similar mechanisms to some CPB machines and some of the short-term devices outlined previously. Once a device has been selected and implanted, patients can often be supported until a donor organ becomes available, while also improving end-organ perfusion and ultimately improving posttransplant prognosis.

DESTINATION THERAPY

Patients who are not candidates for cardiac transplantation may be candidates for DT with a left ventricular assist device (LVAD) or TAH. In 2003 the HeartMate XVE (Thoratec Corp, Pleasanton, CA.) was approved by the FDA for DT and more recently, the HeartMate II (Thoratec Corp, Pleasanton, CA.) was approved in 2010. These are presently the only two VADs approved for DT in the United States. Several devices have supported patients for long periods of time and demonstrated their potential for DT. However, under the current regulatory paradigm, most devices achieve FDA approval as BTT first before completing the approval process for DT. There will likely be several more FDA-approved options for DT in the near future.

TABLE 22–3. List of Current MCS Devices Being Clinically Used or Tested Worldwide (as of October 2010).

Device	Manufacturer	Type	Implantation Method	Duration of Support	Type of Support	Approval Status (as of July 2009)	Current Usage
Abiomed AB5000	Abiomed	First generation (pulsatile)	Extracorporeal	Short term	Biventricular	FDA approved for short term single or biventricular support	Bridge to recovery/decision
Abiomed BVS 5000	Abiomed	First generation (pulsatile)	Extracorporeal	Short term	Biventricular	FDA approved for short term single or biventricular support	Used rarely in post-cardiotomy support
Tandemheart	CardiacAssist, Inc.	Third generation (centrifugal flow)	Extracorporeal	Short term	Biventricular	FDA approved for extracorporeal circulatory support for up to six hours for procedures not requiring full cardiopulmonary bypass	Short-term support (2,000th implant in 4/2010)
Impella	Abiomed	Second generation (axial flow)	Extracorporeal	Short term	Left ventricular	FDA approved for circulatory support of periods up to six hours (April 2009).	Short-term support
Centrimag	Thoratec	Third generation (centrifugal flow)	Extracorporeal	Short term	Biventricular	A clinical trial is currently underway in the United States to investigate CentriMag use as a VAD for support for up to 30 days; Investigational device for left or biventricular support for periods over six hours.	Short-term support
Thoratec PVAD (Paracorporeal Ventricular Assist Device)	Thoratec	First generation (pulsatile)	Extracorporeal	Long term	Biventricular	CE Mark Authorized. Received FDA approval for BTT in 1995 and for post-cardiotomy recovery in 1998.	Rarely used to left ventricular support. Used for long term right sided or biventricular support and as BTT for pediatric support in appropriate cases.
IVAD – Implantable Ventricular Assist Device	Thoratec	First generation (pulsatile)	Intracorporeal	Long term	Biventricular	CE Mark Authorized. Received FDA approval for BTT in 2004. Authorized only for internal implant, not for paracorporeal implant due to reliability issues.	Rarely used due to newer-generation technology
EXCOR	Berlin Heart	First generation (pulsatile)	Extracorporeal	Long term	Biventricular	Pending FDA approval as Humanitarian Device Exception (HDE) for BTT and Bridge to Recovery	Clinical trials
Syncardia TAH	Syncardia Systems	First generation (pulsatile)	Intracorporeal	Long term	Biventricular	FDA approval and CE Mark Authorized for use as BTT in cardiac transplant-eligible candidates at risk of imminent death from biventricular failure	BTT

Device	Manufacturer	Generation	Location	Duration	Support	Regulatory approval	Status
AbioCor® Implantable Replacement Heart	Abiomed	First generation (pulsatile)	Intracorporeal	Long term	Biventricular	Food and Drug Administration approval under a Humanitarian Device Exception (HDE) for DT	Implanted in a limited number of centers
Novacor	World Heart	First generation (pulsatile)	Intracorporeal	Long term	Left ventricular	Previously approved for BTT in North America, European Union and Japan	Taken off the market
HeartMate XVE	Thoratec	First generation (pulsatile)	Intracorporeal	Long term	Left ventricular	FDA approval for BTT in 2001 and DT in 2003. CE Mark Authorized.	Rarely used due to newer generation technology
HeartMate II	Thoratec	Second generation (axial flow)	Intracorporeal	Long term	Left ventricular	Approved for use in North America and EU. CE Mark Authorized. FDA approval for BTT (April 2008) and DT (January 2010).	BTT, DT, and BTD
Jarvik-2000	Jarvik Heart	Second generation (axial flow)	Intracorporeal	Long term	Left ventricular	In Europe, the Jarvik 2000 has earned CE Mark certification for both bridge-to-transplant and lifetime use. Child version currently being developed.	Under FDA-approved clinical investigation for BTT
MicroMed DeBakey VAD	MicroMed	Second generation (axial flow)	Intracorporeal	Long term	Left ventricular	Approved for use in Europe under HDE for BTT and BTD in children. The child version is approved by the FDA for use in children in USA.	Under FDA consideration for BTT trial in US
Synergy® Pocket Micro-Pump	Circulite	Third generation (centrifugal flow)	Intracorporeal	Long term	Left ventricular	Began enrollment in our CE Mark Trial in June 2007	Clinical trials
VentrAssist	Ventracor	Third generation (centrifugal flow)	Intracorporeal	Long term	Left ventricular	Approved for use in European Union and Australia.	Company declared bankruptcy while clinical trials for FDA approval were underway in 2009.
Incor	Berlin Heart	Third generation (axial flow)	Intracorporeal	Long term	Left ventricular	Approved in Europe.	Entered clinical trials in the US in 2009.
HVAD	HeartWare	Third generation (centrifugal flow)	Intracorporeal	Long term	Left ventricular	Obtained CE Mark for distribution in Europe, January 2009.	Completed United States BTT trials in 2009.
DuraHeart	Terumo	Third generation (centrifugal flow)	Intracorporeal	Long term	Left ventricular	CE approved, US FDA trials underway as of January 2010.	Clinical trials
World Heart	Levacor	Third generation (centrifugal flow)	Intracorporeal	Long term	Left ventricular	Limited by Federal (United States) Law to Investigational Use for a BTT Indication under an IDE Application. Not currently available outside the United States.	Clinical trials
Evaheart Medical	EVAHEART LVAS	Third generation (centrifugal flow)	Intracorporeal	Long term	Left ventricular	Approved to initiate an US clinical trial in 2010 for use as BTT from the FDA.	Clinical trials

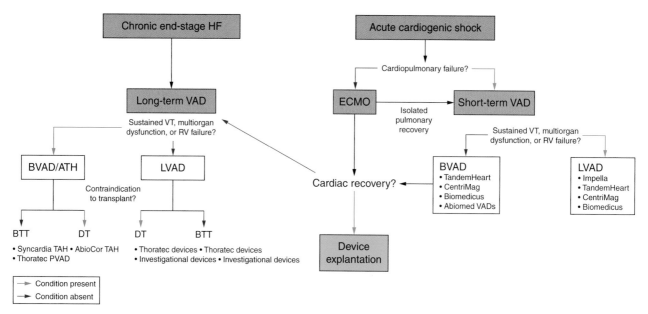

FIGURE 22–2. Decision-making algorithm for deciding on the best mechanical circulatory support (MCS) option for a given clinical scenario.

Patient selection for DT requires similar considerations to BTT devices. However, additional thought must be given to lifestyle, psychosocial issues, and overall ability of the patient and family to tolerate and maintain permanent mechanical ventricular assistance.

In addition to VADs, TAH devices are available for BTT or DT. The first totally implantable TAH to be used clinically was the AbioCor TAH (Abiomed Inc, Danvers, MA) with initial clinical investigation beginning in 2001.[15] Since Cooley's first implant of a TAH in a human being in 1969,[16] numerous TAH devices have been developed with varying results.[10] To date, there is no totally implantable TAH that has achieved widespread clinical use, but the CardioWest (Syncardia Systems Inc., Total Artificial Heart, Tucson, AZ) TAH has FDA approval for BTT and has extensive clinical experience in that role. With continued investigation and technological improvement, a totally implantable TAH will likely be available for biventricular support in the future.

BRIDGE-TO-RECOVERY

With increasing experience with MCS, a third category of bridge-to-recovery (BTR) has developed. Initially, devices were explanted for either mechanical failure or device infection with unexpected recovery of cardiac function.[17] With this observation, several authors have investigated the possibility of device explantation after sufficient myocardial recovery. This is based on the concept of reverse remodeling with regression of fibrosis and hypertrophy as well as evidence at the cellular and molecular level.[18,19] Although some have attempted to define an algorithm for device explantation, there is not yet a well-defined cohort of patients who will benefit from this approach. Presently, BTR is appropriate for a very small subset of chronic heart failure patients supported by VADs. BTR may play a more prominent role in the future as further experience is obtained.

CONCLUSION

Heart failure is a very complex cohort of diseases that range from acute, recoverable decompensation to chronic end-stage disease. Medical management, despite continuing advances, is often insufficient to support acutely decompensated patients or prevent death. Once limited to gravely ill heart failure patients who have exhausted all other options, MCS is increasingly becoming a common treatment modality. There are a wide variety of devices, for an even broader spectrum of disease. With continued clinical experience and technological advancement, MCS devices will continue to expand their utilization reaching beyond tertiary transplant centers. It is thus important for clinicians to have a general understanding of these devices and their clinical applicability. The decision-making algorithm for deciding on the best MCS option for a given clinical scenario can be complicated, but may be simplified by considering the decision based on the needs of the patient with respect to short- versus long-term, single versus biventricular assist, and transplant versus permanent therapy (Fig. 22–2). As more devices are approved for clinical use, the patient will play a larger role in choosing which device to implant, often based on such issues as the difference in the external components and how the patient envisions these will fit into his/her day-to-day activities or the type of anticoagulation required.

REFERENCES

1. Debakey M. Left ventricular bypass pump for cardiac assistance. *Am J Cardiol.* 1971;27:3-11.
2. Garatti A, R. C. Mechanical circulatory support for cardiogenic shock complicating acute myocardial infarction: an experimental and clinical review. *ASAIO J.* 2007;53(3):278-287.
3. Acker M. Mechanical circulatory support for patients with acute-fulminant myocarditis. *Ann Thorac Surg.* 2001;3(Suppl):S73-S76.

4. Thomas JL, A.-A. H. Use of a percutaneous left ventricular assist device for high-risk cardiac interentions and cardiogenic shock. *J Invasive Cardiol.* 2010;22(8):360-364.

5. Kar B, F. M. Use of the TandemHeart percutaneous ventricular assist device to support patients undergoing high-risk percutaneous coronary intervention. *J Invasive Cardiol.* 2006;18(4):A6.

6. Kar B, D. R. Temporary support with TandemHeart pVAD during percutaneous aortic valve replacement in an animal model: rationale and methodology. *Tex Heart Inst J.* 2005;32(3):283-286.

7. Akay MH, F. O. Impella Recover 5.0 assisted coronary artery bypass grafting. *J Card Surg.* 2010.

8. Goldberg R. Recent magnitude of and temporal trends (1994-1997) in the incidence and hospital death rates of cardiogenic shock complicating acute myocardiacl infarction: the second national registry of myocardial infarction. *Am Heart J.* 2001;141(1):65-72.

9. Herskowitz A, C. S. Demographic features and prevalence of idiopathic myocarditis in patients undergoing endomyocardial biopsy. *Am J Cardiol.* 1993;71:982-986.

10. Gemmato CJ, F. M. Thirty-five years of mechanical circulatory support at the Texas Heart Institute. *Tex Heart Inst J.* 2005;32(2):168-177.

11. Marasco SF, L. G. Review of ECMO (estracorporeal membrane oxygenation) support in critically ill adult patients. *Heart Lung Circ.* 2008;4:S41-S47.

12. Rose E. Long-term mechanical left ventricular assistance for end-stage heart failure. *N Engl J Med.* 2001;345(20):1435-1443.

13. Frazier O. Improved mortality and rehabilitation of transplant candidates treated with a long-term implantable left ventricular assist device. *Ann Surg.* 1995;222(327).

14. Gammie JS, E. L. Optimal timing of cardiac transplantation after ventricular assist device implantation. *J Thorac Cardiovasc Surg.* 2004;127(6):1789-1799.

15. R, S. Cardiovascular news: totally contained AbioCor artificial heart implanted July 3, 2001. *Circulation.* 2001;104:E9005.

16. Cooley DA, L. D. Orthotopic cardiac prosthesis for two-staged cardiac replacement. *Am J Cardiol.* 1969;24:723.

17. Frazier OH, M. T. Left Ventricular assist system as a bridge to myocardial recover. *Ann Thoracic Surg.* 1999;68:734-741.

18. Bick RJ, P. B. Improved sarcoplasmic reticulum function after mechanical left ventricular unloading. *Cardiovasc Pathobiol.* 1998;2:159-166.

19. Dilulio NA, D. N. Reversal of heart failure phenotype by mechanical unloading. *J Heart Lung Transplant.* 1999;18:89.

CHAPTER 23
THE IMPELLA 2.5 CATHETER-BASED CARDIAC ASSIST DEVICE

Daniel H. Raess and David M. Weber

The Impella 2.5 Percutaneous Cardiac Support System (Abiomed, Danvers, MA) is intended for partial circulatory support using an extracorporeal bypass control unit for periods up to 6 hours. It is also intended to be used to provide partial circulatory support (for periods up to 6 hours) during procedures not requiring cardiopulmonary bypass (CPB). It also provides pressure measurements, which are useful in determining intravascular pressure. The Impella 5.0 catheters are intended for circulatory support using an extracorporeal bypass control unit, for periods up to 6 hours. They are also intended to be used to provide circulatory support (for periods up to 6 hours) during procedures not requiring CPB. They also provide pressure measurements, which are useful in determining intravascular pressure.

The ideal cardiac assist device for the catheterization laboratory provides effective support for both elective high-risk patients, as well as acute or emergent patients, and has a safety and ease-of-use profile appropriate to each procedure setting. For elective high-risk percutaneous coronary interventions (HR-PCI), the clinical goals of the ideal device are (1) to maintain stable systemic hemodynamics while avoiding disruptions in cardiac output, clinical challenges to end-organ function, and neurological instabilities that disrupt patient compliance; (2) to provide more time for complex percutaneous coronary intervention (PCI) by raising the patient's ischemic threshold to minimize myocardial cell damage from balloon inflation or coronary dissection; and (3) to provide a prophylactic safety and ease-of-use profile—minimizing complications such as bleeding (arising from large sheaths and the need for full anticoagulation) or embolization to end organs (such as stroke or limb ischemia). In short, it provides a low-risk, simple-to-use "safety net" that ensures its success, improves its outcome, and extends the PCI procedure to a broader range of patients who would otherwise be denied revascularization due to excessive risk either in surgery or the catheterization laboratory.

In the emergent setting of acute myocardial infarction (AMI), the roles of the ideal assist device to augment systemic hemodynamics and improve the myocardial ischemic environment are also of prime importance. However, unlike the prophylactic role they play in HR-PCI for AMI patient care, assist devices are needed to provide prompt therapeutic benefit with the shortest delay possible because clinical outcome in AMI, with or without hemodynamic compromise, is strongly correlated with time to therapy.[1] In AMI, the "time is muscle" paradigm remains, and in the case of hemodynamic shock there is also a strong relationship between duration of shock and clinical outcome.[1] The clinical goals of the ideal assist device for the AMI patient are (1) to restore and stabilize systemic hemodynamics to reverse the decline of end-organ perfusion, reduce the risk of end-organ failure, and break the deadly cycle of cardiogenic shock; (2) to minimize residual infarct size by reducing the level of myocardial ischemia, halting further cell damage, maximizing residual cardiac function ,and reducing the overall risk of cardiogenic mortality; and (3) to provide an ease-of-use and safety profile consistent with the critical treatment time scenarios and the risk-benefit considerations of emergency care.

The ideal assist device, therefore, spans the needs of both elective and emergent patient settings, provides systemic hemodynamic support and myocardial protection, and is safe and simple to use. We discuss herein a brief history of cardiac assist technologies in the catheterization laboratory that have struggled to achieve these goals, and we introduce Impella technology (Abiomed, Inc., Danvers, MA), which is the first cardiac assist technology designed to attain this comprehensive ideal.

THE EVOLUTION OF CARDIAC SUPPORT IN THE CATHETERIZATION LABORATORY

Evolving from Gibbon's[2] pioneering roller pump-oxygenator work in the 1950s, cardiac assist in the catheterization laboratory had its origins in the form of extracorporeal membrane oxygenators (ECMO), which were used to support children in respiratory failure. However, because the catheterization laboratory was predominately a diagnostic venue at this time, there was limited need in this environment for a therapeutic technology. With the clinical introduction of an intra-aortic balloon pump (IABP) by Kantrowitz et al in 1968,[3] cardiologists diagnosing and treating patients with acute coronary syndromes began applying IABP therapy in the catheterization laboratory but usually in concert with the surgeons, largely because of the need for a graft on the femoral artery to prevent limb ischemia. Although gradually accepted, there was little clinical evidence of improved survival or function during shock secondary to AMI.[4,5] Specifically, studies comparing the safety and effectiveness of the IABP to nonassisted care in patients with AMI reported no improvement in mortality or composite major adverse cardiac and cerebrovascular events (MACCE), yet there was a significant increase in the incidence of stroke and bleeding. Widespread application of IABP followed the introduction of truly percutaneous systems that employed 8.5- to 9-Fr sheaths (circa 1975). At the close of the 1970s and with the birth of PCI in the early 1980s, the IABP offered cardiologists a truly percutaneous system that could be employed during an intervention or whenever circulatory support was needed. Although deployment of an IABP is relatively simple and does not require a surgeon for implantation or removal, a steady and reliable electrocardiogram (ECG) and/or pressure signal (to ensure its proper deflation right before the onset of the systolic period) is required due to its placement in the descending aorta. When supporting patients undergoing HR-PCI or compromised by AMI (which is usually diagnosed by changes in the ECG), the difficulty of maintaining a steady and reliable ECG timing signal adds complexity to IABP use. The safety and effectiveness of an IABP depends on predictable rhythms and is affected when timing signals are compromised.[6,7] The IABP movement (inflation/deflation) can also interfere with the movement and guidance of the therapeutic catheter and compromise the quality of the intervention. Although IABP use has been found to augment coronary perfusion,[8] overall myocardial ischemic improvements are limited by the fact that it provides little or no reduction in native ventricular work and myocardial oxygen demand.[9,10] Furthermore, it should be recognized that the IABP is not an active forward-flow pump; it is a volume displacement device. Therefore, any improvements in forward flow (ie, cardiac output) in the presence of IABP support are accomplished by the native heart itself and have been demonstrated in failing hearts to be only modest improvements of approximately 0.2 L/min.[11] For this reason, it is typical to combine IABP support with the administration of multiple doses of inotropic drugs that induce higher output from the failing native heart to maintain adequate systemic circulation. This pharmacologic induction increases ventricular work and myocardial oxygen demand, further challenging the myocardial ischemic balance and feeding a downward cycle of increased ischemia, heart failure, and ultimately cardiogenic shock. In a study of more than 3000 patients with postoperative cardiogenic shock, Reesink et al[11] demonstrated a linear relationship between in-hospital mortality and the level of inotropic support. They reported a 21% mortality rate for patients on a high dose of a single inotrope, 42% for a high dose of two inotropes, and 80% for a high dose of three inotropes. Therefore, although the IABP gained widespread use in the catheterization laboratory based on its relative ease of insertion, its lack of hemodynamic impact leading to a reliance on inotropic drug support limited its ability to meet the ideals described previously. Cardiopulmonary support (CPS) systems were introduced in the 1970s,[12] filling a void between what the IABP could provide in the catheterization laboratory and what full CPB provided in the surgical suite. Essentially, CPS systems were an iteration of ECMO that was mobile, supported percutaneous implantation, and was limited to short durations of use. CPS systems consisted of a mobile pump (either roller type or centrifugal) on a moveable cart containing an oxygenator, a portable oxygen supply, a small heat exchanger, a mobile power supply, and all the needed cannula for rapid percutaneous cannulation. These devices employed a femoral cannulation strategy that drew femoral venous blood into the pump and deposited the newly oxygenated blood volume into the femoral artery. Although this support strategy was more effective at

augmenting systemic hemodynamics than the IABP, it had little or no effect on the myocardial ischemic balance, providing no support of coronary perfusion or reduction in ventricular work. Another disadvantage was its safety profile. Even in circuits using heparin-coated tubing, complications remained high and included renal failure requiring dialysis (47%), bacteremia or mediastinitis (23%), six strokes (10%), leg ischemia (70%), oxygenator failure (43%), and pump change (13%).[13] Although CPS allowed longer inflations in the percutaneous transluminal coronary angioplasty era, the vascular complications and the need for frequent transfusion limited widespread use.[14] From the perspective of ease-of-use, some form of vascular repair was typically needed upon completion of the procedure (due to the relatively large cannula size), and use of the CPS system required a perfusionist to be in constant attendance in the catheterization laboratory and in all other departments. Therefore, despite the fact that this technology was the first to provide a moderate level of hemodynamic support in the catheterization laboratory, it also fell short of the ideal in a number of ways. The Hemopump (Medtronic, Inc, Minneapolis, MN), introduced in the late 1980s,[15] was an application of an Archimedes screw, or axial pump, with the motor residing outside the body. The axial pump head was positioned in the left ventricle, and the external motor transferred energy to the pump head through a high-speed, rotating shaft running inside an arterial steering catheter. The Hemopump was attractive to cardiologists because it was implanted via femoral artery access in a nearly percutaneous fashion (although similar to the early days of the IABP, it was usually in concert with a surgeon due to the need for a graft on the femoral artery to prevent limb ischemia), and it was the first active forward-flow pump that did not require an extracorporeal transit of the blood. Furthermore, the clinical goal of HR-PCI support was evolving beyond just providing systemic circulatory support during the procedure to an increased emphasis on protecting the heart muscle from the ischemic insult of the PCI procedure itself. The Hemopump, with its direct left ventricular access, theoretically provided a high level of myocardial ischemic protection due to the efficient unloading of left ventricular work (reducing myocardial oxygen demand), while its outflow, which was at or near the aortic root, held promise of also augmenting coronary flow (increasing myocardial oxygen supply). Despite its conceptual advantages over the currently available systems and the coincidence with many of the ideal goals of cardiac assist in the catheterization laboratory, the Hemopump never reached significant application and fell into disuse in the catheterization laboratory and market due to design flaws (mostly related to the long high-speed rotating drive shaft) that limited its reliability in clinical practice. Development of cardiac assist in the catheterization laboratory has, therefore, progressed through a number of iterations during the last 50 years. With each generation, the technology has attempted to address the challenges of becoming easy to implant, safer for the patient, and/or more effective in providing circulatory support and myocardial protection. The Impella technology is the latest generation of cardiac assist and represents a significant step in the history of technology development described previously. Its design facilitates a support strategy that is safe and simple to use consistent with both elective and emergent clinical environments, while supporting systemic hemodynamics and protecting the myocardium from ischemic damage.[8,10,11,16-20] Impella achieves safety and simplicity by its percutaneous placement combined with an independence from both physiologic timing signals and the consistent need for supplemental inotropic drug support.[8,15-19,21-28] Its hemodynamic support results from the design feature that provides active forward flow[17,29] that increases net cardiac output,[8,11,16-19] and its ability to address the needs for myocardial protection stems from simultaneously unloading the ventricle (decreasing myocardial oxygen demand)[10,11,16-18] and augmenting coronary flow (increasing oxygen supply).[10,20] We provide a brief description of the Impella technology, review its experience with regard to clinical usability and patient safety, discuss its fundamental principles of action, and review the scientific and clinical investigations that have demonstrated these principles.

DEVICE DESCRIPTION

The Impella 2.5 is a catheter-mounted microaxial flow pump capable of pumping up to 2.5 L/min of blood from the left ventricle, across the aortic valve, and into the aortic root. The cannula portion of the device, which sits across the aortic valve, is contiguous to the integrated motor that comprises the largest-diameter section of the catheter (12 Fr) (Fig. 23–1). The small diameter of the cannula is designed to allow easy coaptation of the aortic valve leaflets around it, resulting in the lack of aortic valve insufficiency. A repositioning device allows removal of the introducer sheath after placement, leaving the 9-Fr catheter at the arterial access site. The Impella catheter is powered and controlled by the Impella console (Fig. 23–2), which is also used for the entire family of Impella devices, both existing and in development. An infusion pump controls a purge system designed to keep blood from entering the motor compartment by creating a pressure barrier against the blood that the device is exposed to. Future controllers will incorporate the purge function into the console itself. Unlike the IABP, the device control does not require synchronization with ventricular activity. There is no need for timing of the device cycle and for ECG or pressure triggering. ECG signal deterioration typically seen in sick patients, such as those with atrial tachycardia, ST-segment changes, fibrillation, or intractable arrhythmia, does not compromise device function and efficacy as it frequently can with the IABP.[6,7] Impella 2.5 has been available for general use in the United States since June 2008 and is available in more than 40 countries, including Europe and Canada. The Impella 5-L/min devices (Impella 5.0 and Left Direct [LD]) have been cleared for general use in the United States since April 2009. The

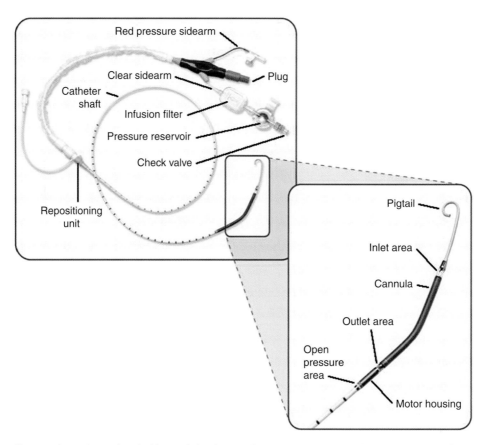

FIGURE 23–1. The Impella 2.5 catheter. (Reproduced with permission from Weber DM, Raess DH, Henriques JPS, Siess T, eds. Principles of Impella cardiac support: the evolution of cardiac support technology toward the ideal assist device. Supplement to *Cardiac Interventions Today. Principles of Hemodynamics.* August/September 2009. Fig. 4. Sponsored by Abiomed, Inc.)

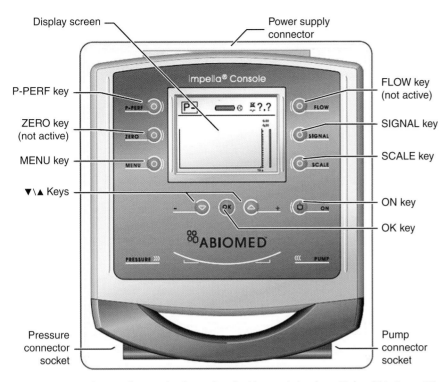

FIGURE 23–2. The Impella console. (Reproduced with permission from Weber DM, Raess DH, Henriques JPS, Siess T, eds. Principles of Impella cardiac support: the evolution of cardiac support technology toward the ideal assist device. Supplement to *Cardiac Interventions Today. Principles of Hemodynamics.* August/September 2009. Fig. 5. Sponsored by Abiomed, Inc.)

the performance level on the Impella console is started at its minimum setting (just enough to counteract physiologic forces and stabilize the device position). Once positioned across the aortic valve, the console can be used to confirm that the device placement is proper and stable. At this point, the device performance is typically adjusted to a higher level.

SAFETY AND USE PROFILE

The safety and ease-of-use of Impella technology is founded on three principles. The first is its size. Impella's 12-Fr pump head and 9-Fr catheter enable percutaneous placement with a single vascular access point, requiring no cardiac wall puncture and imparting no damage to the aortic valve.[8,16,17,22,29] In short, its size and implantation methods are designed to facilitate reduced complications relative to its predecessor technologies. Second, Impella is an active flow pump that, unlike the IABP, provides hemodynamic support without the need for inotropic drug support and its associated mortality risks.[1] Third, Impella provides support independent of the need for ECG or pressure waveform synchronization, limiting the overall complexity of the setup and support maintenance. Impella implantation time compared to the IABP has been reported by Seyfarth et al.[8] Figure 23–4 summarizes these results. In this cardiogenic

entire family of Impella products has been CE Mark approved and approved by Health Canada. The Impella 2.5 duration of support specified under the CE Mark is 5 days. In parallel to its general-use clearance in the United States (which is for partial circulatory up to 6 hours), the Impella 2.5 is also the subject of a number of ongoing clinical trials (involving up to 5 days of support).

DEVICE INSERTION

Impella 2.5 is inserted using a modified monorail technique under direct fluoroscopic control. It uses both a pressure lumen adjacent to the motor, as well as motor current monitoring to give positioning verification to the operator. The device is placed using fluoroscopic control to avoid kinking the catheter and compromising the purge lumen. Transesophageal echocardiography is used as an adjunct only and is useful to confirm device position. After arterial access is achieved, the 13-Fr peel-away sheath is positioned. A coronary guiding catheter (typically a multipurpose or pigtail) and, subsequently, a 0.018-in guidewire are placed across the aortic valve into the left ventricle. Once the guidewire is across the aortic valve, the guiding catheter is removed, and the Impella catheter is threaded onto the wire. Several guidewires have been certified by Abiomed for use with the Impella system (see Abiomed Impella Instructions for Use and Technical Bulletin 9 for details). With the device positioned in the ventricle (Fig. 23–3), the wire is removed and

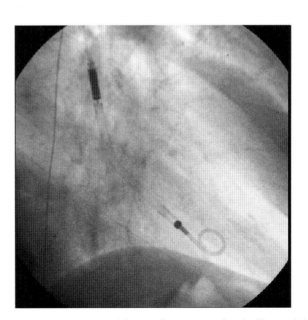

FIGURE 23–3. Placement of the Impella 2.5. (Reproduced with permission from Weber DM, Raess DH, Henriques JPS, Siess T, eds. Principles of Impella cardiac support: the evolution of cardiac support technology toward the ideal assist device. Supplement to *Cardiac Interventions Today. Principles of Hemodynamics.* August/September 2009. Fig. 6. Sponsored by Abiomed, Inc.)

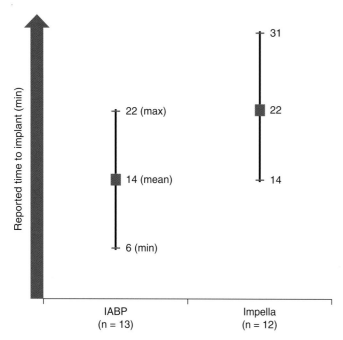

FIGURE 23–4. Reported Impella implantation times compared to IABP (*P* = .4) in AMI cardiogenic shock patient population. (Reproduced with permission from Weber DM, Raess DH, Henriques JPS, Siess T, eds. Principles of Impella cardiac support: the evolution of cardiac support technology toward the ideal assist device. Supplement to *Cardiac Interventions Today. Principles of Hemodynamics.* August/September 2009. Fig. 7. Sponsored by Abiomed, Inc.)

shock patient population, IABP implantation times range from 6 to 22 minutes, with a mean of 14 minutes. Impella implantation times were reported to range from 14 to 31 minutes, with

a mean of 22 minutes with no statistical difference between the mean implantation times (*P* = .4). It is also noteworthy that this investigation represented early experience with Impella implantation. Several studies have reported an extremely low incidence of failure to implant or achieve support, as well as a very low incidence of complications, including groin issues, hemolysis, or any evidence of acute or chronic complications relating to the aortic valve or aortic insufficiency.[16-29] Table 23–1 summarizes reported adverse event rates for Impella 2.5 in five key studies spanning both HR-PCI and AMI patients.

FUNDAMENTAL PRINCIPLES OF ACTION

In addition to the safety and ease-of-use aspects described previously, Impella is designed to address the other two ideals of cardiac assist—hemodynamic support and myocardial protection. The innate ability of Impella to simultaneously provide systemic hemodynamic support and myocardial protection is based on its fundamental principles of support. In short, Impella is designed to replicate the natural function of the heart—moving blood from the ventricle, through the aortic valve, and into the aortic root. For the heart, this flow path is essential to accomplishing its native function because blood flow is conveyed from the aortic root to the systemic circulation through the ascending aorta, and to the myocardial circulation through the coronary ostia. Because Impella's flow path mimics this natural direction of forward flow, it too conveys blood flow to the systemic and coronary circulation. With the outflow of the Impella device in the aortic root, it provides both an active flow and systemic pressure (AOP) contribution leading to increased cardiac power output (Fig. 23–5). Furthermore, with the inflow of the device drawing blood directly from the ventricle, it reduces ventricular

TABLE 23–1. Reported Adverse Event Rates for Impella 2.5 HR and AMI Studies

Study	Device	N	Aortic Regurgitation	Valve/ Trauma	Limb Ischemia	Device-Related Bleeding	Intrasupport Modality
HR PCI							
Burzotta et al (2008)[17]	2.5	10	0%	0%	0%	0%	0%
Dixon et al (2009)[29]	2.5	20	0%	0%	0%	0%	0%
Henriques et al (2006)[16]	2.5	19	0%	0%	0%	6%	0%
AMI							
Seyfanh et al (2008)[8]	2.5	13	0%	0%	8%	0%	23%[a]
Spuw et al (2008)[22]	2.5	10	0%	0%	0%	0%[b]	0%

[a]*Cardiogenic shock patients.*

[b]*After implementing adjusted heparin protocol.*

Reproduced with permission from Weber DM, Raess DH, Henriques JPS, Siess T, eds. Principles of Impella cardiac support: the evolution of cardiac support technology toward the ideal assist device. Supplement to *Cardiac Interventions Today. Principles of Hemodynamics.* August/September 2009. Table 2. Sponsored by Abiomed, Inc.

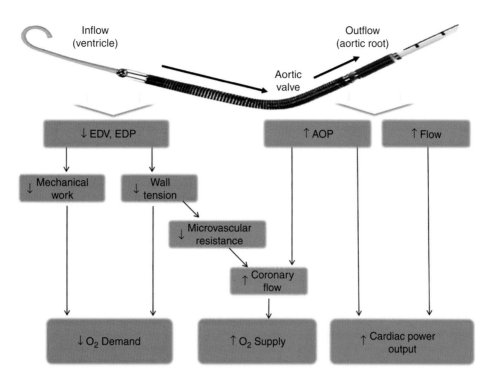

FIGURE 23–5. Schematic of the hemodynamic design principles of Impella. (Reproduced with permission from Weber DM, Raess DH, Henriques JPS, Siess T, eds. Principles of Impella cardiac support: the evolution of cardiac support technology toward the ideal assist device. Supplement to *Cardiac Interventions Today. Principles of Hemodynamics.* August/September 2009. Fig. 8. Sponsored by Abiomed, Inc.)

end-diastolic volume and pressure (EDV, EDP).[21] Reducing EDV and EDP leads to a reduction in mechanical work and myocardial wall tension, both of which reduce myocardial oxygen demand.[30-33] Additionally, the increased AOP combined with reduced wall tension leads to increased coronary flow, which increases myocardial oxygen supply. In total, Impella favorably alters the balance of myocardial oxygen demand and supply, improving the muscle's ability to survive ischemic challenges.[10,11] Impella technology is, therefore, the first clinically viable cardiac assist technology to provide this natural forward flow from the ventricle, through the aortic valve, and into the aortic root, simultaneously supporting systemic hemodynamics and protecting the myocardium from ischemic damage (by increasing myocardial oxygen supply and decreasing myocardial oxygen demand).[8,10,11,16-20] These principles, combined with its established safety profile[8,16-19,21-28] and ease of use, comprise a comprehensive approach to all of the ideals described earlier. We now discuss these principles in more detail and review the scientific and clinical investigations through which they have been demonstrated (Table 23–2).

TABLE 23–2. Summary of Impella Studies Demonstrating Systemic Hemodynamic Support and Myocardial Protection

Impella Study	Systemic Hemodynamic Support	Myocardial Protection	
		Increased O_2 Supply (Coronary Flow)	Decreased O_2 Demand (LV Unloading)
Burzotta et al (2008)[17]	√		
Sauren et al (2007)[10]		√	√
Valgimigli et al (2005)[21]	√		√
Meyns et al (2003)[20]	√		√
Meyns et al (2003)[23]			√
Remmelink ec al (2007)[38]	√	√	
Reesink et al (2004)[11]	√		√
Dixon et al (2009)[29]	√		
Seyfarth et al (2008)[8]	√		

Reproduced with permission from Weber DM, Raess DH, Henriques JPS, Siess T, eds. Principles of Impella cardiac support: the evolution of cardiac support technology toward the ideal assist device. Supplement to *Cardiac Interventions Today. Principles of Hemodynamics.* August/September 2009. Table 3. Sponsored by Abiomed, Inc.

SYSTEMIC HEMODYNAMIC SUPPORT

The hemodynamic support provided by Impella stems from both a flow and pressure augmentation that leads to improved cardiac power output. Beginning with the flow contribution, Impella is an active forward-flow pump that is designed to provide up to 2.5 L/min (Impella 2.5) or up to 5 L/min (Impella 5.0 and Impella LD) of flow support. Actual forward flow achieved is dependent on pump performance level ("P" level) and the pressure gradient between the aorta and left ventricle. Higher P-level settings or lower pressure gradients result in higher flow augmentation. The relationship between P-level setting, pressure, and flow through the Impella 2.5 pump is illustrated in Fig. 23–6. This active forward flow was measured and reported by Reesink et al[11] and Meyns et al[20] in acute animal models, and by Burzotta et al,[17] Valgimigli et al,[21] and Dixon et al[29] in humans. Valgimigli et al also reported a total net cardiac output increase associated with Impella 2.5 support of 23%. It is important to clarify, however, that this cardiac output increase was the net effect of (1) a native or true cardiac output reduction (the result of ventricular unloading discussed below) and (2) the forward-flow contribution of the Impella pump leading to a systemic observed cardiac output increase. Furthermore, when properly placed, the outflow of the Impella device resides in the aortic root just above the valve plane (Fig. 23–7A) and provides a sustained augmentation of the diastolic aortic pressure in correlation to the level of Impella support. This systemic pressure augmentation was demonstrated by Remmelink et al,[34] who reported a correlation between Impella 2.5 support level and mean AOP (Fig. 23–7B).

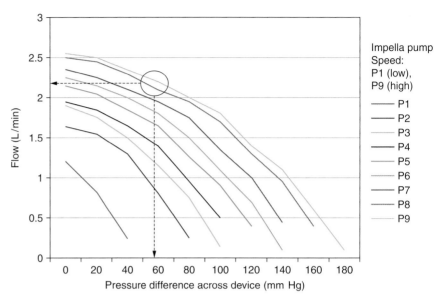

FIGURE 23–6. Impella 2.5 flow-pressure relationship. Active forward flow through the device depends on the pressure difference across the device (the difference between left ventricular and aortic pressure) and the pump support level (*P* value). (Reproduced with permission from Weber DM, Raess DH, Henriques JPS, Siess T, eds. Principles of Impella cardiac support: the evolution of cardiac support technology toward the ideal assist device. Supplement to *Cardiac Interventions Today. Principles of Hemodynamics.* August/September 2009. Fig. 9. Sponsored by Abiomed, Inc.)

ventricular volume and pressure reduces myocardial wall tension and microvascular resistance. The maximum ventricular wall tension (T) occurs at end diastole and can be estimated using the Law of LaPlace as:

$$T \propto \frac{(\text{EDP} \times \text{EDV})}{w} \propto \text{Microvascular Resistance}$$

MYOCARDIAL PROTECTION

■ AUGMENTING CORONARY FLOW: INCREASING O₂ SUPPLY

Flow through any particular coronary artery is dependent on both the pressure gradient across the coronary artery and the vascular resistance. If we assume the venous (distal) pressure and the resistance of the primary artery are fixed, the flow through the coronary artery will be proportional to the ratio of the aortic pressure and the resistance of the microvasculature into which the coronary artery flows. In addition to the augmentation of the aortic pressure demonstrated by Remmelink et al, the Impella-induced reduction in the left

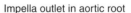

Impella outlet in aortic root

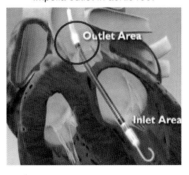

Mean AOP, mm Hg (*P* = .001)

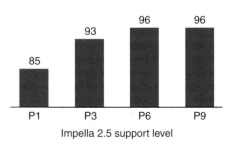

FIGURE 23–7. Outflow of Impella in the aortic root augments aortic pressure. Mean AOP is demonstrated to correlate with increasing Impella support level (*P* = .001). (Reproduced with permission from Weber DM, Raess DH, Henriques JPS, Siess T, eds. Principles of Impella cardiac support: the evolution of cardiac support technology toward the ideal assist device. Supplement to *Cardiac Interventions Today. Principles of Hemodynamics.* August/September 2009. Fig. 11. Sponsored by Abiomed, Inc.)

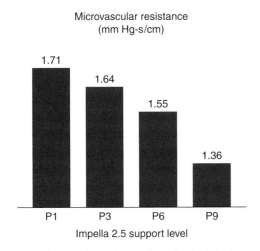

Microvascular resistance
(mm Hg-s/cm)

FIGURE 23–8. Microvascular resistance (mm Hg-s/cm) is demonstrated to decrease with increasing Impella support level (*P* = .005). (Reproduced with permission from Weber DM, Raess DH, Henriques JPS, Siess T, eds. Principles of Impella cardiac support: the evolution of cardiac support technology toward the ideal assist device. Supplement to *Cardiac Interventions Today. Principles of Hemodynamics.* August/September 2009. Fig. 13. Sponsored by Abiomed, Inc.)

in which EDP is the end-diastolic pressure, EDV is the end-diastolic volume, and *w* is the ventricular wall thickness. As Impella draws blood directly from the ventricle, the EDP and EDV are reduced, thereby reducing the maximum wall tension and microvascular resistance. This effect was also demonstrated by Remmelink et al in patients undergoing increasing levels of Impella support (Fig. 23–8). It follows that the combination of

the increase in AOP and the reduction in microvascular resistance with increasing Impella support levels would lead to a subsequent augmentation of the coronary flow, and this effect has been well demonstrated by a variety of investigators.[10,34] Hunziker, using results from a sophisticated hemodynamic simulator model, predicted an increase in diastolic aortic pressure and coronary flow with Impella 2.5 support (personal communication, October 2008). This model was used to compare the predicted pressure and subsequent coronary flow augmentation of the Impella compared to the IABP (Fig. 23–9). The simulation results demonstrated coronary flow augmentation (blue line) from both devices but a more sustained augmentation with Impella throughout the diastolic period (black circles). This is attributed to the constant flow of the Impella, which sustains an elevated diastolic pressure. Because of the required deflation of the IABP in late diastole, it provides only a transient pressure increase early in diastole but reverses this augmentation just before systole, lowering the end-diastolic pressure. IABP deflation in late diastole has been postulated to result in late diastolic flow reversal over and above that seen with physiologic normal pulsatile flow. This has been thought to create a coronary or possibly cerebral steal phenomenon, robbing the heart and brain circulation of much-needed blood flow. This effect has been observed in animal models, and Sjauw et al's meta-analysis of IABP literature[5] showed evidence of more central nervous system complications in patients treated with IABP therapy. Hunziker's predictions were validated in animals by Sauren et al,[10] who reported a maximum 47% increase in coronary flow with Impella (Impella 5.0 operated at 3.8 L/min) compared to a 13% increase with IABP. Finally, Remmelink et al[34] demonstrated this coronary flow augmentation in Impella

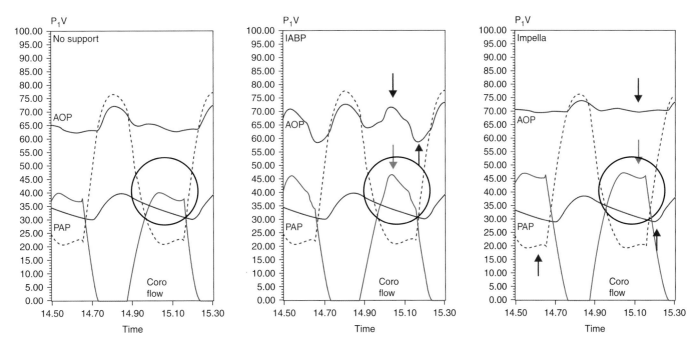

FIGURE 23–9. Hemodynamic simulator-predicted coronary flow enhancement (blue line) with Impella (right) compared to baseline (left) and IABP (center). (Reprinted with permission from Hunziker et al. Personal communication, 2006.)

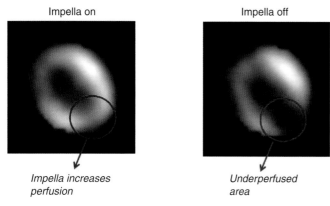

Impella on   Impella off

Impella increases perfusion   *Underperfused area*

FIGURE 23–10. Improvement in myocardial perfusion with Impella support (technetium-99m sestamibi imaging). (Reprinted with permission from Aqel et al.[35])

patients, reporting a significant correlation between the level of Impella 2.5 support and the hyperemic coronary flow velocity. Additionally, Aqel et al[35] used technetium-99m sestamibi myocardial perfusion imaging to demonstrate the effects of Impella support on the microcirculation (Fig. 23–10). In this case study of a patient with triple-vessel disease, prophylactic

Impella support was used during PCI of the primary left anterior descending artery stenosis. Secondary stenoses remained untreated. Technetium-99m sestamibi perfusion imaging was performed after revascularization while remaining on Impella support (see Fig. 23–10A) and then again after removal of the Impella device (see Fig. 23–10B). Comparison of these images illuminates an area of focal hypoperfusion after removal of the Impella that had remained adequately perfused while on Impella support. One explanation of this is that Impella support augmented the blood flow through the collateral pathways supplying this area of the myocardium. This explanation is consistent with the observations of the Remmelink study that reported increased intracoronary pressure and decreased microvascular resistance while on Impella support, both of which will result in increased collateral circulation.

■ VENTRICULAR UNLOADING: DECREASING O_2 DEMAND

Ventricular unloading is often characterized by the PV loop (Fig. 23–11). The PV loop depicts the dynamics of the ventricular pressure and volume during one complete cardiac cycle. At point A, the heart begins its contraction and pressure builds up rapidly prior to any change in volume. At point B, the aortic valve opens and a volume of blood is ejected into

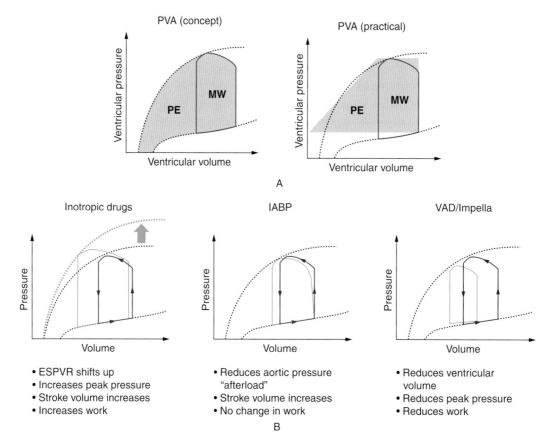

FIGURE 23–11. A. Pressure-volume (PV) loop of the cardiac cycle in baseline and unloaded conditions. **B.** PV loop changes with treatment. (Reproduced with permission from Weber DM, Raess DH, Henriques JPS, Siess T, eds. Principles of Impella cardiac support: the evolution of cardiac support technology toward the ideal assist device. Supplement to *Cardiac Interventions Today. Principles of Hemodynamics.* August/September 2009. Figs. 18 and 19. Sponsored by Abiomed, Inc.)

the ascending aorta. Beyond point B, the pressure continues to build to its maximum until; at point C, the aortic valve closes and the pressure falls rapidly to point D, where the mitral valve opens and the chamber begins filling with a new volume of blood for the next heart cycle. The PV loop is bounded below by the end-diastolic pressure-volume (PV) relationship curve and on top by the end-systolic PV relationship curve. Because one expression of mechanical work is the product of pressure and volume, the area circumscribed by the PV loop is equal to the mechanical work (sometimes called the "external" work) of the heart during each cycle. There are a variety of ways to affect the PV loop, depending on what type of treatment or assist device is applied. Inotropic drugs, for example, have the effect of shifting the end-systolic PV relationship up, thereby increasing the peak pressure and stroke volume. This increases the area of the PV loop and increases the overall work of the muscle. An IABP has the effect of reducing the pressure at which the aortic valve opens (point B on the PV loop), also known as the *afterload*, but that often comes with an increased overall stroke volume. This offsets the pressure reduction, leaving little or no change in the overall area of the PV loop. Note also that because of their limited improvement in cardiac output, IABPs are most often used in conjunction with inotropic drugs, offsetting any IABP-induced reduction in afterload with the significant increase in mechanical work caused by the inotropes. Active unloading devices, such as traditional ventricular assist devices and Impella, pull blood from the ventricle, which reduces the overall filling volume and pressure. According to the Frank-Starling curve,[36] this reduction in filling volume and pressure leads to a reduction in stroke volume (if the heart fills less, it expands less and reduces its subsequent stroke output). In terms of the PV loop, this is expressed as a reduction in its overall area, corresponding to a reduction in its mechanical work, and is one aspect of unloading. The ultimate goal of unloading with an assist device is to reduce the inherent oxygen demand of the myocardium. Reducing oxygen demand places the muscle in a more protective state in the event of an ischemic insult (eg, AMI, PCI, coronary dissection). The amount of mechanical or kinetic work the muscle produces is one component that determines its oxygen demand, but, as discussed by a number of authors,[10,30,37] an additional determiner of myocardial oxygen demand is the amount of potential energy in the myocardium. The myocardial potential energy is related to the amount of wall tension that is present in the muscle, which has been shown to be highly correlated with myocardial oxygen demand.[30-33] As discussed previously, maximum wall tension is related to the EDP and EDV through the Law of LaPlace, and reductions in these parameters lead to reduced microvascular resistance and increased myocardial perfusion. It is important to note that in addition to this perfusion effect (increasing myocardial oxygen supply), Impella-induced reductions in EDP, EDV, and wall tension (T) lead to reduced myocardial oxygen demand: The EDP and EDV, which comprise point A on the PV loop (see Fig. 23–17), are significant determiners of the myocardial oxygen balance because, through their relationship to wall tension, they impact both sides of the demand-supply equation. Myocardial oxygen demand has, therefore, two components: mechanical

work and potential energy (wall tension). Conceptually, the sum of the MW and PE is known as the *pressure-volume area* (PVA) and is proportional to the total myocardial oxygen demand. In order to practically estimate the sum of these areas, Sauren and others have employed a simple expression of the PVA as a method of characterizing the total oxygen demand based on simple hemodynamic points on the PV loop: in which ESV is the end-systolic volume and peak is the maximum pressure. In summary, ventricular unloading is ultimately reducing myocardial oxygen demand. It is possible to characterize the oxygen demand of the myocardium in terms of hemodynamic variables, and the PV loop provides a convenient expression of hemodynamics. In particular, the position of the PV loop in the PV space, as well as the area circumscribed by it, correlates well with myocardial oxygen demand, and the unloading impact of a cardiac assist device is expressed in the PV loop by a leftward shift in its position and an overall reduction in its area. Valgimigli et al[21] observed these types of Impella-induced changes in the PV loop in the clinical realm. It is important to note that although some investigators have also reported on the combined hemodynamic impact of the simultaneous use of the Impella and the IABP, this practice is not recommended due to uncertainties in device interactions that have yet to be characterized. Going beyond the demonstration of unloading in the PV loop, Meyns et al[23] further demonstrated a reduction in myocardial oxygen demand in an Impella-supported acute animal model (Fig. 23–12A), and that the reduction in oxygen demand correlates with a reduction in eventual infarct size (Fig. 23–12B).

◼ IMPROVING OXYGEN DEMAND-SUPPLY RATIO

From the perspective of the myocardium, the net desired impact of the Impella cardiac assist device is, therefore, to decrease myocardial oxygen demand (unload) and to augment oxygen supply through an increase in coronary flow. Reesink et al[11] investigated this combined effect in an acute animal model. Considering only the kinetic work component of oxygen demand, they characterized the demand supply balance as the ratio of the mechanical work to the coronary flow (MW [mechanical work]/QCOR [myocardial blood flow]) and demonstrated a 36% improvement with Impella compared to an 18% improvement with the IABP. These results also illustrated a dependence of this difference on the baseline (presupport), or native cardiac output, with the Impella benefit more pronounced at lower native cardiac output. Sauren et al[10] also investigated the net change in this oxygen demand-supply ratio, this time, however, taking into account the potential energy component. Characterizing the ratio using the pressure-volume area and the coronary flow (PVA/QCOR), they reported a 69% improvement with Impella compared to a 15% improvement with IABP alone. It is important to note that both of these studies employed an Impella 5.0 device operating at 3.8 and 4.2 L/min, respectively.

CLINICAL EXPERIENCE

The first clinical activity in the United States with Impella 2.5 was in the context of the PROTECT I (A Prospective Feasibility Trial Investigating the Use of the Impella 2.5 System in Patients

Impact of unloading on O$_2$ demand and infarct size

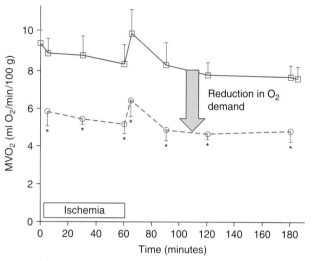

(a) Ventricular unloading during ischemia & reperfusion decreases O$_2$ demand

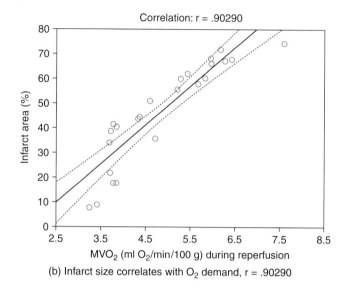

(b) Infarct size correlates with O$_2$ demand, r = .90290

A

Reduction in infarct size with impella

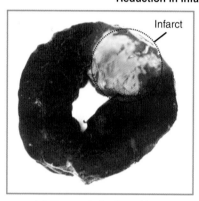

(a) Revascularization without impella support

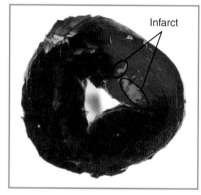

(b) Revascularization with impella support

B

FIGURE 23–12. A. Impact of unloading on O$_2$ demand and infarct size. Ventricular unloading during ischemia and reperfusion decreases O$_2$ demand (a). Infarct size correlates with O$_2$ demand (r = 0.90290) (b). *Animals supported with Impella 5.0 device. (Adapted with permission from Meyns et al.[23] Copyright © Elsevier.) **B.** Impella 5.0 device. Reduction in infarct size with Impella. Revascularization without Impella support (a). Rearization with Impella support (b). (Adapted with permission from Meyns et al.[23] Copyright © Elsevier.)

Undergoing High-Risk Percutaneous Coronary Intervention) clinical trial. PROTECT I (20 patients) established the safety and feasibility of Impella 2.5 for a HR-PCI patient population and was completed in 2007.[29] Before PROTECT I, there was already extensive use of Impella in Europe. In addition to use in the context of clinical trials in the United States, Impella 2.5 was granted FDA clearance under 510(k) in June 2008 for up to 6 hours of partial circulatory support. Since this clearance, more than 300 institutions have adopted the 2.5, and it has been used to support more than 1000 patients. Thus far, physicians have decided to treat the HR-PCI population (64% of Impella general use), followed by hemodynamically unstable AMI patients (16% of Impella general use). Other patient groups that physicians have decided (on a case-by-case basis) could potentially benefit from the Impella include cardiomyopathy with acute decompensation, postcardiotomy shock,

off-pump coronary artery bypass graft surgery, transplant rejection, and support for high-risk electrophysiology (EP) ablation procedures.[38] Outside of the catheterization laboratory, the surgical experience with Impella has predominantly been in Europe and Canada, and has mostly involved the Impella 5.0 and LD (5-L devices). The Impella 5.0 devices were granted 510(k) clearance in the United States in April 2009. Before this clearance, North American surgeons had been using the Impella 2.5 device in greater numbers than their European counterparts. These applications have also been encouraging and are similar to the Canadian experience recently reported by Cheung et al.[39] As with all devices, partial circulatory support (< 5.0 L/min) must be escalated to full-support and/or biventricular devices should the clinical situation warrant. Guidelines for monitoring adequacy

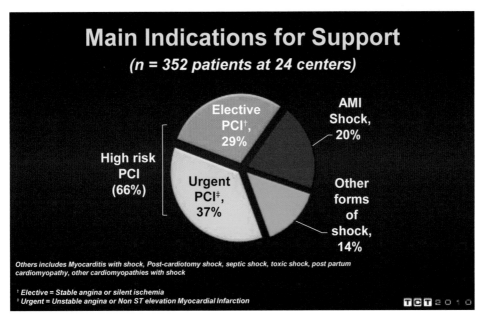

FIGURE 23–13. Indications for support in the USpella registry. (Reproduced with permission from Impella 2.5: From High Risk PCI to Shock [as presented at Transcatheter Cardiovascular Therapeutics, 2010].)

of circulatory support include freedom from large-dose inotropic administration, maintenance of normal acid-base status (lactate levels), evidence of continued systemic end-organ function, and overall survival. With the success of the PROTECT I trial in the United States, two pivotal trials have been initiated and are ongoing in parallel with Impella general use under the 510(k) clearance. PROTECT II and RECOVER II are randomized studies comparing Impella 2.5 to IABP in HR-PCI and in AMI with hemodynamic compromise, respectively. Note that favorable reimbursement exists for hospitals using Impella, and both clinical trials receive reimbursement as class II-B trials. An additional study in Europe is evaluating Impella in post-MI patients compared to IABP treatment (IMPRESS in ST-segment elevation myocardial infarction).

■ USPELLA REGISTRY

USpella is a prospective registry for Impella 2.5 patients in North America. Data are obtained after IRB submission and include all comers at included sites. Thus far, 64 centers with more than four Impella cases have been invited with 24 centers now reporting 352 patients. There is a Clinical Events Committee (CEC) to adjudicate all of the events as well as a core laboratory used to correlate angiographic success and calculation of Syntax score. The CEC adjudicated events per the FDA Impella 2.5 trial definitions.

The latest report of the data was made at the Transcatheter Cardiovascular Therapeutics (TCT) Conference by Dr William O'Neill. HR-PCI now represents 66% of the use with urgent PCI (37%) (unstable angina or non–ST segment elevation MI) and 29% were cases used during HR elective PCI. It is interesting to note that 20% of the use was acute myocardial infarction shock (AMI-shock), which was increased from 17% in an earlier harvest. The remaining 14% were used in other forms of shock such

as myocarditis, postcardiotomy shock, and a variety of other cardiomyopathies with shock (Fig. 23–13).

HIGH-RISK PCI

The report at TCT was divided primarily into two major categories: HR-PCI and AMI-shock. In the HR-PCI group, nonemergent PCI were reported, excluding patients in shock or in need of inotropes. Inclusion criteria were functional (low EF) or anatomical (left main, three vessel disease, last remaining conduit) risk with prophylactic pump placement in either elective stable patients or urgent unstable angina or non-STEMI. The primary Endpoint was major adverse cardiac events (MACE) at 30 days, and currently the longest follow-up was up to 1 year.

The HR-PCI patient demographics are depicted in Fig. 23–14. Most notable is the Syntax score of 36 ± 15 and an STS (Society of Thoracic Surgeons) score of 5.6 ± 6.5. In Fig. 23–15, the baseline patient morbidity for the HR-PCI group is depicted with 66% of the patients exhibiting either New York Heart Association (NYHA) class IV (28%) or class III (38%) symptoms. Fifty-four percent of the patients had been declined coronary artery bypass graft (CABG) surgery based on excessive mortality risk. Procedural data showed that 49% had three or more segments revascularized with 2.0 stents per patient with 13.4% of patients undergoing rotational atherectomy with 2.0 rotoblated segments per patient. Left ventricular ejection fraction (LVEF) gain was 17% (30 ± 15-35 ± 15) which was consistent with other previous studies and is likely be related to completeness of revascularization.[29,17] Thirty-day MACE as adjudicated by the independent CEC was 8.2% with nine deaths (3.9%), three MI (1.3%), revascularization at 0.9% (n = 2), and 1 CVA (0.4%). In summary, the HR-PCI cohort showed a 17% increase in LVEF post-supported PCI ($P < .05$). There was

High Risk PCI Demographics

(n = 231)

Patient Characteristics	Mean ± SD or %
Age (y)	70 ± 11
Gender (Male in %)	74%
Procedure (Elective vs Urgent)	45% vs 55%
LVEF (%)	30 ± 16
LVEF ≤ 35%	71%
Unprotected LM	51%
Unprotected LM or LPC	52%
Multivessel Disease	88%
Nb of Segments Treated	2.5 ± 1.2
STS Score	5.6 ± 6.5
Syntax Score	36 ± 15

TCT 2010

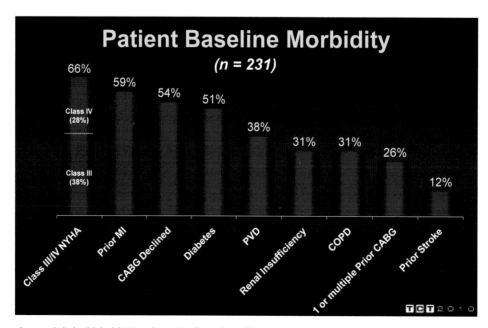

FIGURE 23–14. Demographics for high risk PCI cohort of USpella registry. (Reproduced with permission from Impella 2.5: From High Risk PCI to Shock [as presented at Transcatheter Cardiovascular Therapeutics, 2010].)

significant improvement in NYHA class (49% of patients) with a 61% reduction in NYHA class IV patients ($P < .05$). There was a 25% reduction in the implantable cardioverter defibrillator (ICD) target population leading to potential system-wide cost savings, and a low mortality and MACE event rate compared to HR-PCI literature.

ACUTE MYOCARDIAL INFARCTION SHOCK

The acute myocardial infarction shock (AMI-shock) group excluded patients with stable hemodynamics and other forms of shock without AMI. Shock was defined as systolic blood pressure (SBP) less than 90 for more than 30 minutes or need of inotropes to maintain SBP, or CI less than 2.2 L/min/m^2. In all cases the pump was placed emergently to restore hemodynamics. Survival was to discharge or 30 days. One of the biggest differences in the 2010 data harvest compared to 2009 was the increase in the patients having Impella placed prior to first balloon inflation (Fig. 23–16).[38] Now 33% of the patients had the Impella placed prior to PCI while in 2009 only 18% had achieved early support. Impella 2.5 significantly impacted CI from 1.9 ± 0.6 to 2.7 ± 0.9 L/min/m^2 ($P = .002$) while increasing

FIGURE 23–15. Patient characteristic for high risk PCI cohort USpella registry. (Reproduced with permission from Impella 2.5: From High Risk PCI to Shock [as presented at Transcatheter Cardiovascular Therapeutics, 2010].)

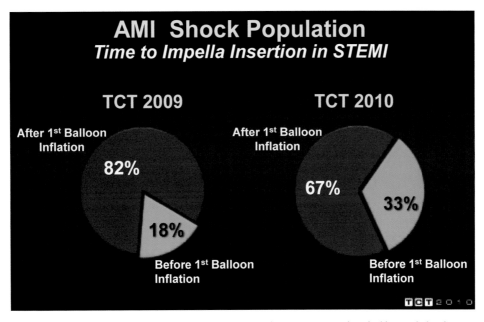

FIGURE 23–16. Variance in Impella insertion in AMI shock population from 2009 to late 2010. (Reproduced with permission from Impella 2.5: From High Risk PCI to Shock [as presented at Transcatheter Cardiovascular Therapeutics, 2010].)

mean arterial pressure 62 ± 17 to 92 ± 21 ($P = .0001$). More importantly, Cardiac power output (CPO) increased from 0.5 ± 0.2 W pre-Impella to 1.0 ± 0.2 W on Impella. Fincke et al found that in analyzing shock trial patients the CPO had the highest correlation with mortality in AMI shock patients.[40] Twenty patients[20] had Impella placed after an IABP was first used. Mean arterial pressure (MAP) improved 41% ($P < .001$) when the pre-Impella blood pressure was compared to the pressure with Impella on and running. Pressure increased from 59 ± 15 to 83 ± 17 with Impella. The most impressive difference between the

Impella before PCI and Impella after PCI group was the difference in the 30-day mortality with the pre-PCI group (n = 22) having a 23% and the post-PCI group (n = 34) having a 56% 30-day mortality ($P = .01$). The hemodynamic presentation of both groups was very similar and is shown in Fig. 23–17. The overall survival was 58% with an expected in-hospital survival based on the CPO predictor of less than 50%.[40] Three patients were bridged to bridge devices (7%) and one patient (3%) was transplanted directly from Impella 2.5. Ninety percent of survivors (37/41) recovered native heart function. Additionally, there

Timing of Impella Support vs Outcome

Baseline Characteristics	Impella ON "Pre-PCI" (n = 22)	Impella ON "Post-PCI" (n = 34)	P-value
Age (Median, range in years)	64 (53-84)	63 (19-83)	0.4
Cardiac index pre-impella (L/m2)	2.0 ± 0.2	2.0 ± 0.6	0.9
Heart rate pre-impella (beat/min)	73 ± 24	77 ± 26	0.6
MAP pre-impella (mm Hg)	54 ± 22	50 ± 17	0.4
LVEF pre-impella (%)	26 ± 11	26 ± 12	0.9
STEMI presentation (%)	60	80	0.2
Outcome			
30-day mortality	**23%**	**56%**	**0.01**

FIGURE 23–17. Timing of Impella support versus outcome, 2010. (Reproduced with permission from Impella 2.5: From High Risk PCI to Shock [as presented at Transcatheter Cardiovascular Therapeutics, 2010].)

was a 19% improvement in LVEF in patients who had EF measurements pre- and post-Impella support (n = 35). In summary, the latest USpella registry for AMI-shock patients demonstrated excellent hemodynamic support with Impella 2.5, significantly better than IABP. There was a 19% improvement in LVEF at discharge, with a significant reduction (59%) in mortality in the group that received Impella before PCI. The vast majority of survivors (90%) recovered native heart function and were discharged with their own heart.

CONCLUSION

Impella 2.5 is now available for widespread general use outside of the ongoing clinical trials and is being applied by treating physicians with growing frequency in HR-PCI, AMI, and other patient groups. It is the first catheter-based therapy of its kind available to cardiologists and has been well established in the literature to be hemodynamically superior to the IABP. Within the landscape of circulatory support, it is the only available device designed to safely and effectively support the natural transport of blood from the ventricle through the aortic valve to the aortic root, simultaneously improving systemic cardiac output, augmenting coronary flow (increasing myocardial oxygen supply), and unloading ventricular work (reducing myocardial oxygen consumption). Along with an established safety profile of low adverse events and independence from the detrimental effects of supplemental inotropic drugs, as well as an ease-of-use profile appropriate for both elective and emergent patient settings, Impella addresses the ideal criteria for circulatory support in the catheterization laboratory. In the HR-PCI study (PROTECT II), Impella support is expected to demonstrate the ability to provide stable hemodynamics during significant ischemic challenges, allow more time for balloon inflation and stent placement, and extend PCI therapy to patients who would otherwise be denied revascularization due to excessive surgical risk relative to existing treatment modes. In the AMI patient population, RECOVER II is expected to demonstrate the ability to restore stable hemodynamics, reduce infarct size to improve residual cardiac function, and reduce overall mortality from cardiogenic shock relative to existing treatment modes. In short, these randomized clinical trials are designed to demonstrate how the established hemodynamic superiority of Impella over the IABP translates to favorable outcomes in HR-PCI and AMI patient populations.

REFERENCES

1. Samuels LE, Kaufman MS, Thomas MP, et al. Pharmacological criteria for ventricular assist device insertion following postcardiotomy shock: experience with the Abiomed BVS system. *J Card Surg.* 1999;14:288-293.
2. Gibbon JH, Jr. Application of a mechanical heart and lung apparatus to cardiac surgery. *Minn Med.* 1954;37:171.
3. Kantrowitz A, Tjonneland S, Freed PS, et al. Initial clinical experience with intraaortic balloon pumping in cardiogenic shock. *JAMA.* 1986;203:135.
4. Stone GW, Marsalese D, Brodie BR, et al. A prospective, randomized evaluation of prophylactic intraaortic balloon counterpulsation in high-risk patients with acute myocardial infarction treated with primary angioplasty. *J Am Coll Cardiol.* 1997;29:1459-1467.
5. Sjauw KD, Engström AE, Vis MM, et al. A systematic review and meta-analysis of intra-aortic balloon pump therapy in ST-elevation myocardial infarction: should we change the guidelines? *Eur Heart J.* 2009;30:459-468.
6. Osentowski MK, Holt DW. Evaluating the efficacy of the intra-aortic balloon pump timing using the auto-timing mode with the Datascope CS100. *J Extra Corpor Technol.* 2007;39:87-90.
7. Schreuder JJ, Maisano F, Donelli A, et al. Beat-to-beat affects of intra-aortic balloon bump timing on LV performance on patients with low EF. *Ann Thorac Surg.* 2005;79:872-880.
8. Seyfarth M, Sibbing D, Bauer I, et al. A randomized clinical trial to evaluate the safety and efficacy of a percutaneous left ventricular assist device versus intra-aortic balloon pumping for treatment of cardiogenic shock caused by myocardial infarction. *J Am Coll Cardiol.* 2008;52:1584-1588.
9. Nanas JN, Moulopoulos SD. Counterpulsation: historical background, technical improvements, hemodynamic and metabolic effects. *Cardiology.* 1994;84:156-167.
10. Sauren LD, Accord RE, Hamzeh K, et al. Combined Impella and intra-aortic balloon pump support to improve both ventricular unloading and coronary blood flow for myocardial recovery: an experimental study. *Artif Organs.* 2007;31:839-842.
11. Reesink KD, Dekker AL, van Ommen V, et al. Miniature intracardiac assist device provides more effective cardiac unloading and circulatory support during severe left heart failure than intraaortic balloon pumping. *Chest.* 2004;126:896-902.
12. von Segesser LK. Cardiopulmonary support and extracorporeal membrane oxygenation for cardiac assist. Ann Thorac Surg. 1999;68:672-677.
13. Kolobow T, Rossi F, Borelli M, et al. Long-term closed chest partial and total cardiopulmonary bypass by peripheral cannulation for severe right and/or left ventricular failure, including ventricular fibrillation. *ASAIO Trans.* 1988;34:485.
14. Schreiber TL, Kodali UR, O'Neill WW, et al. Comparison of acute results of prophylactic intraaortic balloon pumping with cardiopulmonary support for percutaneous transluminal coronary angioplasty (PTCA). *Cathet Cardiovasc Diagn.* 1998;45:115-119.
15. Sweeney M. The Hemopump in 1997: a clinical, political, and marketing evolution. *Ann Thorac Surg.* 1999;68:761-763.
16. Henriques JP, Remmelink M, Baan J, Jr, et al. Safety and feasibility of elective high-risk percutaneous coronary intervention procedures with left ventricular support of the Impella Recover LP 2.5. *Am J Cardiol.* 2006;97:990-992.
17. Burzotta F, Paloscia L, Trani C, et al. Feasibility and long-term safety of elective Impella-assisted high-risk percutaneous coronary intervention: a pilot two-centre study. *J Cardiovasc Med.* 2008;9:1004-1010.
18. Strecker T, Fischlein T, Pfeiffer S. Impella Recover 100: successful perioperative support for off pump coronary artery bypass grafting surgery in a patient with end-stage ischemic cardiomyopathy. *J Cardiovasc Surg (Torino).* 2004;45:381-384.
19. Jurmann MJ, Siniawski H, Erb M, et al. Initial experience with miniature axial flow ventricular assist devices for postcardiotomy heart failure. *Ann Thorac Surg.* 2004;77:1642-1647.
20. Meyns B, Dens J, Sergeant P, et al. Initial experiences with the Impella device in patients with cardiogenic shock—Impella support for cardiogenic shock. *Thorac Cardiovasc Surg.* 2003;51:312-317.
21. Valgimigli M, Steendijk P, Sianos G, et al. Left ventricular unloading and concomitant total cardiac output increase by the use of percutaneous Impella Recover LP 2.5 assist device during high risk coronary intervention. *Cathet Cardiovasc Interv.* 2005;65:263-267.
22. Sjauw KD, Remmelink M, Baan J, Jr, et al. Left ventricular unloading in acute ST-segment elevation myocardial infarction patients is safe and feasible and provides acute and sustained left ventricular recovery. *J Am Coll Cardiol.* 2008;51:1044-1046.
23. Meyns B, Stolinski J, Leunens V, et al. Left ventricular support by catheter-mounted axial flow pump reduces infarct size. *J Am Coll Cardiol.* 2003; 41:1087-1095.
24. Vlasselaers D, Desmet M, Desmet L, et al. Ventricular unloading with a miniature axial flow pump in combination with extracorporeal membrane oxygenation. *Intensive Care Med.* 2006;32:329-333.
25. Siegenthaler MP, Brehm K, Strecker T, et al. The Impella Recover microaxial left ventricular assist device reduces mortality for postcardiotomy failure: a three-center experience. *J Thorac Cardiovasc Surg.* 2004;127:812-822.
26. Catena E, Barosi A, Milazzo F, et al. Three-dimensional echocardiographic assessment of a patient supported by intravascular blood pump Impella recover 100. *Echocardiography.* 2005;22:682-685.

27. Catena E, Milazzo F, Merli M, et al. Echocardiographic evaluation of patients receiving a new left ventricular assist device: the Impella recover 100. *Eur J Echocardiogr.* 2004;5:430-437.

28. Colombo T, Garatti A, Bruschi G, et al. First successful bridge to recovery with the Impella Recover 100 left ventricular assist device for fulminant acute myocarditis. *Ital Heart J.* 2003;4:642-645.

29. Dixon SR, Henriques JPS, Mauri L, et al. A prospective feasibility trial investigating the use of the Impella 2.5 system in patients undergoing high-risk percutaneous coronary intervention (The PROTECT I Trial): initial US experience. *J Am Coll Cardiol Interv.* 2009;2:91-96.

30. Suga H, Hayashi T, Shirahata M. Ventricular systolic pressure-volume area as predictor of cardiac oxygen consumption. *Am J Physiol.* 1981;240: H39-H44.

31. Suga H. Total mechanical energy of a ventricle model and cardiac oxygen consumption. *Am J Physiol.* 1979;236:H498-H505.

32. Sarnoff S, Braunwald G, Welch R, Jr. et al. Hemodynamic determinants of oxygen consumption of the heart with special reference to the tension-time index. Presented at the XXth International Physiological Congress, Brussels, August, 1956.

33. Braunwald G. Myocardial oxygen consumption: the quest for its determinants and some clinical fallout. *J Am Coll Cardiol.* 1999;34:1365-1368.

34. Remmelink M, Sjauw KD, Henriques JP, et al. Effects of left ventricular unloading by Impella Recover LP2.5 on coronary hemodynamics. *Cathet Cardiovasc Interv.* 2007;70:532-537.

35. Aqel RA, Hage FG, Iskandrian AE. Improvement of myocardial perfusion with a percutaneously inserted left ventricular assist device [published online ahead of print August 15, 2009]. *J Nucl Cardiol.*

36. Braunwald E, Ross J, Sonnenblick EH. Mechanisms of contraction of normal and failing heart. *N Engl J Med.* 1967;277:794.

37. Rodbard S, Williams CB, Rodbard D, et al. Myocardial tension and oxygen uptake. *Circ Res.* 1964;14:139-149.

38. Maini B. High-risk PCI with Impella 2.5: registry perspectives and an ongoing trial. Presented at the Transcatheter Cardiovascular Therapeutics (TCT) 2009, San Francisco, CA.

39. Cheung A, Higgins J, Kaan A, et al. First North American experience do with microaxial percutaneous LVAD for severe cardiogenic shock. *J Heart Lung Transplant.* In press.

40. Finke R, Hochman J, Lowe A, et al. Cardiac power is the strongest hemodynamic correlate of mortality in cardiogenic shock: a report from the SHOCK trial registry. *J Am Coll Cardiol.* 2004;44(2):304-308.

CHAPTER 24

THE TANDEMHEART SYSTEM: DEVICE DESCRIPTION AND CLINICAL RESULTS

Robert G. Svitek

TANDEMHEART DESCRIPTION

The TandemHeart System (CardiacAssist, Inc. Pittsburgh, Pennsylvania) is an extracorporeal circulatory assist device that drains blood from the left atrium (LA) and pumps it back into the femoral artery to bypass the left ventricle. The TandemHeart System (Fig. 24–1) has four major components: (1) an extracorporeal centrifugal pump (2) a 21-Fr transseptal cannula, (3) an arterial cannula, and (4) a microprocessor-based controller. The System can provide up to 5 L/min of blood flow percutaneously and is CE marked for 30 days and approved by the Food and Drug Administration (FDA) for use up to 6 hours.[1-4] The device has been used in over 2000 patients[5] and has undergone several clinical trials.[1,6-8]

The TandemHeart pump is a centrifugal blood pump that has a priming volume of 7 mL, weighs 280 g, and contains a hydrodynamic bearing to support the spinning impeller.[9] The pump has a motor chamber and a blood chamber that are separated by a polymeric seal (Fig. 24–2). The motor is a brushless direct current motor consisting of a laminated stack of stainless steel plates wound with copper wire embedded in a heat-dissipative epoxy. The rotor is centered in the stator, is spun by the motor through an electromagnetic coupling, and is attached directly to the impeller. Saline flows at 10 mL/h through the motor chamber and completely surrounds the rotor.[10] Lift pads in the lower housing of the motor chamber provide thrust forces to stabilize the rotor in the axial direction. The saline flows between a journal and the rotor toward the impeller to provide radial stability. The impeller shaft passes through the center of the seal, and the saline (heparinized with 90,000 U/L) flows around the impeller shaft-seal interface to flush the area to prevent thrombus formation. The impeller contains six blades and rotates between 3000 and 7500 rpm (revolutions per minute) to provide flow rates from 1 to 8 L/min, depending on the size of the cannulae.[9]

The pump is small enough to be surgically implanted in the chest cavity (formerly named the AB-180). In the AB-180 embodiment, the inflow cannula to the pump was inserted into the LA and a 10-mm thin-walled polytetrafluoroethylene (PTFE) graft connected the outflow port of the pump anastomosed to the aorta. The device underwent implantation in 17 patients for the treatment of postcardiotomy cardiogenic shock (CS), decompensated cardiomyopathy, viral myocarditis, and acute myocardial infarction (AMI) with hemodynamic instability. The pump was used for an average of 8 days with 58% of the patients weaned and 29% of the patients survived.[9] The pump and controller were then adapted for extracorporeal and percutaneous use (TandemHeart System) by incorporating the transseptal cannula for the pump inflow and a femoral arterial cannula for the pump outflow.

The transseptal cannula (Fig. 24–3) is made of a smooth polyurethane material and is wire-reinforced to prevent kinking. The insertable length is available in two sizes: 62 cm and 72 cm. The cannula tip distal to the wire-wound portion is 1.2 cm in length, and drainage of the LA is achieved through 14 side holes in addition to being open at the distal end. The tip contains three radiopaque marker disks that can be seen under fluoroscopy to instruct the user of the location of the cannula tip. The insertable portion is 21 Fr and contains centimeter markings for reference as to where the tip is in relationship to the insertion site. A suture wing is included at the proximal end of the cannula to help prevent cannula migration. The arterial cannula is similar in construction to the transseptal cannula and ranges in size from 12 to 17 Fr.

The Escort (Fig. 24–4) is the controller that drives the pump and supplies saline to the pump. The controller includes self-diagnostics and alarm features to ensure patient support without the need for constant operator surveillance. Built-in batteries allow for uninterrupted operation for 60 minutes during patient transport or in the event of an AC power failure. The controller has dual redundant motor control units. In the event of a catastrophic failure of the controller hardware, the controller will automatically switch to an emergency backup mode. Although the system display screen and monitoring functions may not be functional, basic pump operation such as pump start and pump speed control will continue to function. A built-in pressure transducer measures the operating pressure of the infusion system. Alarms are linked to changes in the infusion system operating pressure to alert the user of a problem with the delivery of saline to the pump. The air bubble detector monitors for air in the infusion system. The Escort weighs 21 lb and can be mounted to an IV pole to facilitate transportation.

IMPLANTATION PROCEDURE

The TandemHeart system can be inserted percutaneously in the catheterization laboratory through standard insertion techniques. The femoral vein is accessed for transseptal puncture, which is performed under fluoroscopic guidance using the Brockenbrough needle and a Mullins sheath, as is done during atrial fibrillation ablations.[11] Once the puncture is made in the fossa ovalis, heparin is given to achieve a target activated clotting time (ACT) of more than 300 seconds before inserting the cannula. After confirming the position of the Mullins sheath in the LA, a stiff wire (Inoue Wire TRG-25175, Toray International,

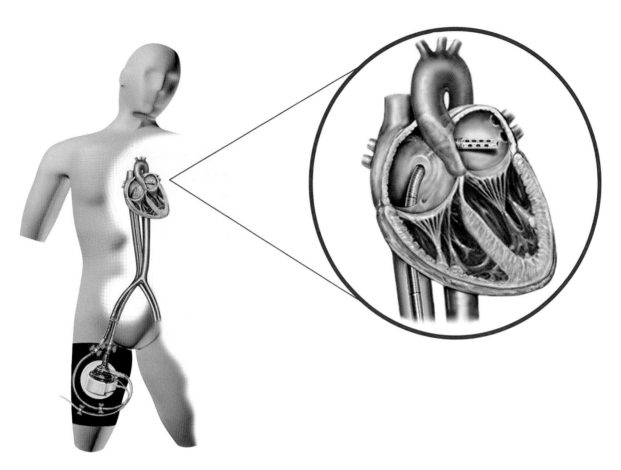

FIGURE 24–1. TandemHeart System including the 21-Fr transseptal venous cannula, the extracorporeal centrifugal pump, and the arterial cannula. Blood is withdrawn from the left atrium and pumped into the femoral artery to bypass the left ventricle. (Reproduced with permission from CardiacAssist, Inc.)

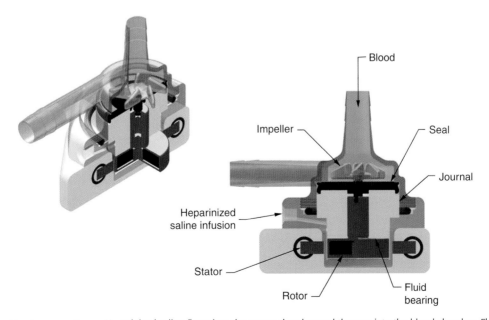

FIGURE 24–2. TandemHeart pump cutaway. Heparinized saline flows into the motor chamber and then up into the blood chamber. Fluid forces in the lower housing act stabilize the rotating impeller axially, and fluid forces in the journal stabilize the impeller radially. (Reproduced with permission from CardiacAssist, Inc.)

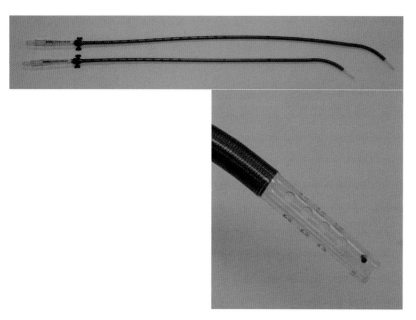

FIGURE 24–3. The TandemHeart transseptal cannula comes in two sizes with insertable lengths of 62 and 72 cm. The cannula features a wire-wound construction for kink resistance, and radiopaque marker discs at the tip to aid in visualization of the tip location in the left atrium under fluoroscopy. (Reproduced with permission from CardiacAssist, Inc.)

Houston, TX) is placed into the LA and the Mullins sheath is exchanged for the TandemHeart 14-Fr/21-Fr two-stage dilator. The dilator increases the septum puncture site diameter and enables the 21-Fr transseptal cannula to be inserted into the LA. The cannula tip contains three radiopaque marker disks that can be viewed under fluoroscopy to confirm that the position

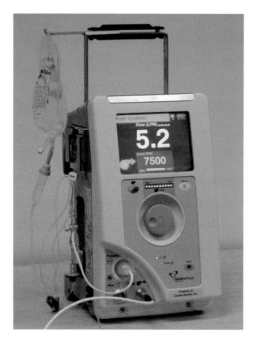

FIGURE 24–4. The TandemHeart Escort is a microprocessor-based controller that powers the pump and has built-in alarms and diagnostics such as flow measurement that help assess pump function. (Reproduced with permission from CardiacAssist, Inc.)

of the cannula tip is in the LA. Transesophageal echocardiography has also been used to help with the insertion and cannula tip placement.[12] The end of the cannula outside of the patient is sutured to the thigh to help prevent cannula dislodgement. Color Doppler has been used to visualize flow through the holes of the cannula tip to verify correct placement.[12]

The arterial cannula is placed in the femoral artery with the distal end sitting above the aortic bifurcation and is also sutured to the thigh to prevent cannula migration or dislodgement. Prior to arterial cannula insertion, the patients should be subjected to a femoral artery angiogram using a 4-Fr arterial sheath dilator before upsizing to a larger French arterial sheath to ensure peripheral vascular disease will not prevent insertion. If the artery is greater than 5 mm, Perclose devices can be deployed to assist in achieving hemostasis following arterial cannula removal.[13] Other preclosure devices have also been used to reduce arterial complications during cannula removal.[14] Additional manual compression can be employed when needed. In some patients the femoral artery is too small or too calcified for insertion of the standard cannula. Therefore, a graft can be sewn onto the femoral artery and connected to the outflow of the pump with a connector. Busch et al describe the procedure where they use a partial occlusion clamp to sew an 8-mm reinforced GORE-TEX graft to the femoral artery in an end-to-side fashion using 5-0 polypropylene sutures.[15] Once the transseptal and arterial cannulae are in place, the pump and cannulae are de-aired and connected via a wet-to-wet connection to remove all air from the circuit. The pump is then connected to the TandemHeart controller, and its speed is adjusted to provide the desired level of support.

UNIQUE INSERTION PROCEDURES AND PATIENT MANAGEMENT OF THE TANDEMHEART SYSTEM

The transseptal cannula can also be inserted surgically allowing the chest to be closed for the device to be removed percutaneously following support.[16,17] The surgical cannulation uses an "open transseptal" technique when a sternotomy has already been performed. The patient is placed on cardiopulmonary bypass (CPB) through bicaval cannulation. The transseptal cannula is inserted into the femoral vein, and the tip is brought into the right atrium (RA) prior to insertion of the inferior vena cava (IVC) cannula. Placing a tourniquet around the IVC ensures adequate occlusion of blood around the CPB and TandemHeart cannulae, which are adjacent to each other. The RA is opened through the appendage, a stab wound is placed through the fossa ovalis with a scalpel, and the tip of the cannula is placed across the septum into the LA by direct visualization. The patient can then be weaned off of bypass, the atrium de-aired, and the patient placed on TandemHeart support. Surgical cannulation of the LA has also been accomplished by placing the cannula through the right superior pulmonary vein into the LA.[17] For failure to wean patients, the IVC cannula is clamped, the snare around the IVC cannula is released, and the transseptal cannula is threaded into the RA. A small incision is made in the atrial septum and the transseptal cannula tip is pushed across. The RA is closed and CPB can be resumed or weaned as TandemHeart flows are increased.

The TandemHeart System has also been placed in the axillary artery and vein to allow for patient mobility.[18] The right axillary artery and vein were exposed in a right thoracotomy. An 8-mm Dacron graft (Hemashield; Boston Scientific, Natick, MA) was sutured in an end-to-side fashion to the axillary artery using 5-0 polypropylene. A wire-reinforced arterial cannula was then inserted through the graft to a point 1 cm close to the anastomosis and secured with silk ties, both within the wound and outside the skin. The pump inflow cannula was tunneled through the axillary vein and into the LA through direct visualization via a right atriotomy. The advantage of the axilloaxillary approach is that it avoids the risk of lower limb vascular complications, avoids infection complications of the groin, and enables the patient to sit in bed at a 45-degree angle.

Bleeding can be an issue with circulatory assist devices.[19-24] For patients with heparin-induced thrombocytopenia (HIT), type II Argatroban has been used successfully with the TandemHeart. Before transseptal cannula insertion, the patient was given a bolus of 3500 μg of Argatroban and during support the Argatroban infusion rate was titrated to maintain an activated partial thromboplastin time (aPTT) at or near 2.5 times normal. A dosage of 7000 μg of Argatroban was used in the 1 L of saline infusate[25] to prevent thrombus and bleeding complications. For non-HIT patients, systemic heparin is given to maintain ACTs of 180 to 220 seconds or partial thromboplastin time (PTT) of 65 to 80 seconds.

TANDEMHEART SYSTEM CLINICAL DATA

Left atrial to femoral artery bypass was first attempted in 1962 and has been investigated by several groups since that time.[26-34] The TandemHeart System was evaluated for the reversal of CS following AMI in 18 patients. The mean flow rate of blood was 3.2 ± 0.6 L/min. The cardiac index (CI) improved from 1.7 ± 0.3 L/min/m^2 at baseline to 2.4 ± 0.6 L/min/m^2 while on support ($P < 0.001$). Mean blood pressure increased from 63 ± 8 to 80 ± 9 mm Hg ($P < 0.001$) and pulmonary capillary wedge pressure (PCWP) decreased from 21 ± 4 to 14 ± 4 mm Hg ($P < 0.001$). The survival rate was 56%.[7] The conclusion of the study was that the TandemHeart could be rapidly deployed to potentially aid in reverting CS.

A randomized follow-up study was conducted by Thiele to compare the use of the intra-aortic balloon pump (IABP) to the TandemHeart for patients with an AMI complicated by CS.[8] The inclusion criteria included the presence of shock complicating AMI and the intention to revascularize the infarcted artery by percutaneous coronary intervention (PCI) as the first-line treatment option. CS was defined as (1) persistent systolic blood pressure less than 90 mm Hg or vasopressors required to maintain blood pressure greater than 90 mm Hg; (2) evidence of end organ failure (eg, urine output < 30 mL/h, cold skin and extremities, and serum lactate > 2 mmol/L); (3) evidence of elevated left ventricular filling pressures PCWP greater than 15 mm Hg; (4) CI less than 2.1 L/min/m^2. Exclusion criteria were age greater than 75 years, mechanical complications of AMI, duration of CS longer than >12 hours, right heart failure, sepsis, significant aortic regurgitation, severe cerebral damage, resuscitation longer than 30 minutes, severe peripheral vascular disease, and other diseases with reduced life expectancy. Twenty patients were enrolled in the IABP arm, and 21 patients were enrolled in the TandemHeart arm. The primary outcome measure of cardiac power index (CPI) was improved more effectively with the TandemHeart from 0.22 W/m^2 preimplant to 0.37 W/m^2 postimplant compared to the balloon pump which only increased the CPI from 0.22 to 0.28 W/m^2 ($P = .004$). The study was not powered to detect differences in mortality between the two groups, and 30-day mortality was similar (IABP 45% vs VAD 43% $P = .86$). Complications such as bleeding and leg ischemia were higher for the TandemHeart group.

In the United States, the TandemHeart was evaluated for safety in a feasibility study consisting of 13 patients with CS from five centers.[6] The enrollment criteria were broader than those of Thiele in that CS was secondary to AMI (n = 8), decompensated idiopathic cardiomyopathy (n = 1), decompensated ischemic cardiomyopathy (n = 1), postcardiotomy syndrome (n = 2), and high-risk intervention (n = 1). As seen in the previous studies, hemodynamic variables including CI, MAP, and PCWP were improved following initiation of TandemHeart support. Survival rate was 54% in this high-risk group of patients.

A randomized multicenter trial was then initiated to compare the TandemHeart to the IABP for patients presenting within 24 hours of developing CS.[1] The primary objective was to test whether the TandemHeart device provided superior hemodynamic benefits compared with the IABP in patients with medically refractory CS. The secondary objective was to compare survival 30 days after randomization. Patients who had a balloon pump and still met the criteria for CS were eligible for the trial. Forty-two patients were enrolled at 12 centers. Of the 42 patients, 26 were diagnosed with AMI, 3 had coronary artery bypass graft (CABG), and 1 underwent a left ventricular assist device (LVAD) implant. Most of the remaining patients had decompensated chronic heart failure. Compared to the IABP, patients with the TandemHeart had significantly greater increases in CI and greater decreases in PCWP. An independent data safety monitoring board (DSMB) reviewed the data and concluded that the hemodynamic effects of the TandemHeart group were superior to those of IABP group and that no definitive conclusion regarding mortality was achievable. Therefore, the study was halted.[1] In a summary of several technologies for treating AMI complicated by CS, Garatti et al cited the TandemHeart to have the highest wean and highest survival rate of 75% and 58%, respectively.[35] Bleeding remained the leading complication of the TandemHeart, and no significant left-to-right shunt has been observed following removal of the transseptal cannula.[36] The small sample sizes in the trial prevented a statistically significant mortality benefit; however, different subgroups of CS patients have been shown to benefit from the TandemHeart more than others.[37-41]

Since the clinical trials, the TandemHeart has been used during cardiac procedures other than patients with CS. Tanaka et al described the use of the TandemHeart on patients turned down by surgery for aortic valvuloplasty.[42] Seven patients underwent insertion of the TandemHeart prior to valvuloplasty and were compared to four patients who had the valvuloplasty without TandemHeart support. The patients with the TandemHeart were able to have to balloon inflated for 37 ± 10 seconds compared to 11 ± 3 seconds for the patients not on TandemHeart. All seven TandemHeart patients survived to at least 30 days whereas only two of the four non-TandemHeart patients survived to 30 days. Rajdev et al used the device to treat a 58-year-old man during an aortic valvuloplasty.[43,44] The patient had a left ventricular ejection fraction of 10%, mitral regurgitation, aortic stenosis, pulmonary artery hypertension, and New York Heart Association (NYHA) class III-IV symptoms of heart failure. He also had triple vessel disease and had been considered too high risk for surgery. The TandemHeart was inserted and the speed adjusted to provide a flow rate of 2.5 L/min. The balloon aortic valvuloplasty was performed, the TandemHeart removed, and the patient was discharged the following day. The TandemHeart has been shown to be effective at several other institutions for assisting with valvuloplasty particularly in patients who have been turned down for surgery.[4,13,42]

CONCLUSION

The TandemHeart System has demonstrated the feasibility of a left atrial to femoral artery bypass circuit. Clinical trials in Europe and the United States provided evidence that the TandemHeart can increase CI, MAP, and decrease PCWP which may be beneficial for patients with depressed cardiac function. Future improvements to the cannula and pump may reduce complications such as bleeding and increase the utility of the device.[45,46]

REFERENCES

1. Burkhoff D, Cohen H, Brunckhorst C, O'Neill WW; TandemHeart Investigators Group. A randomized multicenter clinical study to evaluate the safety and efficacy of the TandemHeart percutaneous ventricular assist device versus conventional therapy with intraaortic balloon pumping for treatment of cardiogenic shock. *Am Heart J.* 2006;152(3):469 e1-e8.
2. Kar B, Forrester M, Gemmato C, et al. Use of the TandemHeart percutaneous ventricular assist device to support patients undergoing high-risk percutaneous coronary intervention. *J Invasive Cardiol.* 2006;18(3):93-96.
3. Ramcharitar S, Vaina S, Serruys PW, Sianos G. Treatment of a distal left main trifurcation supported by the TandemHeart left ventricular assist device. *Hellenic J Cardiol.* 2007;48(2):110-114.
4. Vranckx P, Foley DP, de Feijter PJ, Vos J, Smits P, Serruys PW. Clinical introduction of the TandemHeart, a percutaneous left ventricular assist device, for circulatory support during high-risk percutaneous coronary intervention. *Int J Cardiovasc Intervent.* 2003;5(1):35-39.
5. *Press Release dated April 7, 2010.* www.cardiacassist.com, 2010.
6. Burkhoff D, O'Neill W, Brunckhorst C, Letts D, Lasorda D, Cohen HA. Feasibility study of the use of the TandemHeart percutaneous ventricular assist device for treatment of cardiogenic shock. *Catheter Cardiovasc Interv.* 2006;68(2):211-217.
7. Thiele H, Lauer B, Hambrecht R, Boudriot E, Cohen HA, Schuler G. Reversal of cardiogenic shock by percutaneous left atrial-to-femoral arterial bypass assistance. *Circulation.* 2001;104(24):2917-2922.
8. Thiele H, Sick P, Boudriot E, et al. Randomized comparison of intra-aortic balloon support with a percutaneous left ventricular assist device in patients with revascularized acute myocardial infarction complicated by cardiogenic shock. *Eur Heart J.* 2005;26(13):1276-1283.
9. Magovern JA, Sussman MJ, Goldstein AH, Szydlowski GW, Savage EB, Westaby S. Clinical results with the AB-180 left ventricular assist device. *Ann Thorac Surg.* 2001;71(3 Suppl):S121-S124; discussion S144-S126.
10. Goldstein AH, Pacella JJ, Trumble DR, Clark RE. Development of an implantable centrifugal blood pump. *ASAIO J.* 1992;38(3):M362-M365.
11. Mitchell-Heggs L, Lellouche N, Deal L, et al. Transseptal puncture using minimally invasive echocardiography during atrial fibrillation ablation. *Europace.* 2010;12(10):1435-1438.
12. Kooshkabadi M, Kalogeropoulos A, Babaliaros VC, Lerakis S. Transesophageal guided left atrial positioning of a percutaneous ventricular assist device. *Eur J Echocardiogr.* 2008;9(1):175-177.
13. Rajdev S, Krishnan P, Irani A, et al. Clinical application of prophylactic percutaneous left ventricular assist device (TandemHeart) in high-risk percutaneous coronary intervention using an arterial preclosure technique: single-center experience. *J Invasive Cardiol.* 2008;20(2):67-72.
14. Gimelli G, Wolff MR. Hemodynamically supported percutaneous coronary revascularization improves left ventricular function in patients with ischemic dilated cardiomyopathy at very high risk for surgery: a single-center experience. *J Invasive Cardiol.* 2008;20(12):642-646.
15. Busch J, Torre-Amione G, Noon GP, Loebe M. TandemHeart insertion via a femoral arterial GORE-TEX graft conduit in a high-risk patient. *Tex Heart Inst J.* 2008;35(4):462-465.
16. Gregoric ID, Bruckner BA, Jacob L, et al. Techniques and complications of TandemHeart ventricular assist device insertion during cardiac procedures. *ASAIO J.* 2009;55(3):251-254.
17. Pitsis AA, Visouli AN, Burkhoff D, et al. Feasibility study of a temporary percutaneous left ventricular assist device in cardiac surgery. *Ann Thorac Surg.* 2007;84(6):1993-1999.
18. Anyanwu AC, Fischer GW, Kalman J, Plotkina I, Pinney S, Adams DH. Preemptive axillo-axillary placement of percutaneous transseptal ventricular assist device to facilitate high-risk reoperative cardiac surgery. *Ann Thorac Surg.* 2010;89(6):2053-2055.
19. Kogan A, Berman M, Kassif Y, et al. Use of recombinant factor VII to control bleeding in a patient supported by right ventricular assist device after heart transplantation. *J Heart Lung Transplant.* 2005;24(3):347-349.
20. Letsou GV, Shah N, Gregoric ID, Myers TJ, Delgado R, Frazier OH. Gastrointestinal bleeding from arteriovenous malformations in patients supported by the Jarvik 2000 axial-flow left ventricular assist device. *J Heart Lung Transplant.* 2005;24(1):105-109.
21. Flynn JD, Camp PC Jr, Jahania MS, Ramaiah C, Akers WS. Successful treatment of refractory bleeding after bridging from acute to chronic left ventricular assist device support with recombinant activated factor VII. *ASAIO J.* 2004;50(5):519-521.
22. Potapov EV, Pasic M, Bauer M, Hetzer R. Activated recombinant factor VII for control of diffuse bleeding after implantation of ventricular assist device. *Ann Thorac Surg.* 2002;74(6):2182-2183.
23. Schmid C, Scheld HH, Hammel D. Control of perigraft bleeding during ventricular assist device implantation. *Ann Thorac Surg.* 2000;69(3):958-959.
24. Himmelreich G, Ullmann H, Riess H, et al. Pathophysiologic role of contact activation in bleeding followed by thromboembolic complications after implantation of a ventricular assist device. *ASAIO J.* 1995;41(3):M790-M794.
25. Webb DP, Warhoover MT, Eagle SS, Greelish JP, Zhao DX, Byrne JG. Argatroban in short-term percutaneous ventricular assist subsequent to heparin-induced thrombocytopenia. *J Extra Corpor Technol.* 2008;40(2):130-134.
26. Laschinger JC, Grossi EA, Cunningham JN Jr, et al. Adjunctive left ventricular unloading during myocardial reperfusion plays a major role in minimizing myocardial infarct size. *J Thorac Cardiovasc Surg.* 1985;90(1):80-85.

27. Fonger J, Zhou Y, Matsuura H, Aldea GS, Shemin RJ. Enhanced preservation of acutely ischemic myocardium with transseptal left ventricular assist. *Ann Thorac Surg.* 1994;57(3):570-575.

28. Dennis C, Hall DP, Moreno JR, Senning A. Left atrial cannulation without thoracotomy for total left heart bypass. *Acta Chir Scand.* 1962;123:267-279.

29. Dennis C, Carlens E, Senning A, et al. Clinical use of a cannula for left heart bypass without thoracotomy: experimental protection against fibrillation by left heart bypass. *Ann Surg.* 1962;156:623-637.

30. Dennis JL. Nutritional requirements in preoperative, postoperative and feeding of infants and children. *Pediatr Clin North Am.* 1962;9:911-926.

31. Pavie A, Léger P, Nzomvuama A, et al. Left centrifugal pump cardiac assist with transseptal percutaneous left atrial cannula. *Artif Organs.* 1998;22(6):502-507.

32. Catinella FP, Cunningham JN Jr, Glassman E, Laschinger JC, Baumann FG, Spencer FC. Left atrium-to-femoral artery bypass: effectiveness in reduction of acute experimental myocardial infarction. *J Thorac Cardiovasc Surg.* 1983;86(6):887-896.

33. Catinella FP, Cunningham JN Jr, Laschinger JC, Nathan IM, Glassman E, Spencer FC. Significant reduction of infarct size with left atrial to femoral artery bypass. *Curr Surg.* 1983;40(1):27-29.

34. Laschinger JC, Cunningham JN Jr, Catinella FP, Knopp EA, Glassman E, Spencer FC. "Pulsatile" left atrial-femoral artery bypass. A new method of preventing extension of myocardial infarction. *Arch Surg.* 1983;118(8):965-969.

35. Garatti A, Russo C, Lanfranconi M, et al. Mechanical circulatory support for cardiogenic shock complicating acute myocardial infarction: an experimental and clinical review. *ASAIO J.* 2007;53(3):278-287.

36. Thiele H, Smalling RW, Schuler GC. Percutaneous left ventricular assist devices in acute myocardial infarction complicated by cardiogenic shock. *Eur Heart J.* 2007;28(17):2057-2063.

37. Cheng JM, den Uil CA, Hoeks SE, et al. Percutaneous left ventricular assist devices vs. intra-aortic balloon pump counterpulsation for treatment of cardiogenic shock: a meta-analysis of controlled trials. *Eur Heart J.* 2009;30(17):2102-2108.

38. Brinkman WT, Rosenthal JE, Eichhorn E. Role of a percutaneous ventricular assist device in decision making for a cardiac transplant program. *Ann Thorac Surg.* 2009;88(5):1462-1466.

39. Kar BS, Basra SS, Delgado R, et al. 547: TandemHeart pVAD outcomes based on the intention to treat: a single institution experience. *J Heart Lung Transplant:* the official publication of the International Society for Heart Transplantation. 2009;28(2):S256.

40. Todoran TM, Bangalore S, Bainey KR, et al. Abstract 4372: TandemHeart® percutaneous ventricular assist device for treatment of cardiogenic shock in ischemic versus nonischemic cardiomyopathy: a single-center experience. *Circulation.* 2009;120(18 Meeting Abstracts):S949.

41. Thomas JL, Hazim Al-Ameri, Christina Economides, et al. Use of a percutaneous left ventricular assist device for high-risk cardiac interventions and cardiogenic shock. *J Invasive Cardiol.* 2010;22(8):360-364.

42. Tanaka K, Rangarajan K, Azarbal B, Tobis JM. Percutaneous ventricular assist during aortic valvuloplasty: potential application to the deployment of aortic stent-valves. *Tex Heart Inst J.* 2007;34(1):36-40.

43. Rajdev S, Irani A, Sharma S, Kini A. Clinical utility of TandemHeart for high-risk tandem procedures: percutaneous balloon aortic valvuloplasty followed by complex PCI. *J Invasive Cardiol.* 2007;19(11):E346-E349.

44. Singh IM, Holmes DR, Jr, Rihal CS. Impact of TandemHeart percutaneous left ventricular assist device on invasive hemodynamics. *J Am Coll Cardiol.* 2010. 55(10 Meeting Abstracts):A180.E1684.

45. Lim DS, Cortese CJ, Loree AN, Dean DA, Svitek RG. Left ventricular assist via percutaneous transhepatic transseptal cannulation in swine. *Catheter Cardiovasc Interv.* 2009;73(7):961-965.

46. Svitek RG, Smith DE, Magovern JA. In vitro evaluation of the TandemHeart pediatric centrifugal pump. *ASAIO J.* 2007;53(6):747-753.

CHAPTER 25

LEVITRONIX CENTRIMAG AND PEDIVAS SYSTEMS: APPLICATIONS AND CLINICAL RESULTS

John Marks, Mark Macedo, and Kurt Dasse

INTRODUCTION

Levitronix has developed magnetically levitated ("MagLev") centrifugal pump technologies, CentriMag, and PediVAS systems, to treat both adult and pediatric populations suffering from a wide range of cardiovascular disorders. The CentriMag blood pump has been proven to be highly versatile for the treatment of cardiogenic shock in adults. The device can be used to treat one or both sides of the heart for up to 30 days as a bridge to decision when it is unclear whether the patient will recover or need a longer-term therapy.

Cardiac assist technology for neonatal and pediatric applications has lagged behind those of adults.[1] A variety of devices originally developed for adults have been used to support pediatric patients.[2-6] In practice, the clinical use of such devices is restricted to patients with a relatively large body surface area (0.7 m[2] for extracorporeal devices and 1.4 m[2] for implantable devices) for a relatively short duration of use. Currently, the most commonly used technology for mechanical circulatory support in pediatric patients is the extracorporeal membrane oxygenator (ECMO).[7] However, the use of ECMO is limited by moderate survival rates (approximately 40%), restriction of use to the acute setting (5-10 days) to avoid complications, the complexity of the circuitry requiring labor intensive maintenance, and the lack of regulatory approval from the Food and Drug Administration (FDA) for any ECMO circuit. A multitude of pumps, many designed specifically for the pediatric population, are in various stages of development.[8]

REGULATORY STATUS OF THE CENTRIMAG SYSTEM

The CentriMag System has received regulatory approvals in different parts of the world for various indications for use. In the United States, certain applications discussed in this chapter concern uses that have not been approved or cleared by the FDA.

As of 2010, the CentriMag System is approved in Europe and other parts of the world, except Canada, for the following indications:

- To provide mechanical circulatory support for up to 30 days of use in patients with potentially reversible and recoverable heart failure.
- To provide cardiopulmonary support in an ECMO circuit for up to 30 days when used with other commercially available (CE marked) components approved for this application.

In the United States, as of 2010, the CentriMag System has been cleared or approved by the US FDA for the following indications:

- Approved under a humanitarian device exemption (HDE), to provide temporary circulatory support for use for up to 30 days for patients in cardiogenic shock due to acute right ventricular failure.
- To pump blood through an extracorporeal circulatory support for periods appropriate to cardiopulmonary bypass (CPB) (up to 6 hours) for surgical procedures such as a mitral valve reoperation. It is also indicated for use in extracorporeal support systems (for periods up to 6 hours) not requiring complete CPB (eg, valvuloplasty, surgery of the vena cava or aorta, liver transplants etc).

Also, in the United States, as of 2010, the CentriMag System is undergoing clinical trials for the following indications:

- A pivotal trial to study the safety and effectiveness of the system for use to support one or both sides of the heart for up to 30 days in patients who fail to wean from CPB as a bridge to decision, when it is unclear whether the patient's heart will recover or whether the patient will need alternative, longer-term therapy. The device is specifically indicated to treat failure to wean from CPB patients who are too hemodynamically unstable to be moved from the operating room without mechanical circulatory support.
- A pilot trial to study the safety and effectiveness of the system for use to support one or both sides of the heart for up to 30 days in pediatric patients between 5 and 16 years old who fail to wean from CPB, as a bridge to decision, when it is unclear whether the patient's heart will recover or whether the patient will need alternative, longer-term therapy. The device is specifically indicated to treat failure to wean from CPB patients who are too hemodynamically unstable to be moved from the operating room without mechanical circulatory support.

REGULATORY STATUS OF THE PEDIVAS SYSTEM

Like the CentriMag, the PediVAS System has received regulatory approvals in different parts of the world for various indications for use. In the United States, certain applications discussed in this chapter concern uses that have not been approved or cleared by the FDA. In the United States, the pump is branded as the PediMag when used as part of a cardiopulmonary circuit for up to 6 hours. As of 2010, the PediVAS System is approved in Europe and other parts of the world for the following indication:

- To provide circulatory support in neonatal and pediatric patients. In addition, the PediVAS blood pump may be used in an ECMO circuit to provide cardiopulmonary support when used with other commercially approved (CE marked) components for this application. The PediVAS blood pump may be used for up to 30 days of continuous support.

In the United States, as of 2010, the PediMag has been cleared by the FDA for the following indications:

- To pump blood through an extracorporeal circulatory support for periods appropriate to CPB (up to 6 hours) for surgical procedures such as a mitral valve reoperation. It is also indicated for use in extracorporeal support systems (for periods up to 6 hours) not requiring complete CPB (eg, valvuloplasty, surgery of the vena cava or aorta, liver transplants etc).

In the United States, a pilot clinical trial for the PediVAS is in final stages of review by the US FDA for the following indications:

- For use up to 30 days in a population of patients who fail to wean from CPB as a bridge to decision, when it is unclear whether the patient's heart will recover or whether the patient will need alternative, longer-term therapy. The device is specifically indicated to treat failure to wean from CPB patients who are too hemodynamically unstable to be moved from the operating room without mechanical circulatory support.

TECHNOLOGY OVERVIEW

The CentriMag and PediVAS MagLev centrifugal pumps are driven via bearing-less motor technology. The bearing-less pumps are driven without mechanical bearings, shafts, or seals. The basic principle is shown in Fig. 25–1. An impeller (rotor) is

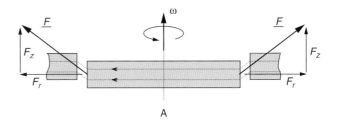

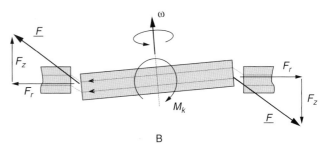

FIGURE 25–2. Axial support (**A**) and stabilization against tilting (**B**) of the rotor by passive magnetic forces in the blood pump. (Reproduced with permission from Levitronix, LLC.)

floating and rotating in the magnetic fields of a stator without mechanical contact. A compact digital signal processor system with a servo amplifier allows precise regulation of the rotor speed. External position sensors actively control the radial rotor position. Processor-controlled electronics regulate the magnetic fields so that the rotor is always centered. The electronics control precise regulation of the radial rotor position and speed. Axial position and tilting of the rotor are passively stabilized (Fig. 25–2). The noncontacting rotor is levitated by magnetic fields through the walls of the blood pump and floats in the center of the pump.

THE CENTRIMAG SYSTEM

The CentriMag Ventricular Assist System (VAS) comprises eight fundamental components: (1) a single-use centrifugal pump, (2) a primary motor, (3) a primary console, (4) a backup motor, (5) a backup console, (6) a flow probe, (7) tubing (drainage and return), and (8) cannulae (drainage and return). The extracorporeal membrane oxygenation (ECMO) configuration for the CentriMag System is virtually identical to the VAS configuration with the exception that an oxygenator may be used as a component of the extracorporeal circuit. Neither peripheral cannulae nor an oxygenator are provided by Levitronix for the ECMO configuration. The primary console is a fully functional VAD/ECMO drive unit equipped with flow and pressure sensing and display capability. The maximum flow of the CentriMag pump is 9.9 L/min (Fig. 25–3).

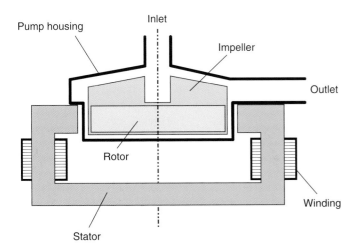

FIGURE 25–1. Schematic illustrating the basic principle of the bearing-less centrifugal pump and motor. (Reproduced with permission from Levitronix, LLC.)

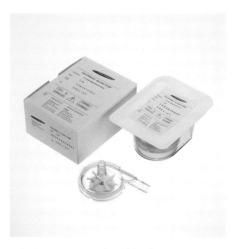
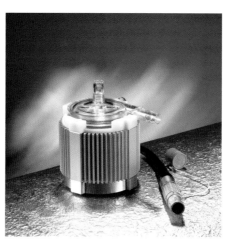
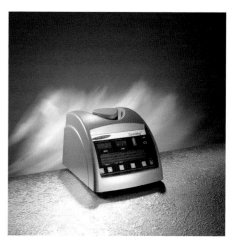

FIGURE 25–3. CentriMag blood pump, motor, and primary console. (Reproduced with permission from Levitronix, LLC.)

THE PEDIVAS SYSTEM

Like the CentriMag System, the PediVAS VAS comprises a single-use centrifugal blood pump, a motor, a primary drive console, a backup drive console and motor, and cannulae (Fig. 25–4). The PediVAS is a direct descendant of the CentriMag VAS with improved hydrodynamic efficiency at lower flows, and reduced size, priming volume, and circuit components. A comparison of the CentriMag and PediVAS pumps are outlined in Table 25–1. The PediVAS is capable of operating over a range of speeds up to 5500 rpm (revolutions per minute) generating flows up to 3.0 L/min (pump alone) and up to 1.7 L/min, using a 12-Fr inlet cannula with a 10-Fr outlet cannula. Compared to currently available technology, the PediVAS blood pump is innovative due to its small size, low priming volume, excellent hemodynamic and hematologic performance, and the elimination of failure modes due to seals and bearings. We believe that these characteristics make PediVAS ideally suited for temporary cardiac support of neonatal and pediatric patients (0.3-1.7 L/min).

CLINICAL APPLICATIONS AND RESULTS OF THE CENTRIMAG SYSTEM

As of mid-2010, over 8000 CentriMag blood pumps have been shipped worldwide since the CentriMag device began to be used clinically in 2003. As seen in Table 25–2, a total of 806 patients were reported in the literature. Five hundred and fifty-five patients were treated with the device when used as a ventricular assist device (VAD). The remaining 251 patients were treated with the system when used with the pump in an ECMO circuit. The average duration of support was 11 days with a range of support from 1 to 111 days. Four hundred and twenty-eight (53%) of the patients were successfully weaned, and 346 (43%) were ultimately discharged from the hospital and survived. When used as a VAD, the average duration of support was 14 days with a range of support from 1 to 111 days. Two hundred and ninety-three (53%) of the VAD patients were successfully weaned, and 263 (47%) were ultimately discharged from the hospital and survived. Seventeen percent of the VAD patients

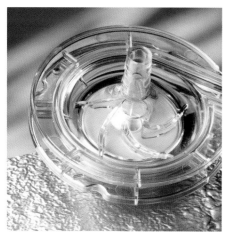
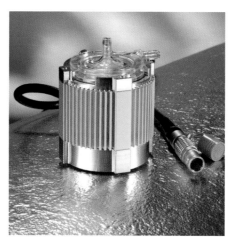
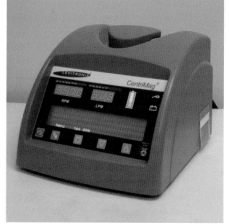

FIGURE 25–4. PediVAS blood pump, motor, and primary console. (Reproduced with permission from Levitronix, LLC.)

Table 25-1. Comparison of the CentriMag and PediVAS Pumps

Attribute	CentriMag Pump	PediVAS Pump
Priming volume	32 mL	14 mL
Operating speed range	0-5500 rpm	0-5500 rpm
Flow range	0-9.9 L/min	0-3 L/min
Cannulae connection size	3/8 in barb	1/4 in barb
Impeller configuration	Open	Closed

were treated with left ventricular support, 35% were supported for right ventricular support, and the remaining 48% needed biventricular assistance.

The results for the patients treated with the CentriMag System in an ECMO circuit were similar but less effective compared to the patients in the VAD group. Of the 251 patients who were treated in the ECMO group, 135 (54%) were successfully weaned and 83 (33%) were ultimately discharged. The average duration of support was 8 days with the range of support from 1 to 45 days. No device failures were reported in any of the studies. The nature and frequency of adverse events were consistent with those reported for other pumps when used as a VAD or for ECMO. The types of adverse events included: multiorgan failure,

Table 25-2. Summary of Clinical Results With the CentriMag Blood Pump (2003-2010) (n = 806 Patients: 555 VAD, 251 ECMO)

- VAD results:
  - 555 patients
  - 17% LVAD; 35% RVAD; 48% BVAD
  - Average duration of support 14 (1-111) d
  - 293 (53%) weaned
  - 263 (47%) discharged
- ECMO results:
  - 251 patients
  - Average duration of support 8 (1-45) d
  - 135 (54%) weaned
  - 83 (33%) discharged
- Combined results:
  - 806 patients
  - Average duration of support 11 (1-111) d
  - 428 (53%) weaned
  - 346 (43%) discharged
  - Zero (0%) failures reported

renal dysfunction, hepatic dysfunction, bleeding, sepsis, hemolysis, thromboembolic complications, and neural dysfunction.

Levitronix is conducting a pivotal clinical trial to evaluate the safety and efficacy of the CentriMag VAS in the United States. Twenty five for this 30-patient study have been enrolled. The data reported in the literature indicate that 47% of the VAD patients were discharged. At present, 56% of the VAD patients enrolled into the current clinical trial in the United States have met the success criterion and survived, consistent with the results reported in the literature. The nature and frequency of the adverse events observed in the United States clinical trial are consistent with those reported in the literature. No device failures have been observed in the clinical trial or in the studies reported in the literature.

The most frequent application for the CentriMag System is when used as a short-term VAS as a bridge to decision for up to 30 days.[9] The patients are supported until they either recover, undergo cardiac transplant, or proceed to be treated with a long-term VAD. In some instances, the CentriMag System has been used as a short-term salvage treatment for primary graft failure (donor heart failure) after heart transplant.[10] In other instances, the device is used immediately following high-risk surgery as a means to stabilize the patients until they can be successfully weaned, or to provide prolonged transcutaneous cardiopulmonary support for postcardiotomy cardiogenic shock.[11]

The CentriMag System has been used to support both adults, as described previously, or to support pediatric patients in cardiac, pulmonary, or cardiopulmonary failure.[12,13] In the latter article, the device was found to be an excellent option for transporting pediatric patients via ground transport from one hospital to another. In this instance, the pediatric patient was supported on ECMO. The device has been used with a wide variety of cannulae and implanted via several unique surgical techniques. In one instance, the CentriMag pump was connected to the patient using the Berlin Heart EXCOR cannulae as new "bridge-to-bridge" approach.[14] The Texas Heart Institute reported implanting the CentriMag left VAS through a right mini-thoracotomy, significantly reducing the degree of surgery to implant the device.[15] Contrary to many previous reports warning against use of a VAD in a patient with a mechanical valve, the CentriMag pump was successfully used as a short-term left ventricular assist device (LVAD) in a patient with a mechanical mitral prosthesis.[16]

The CentriMag pump has also been used in an ECMO circuit to successfully support a patient following lung transplant.[17] Thus, the device has been used both as a VAS and as a respiratory assist device. Recently, the CentriMag System has been used as an LVAD as a "bridge-to-surgery" in postinfarction ventricular septal defect.[18] The concept is to improve the status of the patient in anticipation of high-risk surgery. Based on the positive results summarized previously, use of the CentriMag VAS has been expanded to include prolonged support for bridging patients after salvage from bridge-to-decision directly to transplant.[19] The device has also been used as a mechanical bridge-to-recovery in pheochromocytoma myocarditis.[20]

Right heart failure remains a serious risk for patients suffering from cardiogenic shock or after LVAD implantation.

The CentriMag System has been shown to provide excellent mechanical support for acute right ventricular failure for both scenarios.[21] Occasionally, it is unclear whether a patient will need short- or long-term ventricular assistance. In many instances the neurologic status of the patient is unclear, and there is no means for assessing the status of the patient. The CentriMag System may be used as a low-cost means to stabilize the patient until a decision can be made regarding the neurologic status of the patient to determine whether the patient is a viable transplant candidate or a candidate for a long-term VAD. In one report, the CentriMag System was used to support the patient as a "bridge-to-bridge" to the Berlin Heart EXCOR for patients in refractory cardiogenic shock.[22] A limitation of traditional ECMO circuits is that they tend to be complex with many components, connectors, and tubing sets. A recent report from Hanover, Germany, describes use of the CentriMag System to provide temporary cardiac support in a mini-circuit system consisting of the centrifugal pump and a novel membrane ventilator.[23]

The CentriMag System has been used in a number of additional novel applications. For example, the device has been used for the treatment of massive pulmonary embolism, and in another case as a right ventricular assist device (RVAD) with an oxygenator in combination with the Cardiowest total artificial heart as a bridge-to-transplant.[24,25] In another case, the CentriMag System was used to treat right ventricular failure after LVAD implantation with concomitant pulmonary embolectomy in a patient with terminal heart failure and asymptomatic pulmonary thrombus.[26] Hemolysis has been a significant challenge when pediatric patients are treated with ECMO. A recent report based on the experience with the CentriMag in 33 newborns, infants, and children found the hemolysis associated with the CentriMag device to be remarkably low.[27]

A more recent description of the results obtained when the CentriMag System was used as a VAD to support patients in cardiogenic shock was described by John et al from the University of Minnesota. The authors reported the results for 16 patients who received the CentriMag pump, with 9 of them having suffered cardiogenic shock secondary to massive myocardial infarction. The 1-month and 1-year survival for these nine patients was 78% and 78%, respectively.[28] A report from Harefield and the Royal Brompton Hospitals in the United Kingdom describes pioneering efforts to mobilize patients and to provide physiotherapy to patients supported with a CentriMag device.[29] The authors make the point that mobilization of a patient coupled with improved physiotherapy greatly enhances the well-being of the patient and optimizes the likelihood of recovery. Another publication illustrates the feasibility of biventricular assist device (BiVAD) support with membrane oxygenation using the CentriMag System.[30] There is a growing trend to use the CentriMag System with an oxygenator spliced into the circuit either in a central or peripheral application. Recently, Avalon Laboratories introduced a single access, dual-lumen cannula for use with a pump and oxygenator to provide respiratory assistance. The CentriMag pump was used with the Avalon cannula and a Quadrox polymethylpentene hollow fiber oxygenator to provide ambulatory ECMO. The system supported a 49-year-old patient for 19 days as a new approach for bridge-to-lung transplantation. The patient underwent successful lung transplant.[31] Finally, significant improvements in the pumps and oxygenator components in the ECMO circuit, as well as improved patient management procedures led to improved outcomes as reported by Aziz et al at Penn State Milton Hershey Medical Center.[32] In a series of 10 patients treated for refractory cardiogenic shock, 6 (60%) of them were successfully supported and discharged after being on CentriMag ECMO support for an average of 8 days. Remarkably, CentriMag support was successfully implemented at the bedside in all 10 patients.

CLINICAL APPLICATIONS AND RESULTS OF THE PEDIVAS SYSTEM

As of mid-2010, over 600 patients have been supported with the PediVAS pump. The majority of PediVAS applications outside United States have been ECMO, with a small group of patients supported in a LVAD or BiVAD configuration. The primary indication has been pulmonary support (approximately 65%), followed by cardiac support (approximately 20%), and a combination of cardiopulmonary support (approximately 15%). The longest known duration of support has been 54 days in an ECMO configuration. Overall survival reported by individual clinical centers in Europe has ranged from 47% to 75%.

SUMMARY

The clinical results with the CentriMag and PediVAS systems have been excellent. Novel applications for the systems include, but are not limited to, the following:

- LVAD, RVAD, BiVAD
- Adult, newborn, infant, and pediatric support
- VV, VA ECMO
- Ideal for transport
- Immediate CPB to VAD support for high-risk surgical patients
- Bridge-to-surgery
- Bridge-to-bridge
- Bridge-to-heart transplant
- Bridge-to-lung transplant
- Post–graft failure support
- Mechanical circulatory support that allows for ambulation, mobility, and physical therapy

The applications described previously illustrate the ability of the systems to be used as a tool in some instances or as a therapy in others. When used as a tool, the device is used to stabilize the patient until a known therapy can be performed. When used as a therapy, the device provides the necessary support to unload the heart until it recovers. The device was found to be safe, effective, and reliable in all reports. No device failures were reported.

Historically, the smaller size and anatomical complexity of the pediatric patient have presented unique challenges to clinicians using mechanical circulatory support. Traditional ECMO, one of the most common forms of support in this population, has been fraught with postoperative complications largely due to the use of polypropylene hollow fiber oxygenators and pumps associated with significant hemolysis. Davies and colleagues[33] have found high end-organ failure and mortality rates after implementing ECMO for up to 30 days posttransplantation. The Levitronix PediVAS, built on the successful CentriMag platform, was designed as a short-term circulatory support system to overcome many of the adverse effects associated with use of pumps for circulatory support. The PediVAS pump is approved for use for up to 30 days in Europe in a VAD or ECMO configuration. The pump is also cleared by US FDA for up to 6 hours of use in the United States. A US clinical trial is planned for use of the device as a VAD for up to 30 days.

REFERENCES

1. Hetzer R, Loebe M, Potapov EV, et al. Circulatory support with pneumatic paracorporeal ventricular assist device in infants and children. *Ann Thoracic Surg.* 1998;66:1498-1506.
2. Ashton RC, Oz MC, Michler RF, et al. Left ventricular assist options in pediatric patients. *ASAIO J.* 1995;41:M277-M280.
3. Helman DN, Addonizio LJ, Morales DL, et al. Implantable left ventricular assist devices can successfully bridge adolescent patients to transplant. *J Heart Lung Transplant.* 2000;19:121-126.
4. Korfer R, El-Banayosy A, Arusoglu L, et al. Single-center experience with the Thoratec ventricular assist device. *J Thoracic Cardiovasc Surg.* 2000;119:596-600.
5. Pennington DG. Comments on Circulatory Support in Infants and Children. *Semin Thoracic Cardiovasc Surg.* 1994;6:161-162.
6. Duncan BW. Pediatric mechanical circulatory support. *ASAIO J.* 2005;51: ix-xiv.
7. ECLS Registry Report. Ann Arbor, Michigan: Extracorporeal Life Support Registry Organization, January, 2005.
8. Throckmorton AL, Chopski SG. Pediatric circulatory support: current strategies and future directions. Biventricular and univentricular mechanical assistance. *ASAIO J.* 2008 Sep-Oct;54(5):491-497.
9. De Robertis F, Birks EJ, Rogers P, Dreyfus G, Pepper JR, Khaghani A. Clinical performance with the Levitronix CentriMag short-term ventricular assist device. *J Heart Lung Transplant.* 2006;25(2):181-186.
10. Santise G, Petrou M, Pepper JR, Dreyfus G, Khaghani A, Birks EJ. Levitronix as a short-term salvage treatment for primary graft failure after heart transplantation. *J Heart Lung Transplant.* 2006;25(5):495-498.
11. Westaby S, Balacumaraswami L, Evans BJ, Bertoni GB. Elective transfer from cardiopulmonary bypass to centrifugal blood pump support in very high-risk cardiac surgery. *J Thoracic Cardiovasc Surg.* 2007;133(2):577-578.
12. Saeed D, Kizner L, Arusoglu L, et al. Prolonged transcutaneous cardiopulmonary support for postcardiotomy cardiogenic shock. *ASAIO J.* 2007 May-Jun;53(3):e1-e3.
13. Machin D, Scott R, Hurst A. Ground transportation of a pediatric patient on ECMO support. *J Extra Corpor Technol.* 2007;39:99-102.
14. Maat A, vanThiel R, Dalinghaus M, Bogers A. Connecting the CentriMag Levitronix pump to Berlin Heart Excor cannulae; a new approach to bridge to bridge. *J Heart Lung Transplant.* 2008;27(1)112-115.
15. Gregoric I, Cohn W, Akay M, LaFranchesca S, Myers T, Frazier O. CentriMag left ventricular assist system cannulation through a right mini-thoracotomy. *Tex Heart Inst J.* 2008;35(2):184-185.
16. Mussa S, Large S, Tsui S, van Doorn C, Jenkins D. Mechanical mitral prosthesis with a short term left ventricular assist device. *ASAIO J.* 2008 Jul-Aug;54(4):439-441.
17. Khan N, Al-alouo M, Shad Dl. Early experience with the Levitronix CentriMag device for extra corporeal membrane oxygenation following lung transplantation. *Eur J Cardiothorac Surg.* 2008;34:1262-1264.
18. Pitsis A, Kelpis T, Visouli A, Bobotis G, Filippatos S, Kremastinos D. Left ventricular assist device as a bridge to surgery in post infarction ventricular septal defect. *J Thorac Cardiovasc Surg.* 2008;135:951-952.
19. Haj-Yahida S, Birks E, Armani M, et al. Bridging patients after salvage from bridge to decision directly to transplant by means of prolonged support with the CentriMag short term centrifugal pump. *J Thorac Cardiovasc Surg.* 2009;138:227-230.
20. Westaby S, Shahir A, Sadler G, Flynn F, Ormerod O. Mechanical bridge to recovery in pheochromocytoma myocarditis. *Nat Rev Cardiol.* 2009(6) 482-487.
21. Marquez T, D'Cunha J, John R, Liao K, Joyce L. Mechanical support for acute right ventricular failure: evolving surgical paradigms. *J Thoracic Cardiovasc Surg.* 2009;137:e39-e40.
22. Loforte A, Potapov E, Krabatsch T, et al. Levitronix CentriMag to Berlin heart Excor: a "bridge to bridge" solution in refractory cardiogenic shock. *ASAIO J.* 2009 Sep/Oct;55(5):465-468.
23. Meyer A, Strueber M, Tomaszek S, et al. Temporary cardiac support with a mini-circuit system consisting of a centrifugal pump and a membrane ventilator. *Interact Cardiovasc Thorac Surg.* 2009;9:1980.
24. Griffith K, Jenkins E, Haft T. Treatment of massive pulmonary embolism utilizing a multidisciplinary approach: a case study. *Perfusion.* 2009;24(3): 169-172.
25. Anderson E, Jaroszewski D, Pierce C, DeValeria P, Arabia F. Parallel application of extracorporeal membrane oxygenation and the CardioWest total artificial heart as a bridge to transplant. *Ann Thorac Surg.* 2009;88: 1676-1678.
26. Stepanenko A, Potapov EV, Krabatsch T, Hetzer R. Right ventricular failure after left ventricular assist device implantation with concomitant pulmonary embolectomy needing right ventricular assist device support in a patient with terminal heart failure and asymptomatic pulmonary thrombus. *Interact Cardiovasc Thorac Surg.* 2010;10(1):154-155.
27. Reckers J, Asfour B, Fink C. Goodbye hemolysis! Experience with Levitronix CentriMag in 33 newborns, infants and children. *ASAIO J.* 2008;54:2:39A.
28. John R, Lietz K, Liao K, Miller L, Joyce LD. Short-term circulatory support for cardiogenic shock with Levitronix CentriMag ventricular assist device. *ASAIO J.* 2006 Mar-Apr;52(2):61A.
29. Bindoff C, Dean R, Bashford A, et al. Mobilization and physiotherapy of patients with a Levitronix CentriMag® short-term mechanical circulatory support device. *Heart Lung Transplant.* 2009 Feb;28(25):S280.
30. Yang JA, Takayama H, Kim H, Cohen SA, Naka Y. Feasibility of BiVAD support with membrane oxygenation. *J Heart Lung Transplant.* 2010;29(2S):S181.
31. Garcia J, Iacono A, Kon ZN, Griffith BP. Ambulatory extracorporeal membrane oxygenation: a new approach for bridge-to-lung transplantation. *J Thorac Cardiovasc Surg.* 2010;139(6):e137-e139.
32. Aziz TA, Singh G, Popjes E, et al. Initial experience with CentriMag extracorporeal membrane oxygenation for support of critically ill patients with refractory cardiogenic shock. *J Heart Lung Transplant.* 2009;29(1):66-71
33. Davies RR, Russo JM, Hong KN, et al. The use of mechanical circulatory support as a bridge to transplantation in pediatric patients: an analysis of the United Network for Organ Sharing database. *J Thorac Cardiovasc Surg.* 2008;135:421-427

CHAPTER 26

THE ABIOMED AB5000 CIRCULATORY SUPPORT SYSTEM

Daniel H. Raess

The AB5000 ventricle is a first-generation pulsatile assist device created by Abiomed (Fig. 26–1). The initial Abiomed device, the BVS5000, was a short-term pulsatile device that has been implanted worldwide in over 10,000 patients since it gained initial Food and Drug Administration (FDA) approval in 1993 (Fig. 26–2).[1] The BVS was a short-term device for use up to 14 days. The advantage to the system, which is still in use commercially today, was the totally autonomous pumping mechanism and the simplicity of the patient management at the bedside, which did not require the constant attention of a perfusionist.

During the late 1980 and early 1990s, the AbioCor project was under way. This was a National Institutes of Health (NIH)–funded total artificial heart project utilizing a hydroelectric pump actuating a movable septum and using two ventricles with trileaflet inflow and outflow valves made of polyurethane. The AB5000 project grew out of the excellent design, and preclinical work of these ventricles and each AB5000 is essentially half of the AbioCor design except with a pneumatically actuated ventricle. The trileaflet valves are essentially identical to the AbioCor valves and are very different than the earlier BVS design, incorporating thin-walled laser cut leaflets and excellent washing of the ventricle pumping chamber with a variable vortex washing design. The full to empty device has an active filling component due to the loss of drainage during device systole such as was used in the BVS design. A volume of approximately 100 cc is delivered with each systolic ejection. The vacuum on the device is scalable from −35 to −100 mm Hg. The device is used as either right, left, or biventricular support and is unique among devices as having approval for all recoverable forms of heart failure. The AB5000 ventricle is powered by a variety of iterations of consoles from the AB5000 console and the iPulse (both of which also can be used to power the BVS5000 pump with the iPulse also supporting an intra-aortic balloon pump [IABP]) as well as the new portable driver which is designed for discharge of the patient either to the home or rehab environment to await recovery. Currently, a FDA clinical trial for discharge using the AB5000 in left (LVAD), right (RVAD), or biventricular assist device (BiVAD) configuration with the portable driver is under way. The Voyager trial seeks to compare adverse events in the in-hospital patients with that of the discharged patients.

Although the "5000" in the name is meant to signify 5 L/min of cardiac output from the device, it is not uncommon to see flows over 6 L/min. The device is weaned using a weaning control that allows the operator to choose a target volume from 2 up to 5 L/min. Anticoagulation is usually started within 24 hours of insertion and is targeted at 180-second activated clotting time (ACT). When the flow is below 3 L/min, the ACT target increases to 220 seconds, and, when the flow is below 2 L/min, the ACT is advanced to greater than 350 seconds.

The cannulation has been varied but is surgical with two different sizes of atrial cannula (32 Fr and 42 Fr) and a 10-mm Hemashield graft used for arterial return. The apical sewing cuff is included with every set of cannulae and is sized appropriately to either the 32 Fr or 42 Fr. The cannulae are the same as the BVS system (with the addition of the apical) and this enables transition from the BVS to AB to occur at the bedside, thus avoiding the highly morbid procedure required to change to longer-term support. The apical LV cannulation is the most often used cannulation method and does not require coring of the apex (Fig. 26–3). A shorter apical cannula is used for the apex in order to avoid an excessively long cannulation and to facilitate mobility. One difference that operators who are accustomed to using the BVS will note with the AB design is that the inflow and the outflow cannulae need to be within 5 cm of each other on exit from the body wall due to the proximity of the inflow and outflow ports on the ventricle. Explantation is easy when using the sewing cuff, which allows a simple staple or over sews of the apical sewing cuff, thus minimizing disturbance on the recovered ventricle. The actual configuration of the exit sights will vary depending on patient anatomy and cannulation scheme used. Generally, the apical cannula should either have a gentle curve or as straight a course as possible to the inflow of the ventricle. Some operators prefer to have the left side ventricle faced inward. The ventricle will work the same regardless of the orientation of the ventricle, with the only disadvantage to having the metal base faced up is that the patients complain that everyone is always turning the device over to check the pumping chamber and it can become sore (Fig. 26–4).

One of the most interesting and potentially valuable differences that the AB5000 use has brought to current clinical practice is the use in patients with refractory acute myocardial infarction (AMI) shock. Anderson et al have recently described a series of 100 consecutive AMI-shock patients supported with AB5000.[2] In this group of patients, the AB5000 was used for a longer time than previous short-term devices allowed with the average time on support being 25 days. These were an extremely ill group of patients with over 52% being in shock for longer than 24 hours. These patients were all essentially failing high-dose inotropes and IABP support with 44% of them having been administered cardiopulmonary resuscitation (CPR) for an average of 20 minutes (Fig. 26–5). The patients were split fairly evenly between LVAD (47%) only use and BiVAD (45%) with RVAD used only 8% of the time. A larger group (58%) was implanted

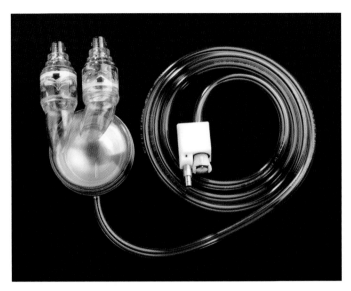

FIGURE 26–1. Shown here is the AB5000 ventricle with the drive line that is attached to the drive console. (Reproduced with permission from Abiomed, Inc.)

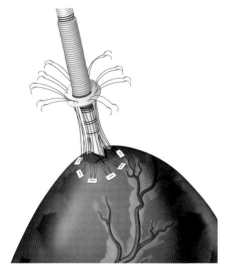

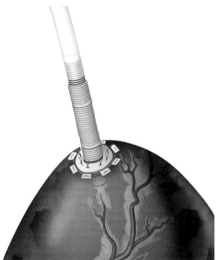

FIGURE 26–3. Use of the apical cuff system allows easy apical cannulation without coring the apex. This system facilitates safe and easy decannulation. (Reproduced with permission from Abiomed, Inc.)

directly with AB5000 as opposed to 42% that were transitioned from BVS5000.

The improvement in hemodynamic status is immediate and profound, with cardiac index (CI) increasing from 1.7 ± 0.5 to 2.6 ± 0.7 L/min/m^2 ($P < .0001$). Aortic systolic blood pressure ($P < 0.0001$), central venous pressure (CVP) ($P = 0.05$), and pulmonary artery (PA) pressure ($P = .001$) were similarly improved. What is perhaps even more impressive is that this improvement

was sustained into the post–ventricular assist device (VAD) explant period. Despite the logistic EuroScore estimate of survival being less than 15%, 40% of these patients survived (with recovery of the native heart the most likely outcome at 63%). Additionally, 10 patients were bridged to transplant using the AB ventricle with 8 of them surviving, and 8 were bridged to a durable device with 7 of them surviving the procedure. An important issue is delineated in (Fig. 26–6). The 90% confidence limits for recovery are presented indicating that 90% of recovery occurs between 2 and 55 days. When factoring in patients who were either transplanted or bridged to another VAD, several fell into the period prior to 55 days. We will not know if any of these patients were recoverable or not, but certainly good practice

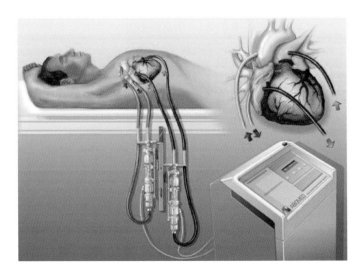

FIGURE 26–2. The Abiomed BVS 5000 system. (Reproduced with permission from Abiomed, Inc.)

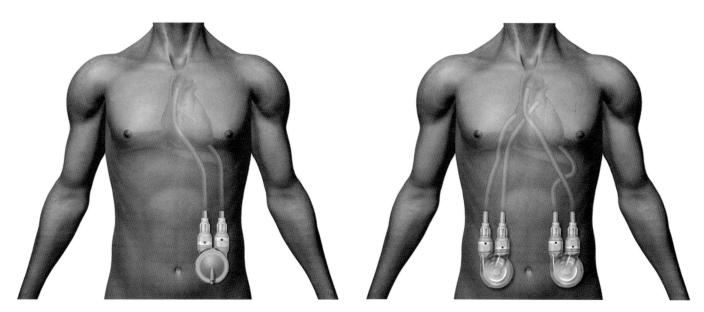

FIGURE 26–4. The exit sites of each side must be within 5 cm of each other to faciliate connection to the AB ventricle. The ventricle will function equally well if it is placed with the clear side up (left) or down (right). (Reproduced with permission from Abiomed, Inc.)

would be to support the patients through this period, which is consistent with the most favorable period for transplantation after LVAD.[3] Kaplan-Meyer survival outlook at 2 years postexplant was 79% (Fig. 26–7). Additional hemodynamic comparisons between a cohort of revascularized SHOCK trial patients[4] and the patients treated with the AB5000 was presented, documenting that the patients in the Anderson study who survived were sicker than the SHOCK trial patients who died. This study, the largest in the literature of AMI patients treated with VAD therapy, concludes that therapy for these patients are often seriously delayed and that this delay with its implications for end-organ functions may be responsible for the long support time required for recovery in these patients. Cardiac recovery does appear to be achievable, sustainable, and preferable when using

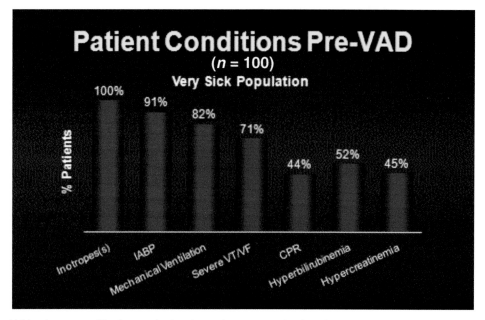

FIGURE 26–5. Co-morbidities demonstrated by the AMI-shock patients prior to AB5000 implantation in Anderson, et al. (Modified with permission from Anderson et al.[2] Copyright © Elsevier.)

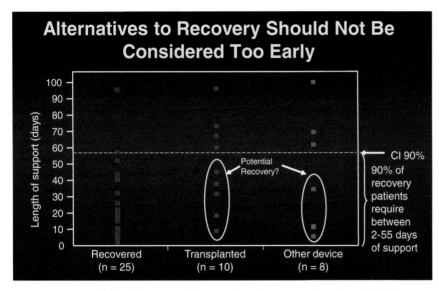

FIGURE 26–6. Multiple patients were either transplanted or converted to a BTT/DT device within the 90% confidence window for recovery. (Modified with permission from Anderson et al.[2] Copyright © Elsevier.)

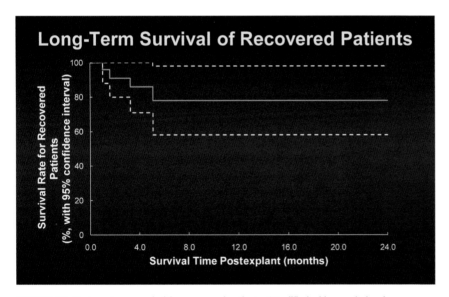

FIGURE 26–7. Long term survival for recovered patients. (Modified with permission from Anderson et al.[2] Copyright © Elsevier.)

a VAD in this manner. Other solutions such as transplantation and durable LVAD therapy should only be considered after a period of adequate ventricular support. Additionally, this report confirms previous findings of the excellent survival of bridge-to-transplantation using the AB5000 which was used initially for a recoverable indication.[5] The differences that we see with the new data from the USpella registry are not at odds with these data since it is hoped that earlier intervention will indeed make recovery of these patients earlier and less morbid. The FDA has awarded the AB5000 a 1-year bench reliability certification.

REFERENCES

1. Guyton Ra, Schonberger JP, Everts PA, et al. Postcardiotomy shock: clinical evaluation of the BVS 5000 Biventricular Support System. *Ann Thorac Surg.* 1993 Aug;56(2):346-56.
2. Anderson M, Smedira N, Samuels L, et al. Use of the AB5000 Ventricular Assist Device in cardiogenic shock after acute myocardial infarction. *Ann Thoracic Surg.* 2010;90(3):706-712.
3. Gammie JS, Edwards LB, Griffith BP, Pierson RN, Tsao L. Optimal timing of cardiac transplantation after ventricular assist device implantation. *J Thorac Cardiovasc Surg.* 2004;127:1789-1799.
4. Hochman J, Sleeper L, Webb J, et al. Early revascularization in acute myocardial infarction complicated by cardiogenic shock. *N Engl J Med.* 1999;341:625-634.
5. Elefteriades J, Madani M, Crumbley AJ, Adams D, Anderson M. Clinical experience with the AB5000 for bridge to transplant: successful cross-over for extended bridge-to-recovery patients. Poster session ISHLT 2007.

CHAPTER 27

THE THORATEC PARACORPOREAL VENTRICULAR ASSIST DEVICE

David J. Farrar and Michael Acker

The Thoratec paracorporeal ventricular assist device (PVAD) can support the function of the left ventricle (LVAD), right (RVAD), or both ventricles (BiVAD) in patients suffering from end-stage heart failure.[1-8] The US Food and Drug Administration (FDA) approved the use of the PVAD in patients as a bridge-to-cardiac transplantation in 1995 and for postcardiotomy support in 1998. More than 4400 patients worldwide with a wide range of ages and body size have been treated with the PVAD. The Thoratec implantable ventricular assist device (IVAD), which shares many of the design features of the PVAD and has an identical flow path, has been implanted in more than 560 patients.[9]

While the prevalence and clinical utilization of newer-generation continuous-flow LVAD devices continues to increase, the PVAD retains its relevance today especially by meeting a critical clinical need—patients requiring biventricular support. These BiVAD PVAD patients are mobile and are commonly discharged home on a portable pneumatic console that allows them the freedom to enjoy a more normal lifestyle at home while they await transplant.[10]

DEVICE DESCRIPTION

The Thoratec paracorporeal ventricular assist device has a 65-mL stroke volume blood-pumping chamber (Thoralon polyurethane) and two mechanical valves (Fig. 27–1). Long-term biostability of ventricular assist device (VAD) blood-pumping sacs removed from human patients has been reported.[11]

Alternating positive and negative air pressure by a console or portable pneumatic driver produces a clinical beat rate range of 40 to 110 beats/min, resulting in a flow-rate of 1.3 to 7.2 L/min.[2] The PVAD is positioned on the anterior abdominal wall, with the cannulae crossing into the chest wall to connect the VAD to the heart and great vessels (Fig. 27–2). Because of the external location, it is suitable for use in smaller patients with body surface area (BSA) > 0.73 m[2].

The PVAD is actuated pneumatically by either the dual-drive console for in-hospital use or the portable TLC-II pneumatic driver for ambulatory use, either in or outside the hospital[10] and a mobile computer is available for changing settings and for diagnostics.[12] The TLC-II was approved by the FDA for home discharge in 2003.

DEVICE IMPLANTATION AND OPERATIVE CONSIDERATIONS

Cardiopulmonary bypass (CPB) is used for most PVAD procedures. To preserve operative options bicaval cannulation is advisable. Normothermic perfusion without cardioplegia or aortic cross-clamping is recommended. The left ventricle is vented and deaired via the left ventricle (LV) apex cannula before it is connected to the VAD. The patient may be ultrafiltrated during bypass to assist in keeping the hematocrit above 30% in case blood-clotting components are needed to assist coagulation.

Several right and left ventricular VAD configurations and cannulation approaches have been employed. The most common configuration is depicted in Fig. 27–2 for either LVAD or BiVAD. The LV apex is the preferred location for the inflow cannula to the LVAD, with return to the ascending aorta. For RVAD support, the right atrium is the site of choice for the venous cannula. A newer multiholed venous cannula has improved the stability and volume of flow. It should be inserted only 1 to 1.5 cm into the right atrium about 2 cm lateral to the atrioventricular groove and just inferior to the origin of the atrial appendage. Right ventricular cannulation technique has been reported to provide greater and more stable flow.[13] However, removal after recovery of the right ventricle (RV) can be problematic since it is difficult to decannulate and repair the site without compromising subsequent myocardial function. Although most implants are performed via standard median sternotomy, an alternative has been reported that utilizes limited access bilateral incisions without entering the thorax.[14]

ANTICOAGULATION

Chronic warfarin anticoagulation (INR 2.5-3.5 U) is required with the PVAD. The recommended anticoagulation protocol begins with heparin 10 U/kg/h, progressing to maintain partial thromboplastin time (PTT) 1.5 times control. However, heparin can cause bleeding and wound hematomas, and several groups have used the option of going directly to warfarin and aspirin. A daily dose of 325-mg aspirin is initiated at approximately 48 hours.

BIVENTRICULAR FAILURE

■ PREOPERATIVE RISK FACTORS FOR RIGHT HEART FAILURE: HEMODYNAMICS

Low cardiac index with high right atrial pressure provides some insight into a poorly functioning RV but does not accurately predict how the RV will perform after implanting an LVAD. Right ventricular function often improves after LVAD ventricular unloading, relief of right-sided congestion, and reduction in right ventricular afterload.[15] It is most important to assess the ability of the right ventricle to generate pressure, with high preoperative pulmonary pressures being a good sign for RV function, while low pulmonary pressures with high central venous pressure (CVP) can identify patients likely to need biventricular

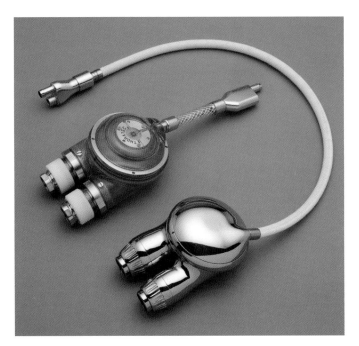

FIGURE 27–1. Thoratec ventricular assist devices. The paracorporeal ventricular assist device (PVAD) is shown (upper left) next to the intracorporeal ventricular assist device (IVAD). The IVAD's blood pump chamber is the same as that of PVAD, but the housing is smooth-polished titanium for implantability. (Reproduced with permission from Thoratec Corporation, Pleasanton, CA.)

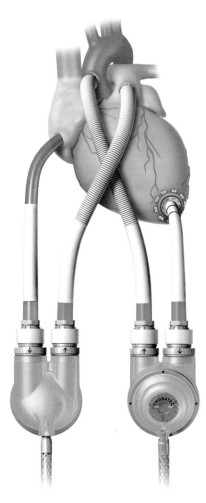

FIGURE 27–2. Illustration of Thoratec paracorporeal ventricular assist devices (PVAD) in a biventricular support configuration. (Reproduced with permission from Thoratec Corporation, Pleasanton, CA.)

support. Perhaps the best way to quantify this characteristic is to calculate the right ventricular stroke work index, which in some studies has been predictive of the need for RVADs.[16,17] In the HeartMate II bridge-to-transplant (BTT) trial in 484 patients, 20% developed right heart failure, including 6% requiring an RVAD and another 7% who required inotropes for more than 14 days post-op.[18] Although right ventricular stroke work index (RVSWI) was a significant univariate predictor of RVF, the most significant hemodynamic risk factor in a multivariate analysis was elevated CVP-to-PCWP ratio (> 0.63).[18]

■ PREOPERATIVE RISK FACTORS FOR RIGHT HEART FAILURE: COMORBIDITIES

Several risk models have recently been published identifying various predictors of right ventricular dysfunction and potentially those patients who may be better suited for BiVAD support.[19-21] The need for biventricular support is highly dependent on the patient's clinical status as well as hemodynamics.[5,22] The earlier LVAD implantation occurs before significant major organ dysfunction, the more likely that only univentricular support will be required. Patients with biventricular failure have had higher preoperative bilirubin[5,20,23,24] and creatinine,[5,20] both of which typically normalize after 2 to 3 weeks of support. Preoperative mechanical ventilation[5,17,18] and emergent implantation predict the need for biventricular support.[5] Intraoperative bleeding and greater transfusion requirements contribute to increased pulmonary vascular resistance and the development of right heart failure. Postoperative bleeding requiring reoperations and transfusions has been more prevalent in patients with

biventricular failure,[5,24] in part related to severity of preoperative hepatic dysfunction. The need for vasopressors has also been identified as a predictor of right ventricular failure.[20,21]

BIVENTRICULAR SUPPORT FOR ACUTE CARDIOGENIC SHOCK

The Thoratec VAD system is a good option for patients presenting in acute cardiogenic shock, especially if several months support duration is anticipated and ambulation and potential patient discharge are desired. Most patients implanted with Thoratec VADs today are in INTERMACS (Interagency Registry for Mechanically Assisted Circulatory Support) clinical profile 1 (so called "crash-and-burn" patient). The planned use of biventricular assistance in these patients provides immediate support of both sides of the circulation, allowing support for weeks or months until cardiac transplantation or recovery without a second bridge to decision procedure required with acute devices. The primary goals in patients who present in extremis with cardiogenic shock should include 1) stabilization of hemodynamics, 2) end-organ perfusion, 3) optimal drainage of pulmonary and right sided circulation and 4) maximizing perfusion pressures to the peripheral organs.

Therapy of focus needs to be acute restoration of perfusion organ function. It is critical to rapidly and successfully reverse shock and restore end-organ perfusion thereby minimizing permanent damage to hepatic, renal, neurologic and GI systems. Maintenance of end-organ function is vital is assuring long term survival and successful bridge to heart transplantation. In our experience biventricular support is often superior to LVAD support alone for unloading of the right ventricle, minimizing central venous pressures, and maximizing perfusion pressures to peripheral organs. The Thoratec PVAD or IVAD properly placed restores perfusion while maximally eliminating venous congestion that adversely impacts end-organ function.   In patients presenting in extremis as a result of acute cardiogenic shock resulting from post infarction and ischemic heart failure, myocarditis, refractory ventricular arrhythmia and biventricular dysfunction Thoratec VADs are indicated.   Institution of biventricular support has repeatedly been demonstrated to provide improved survival compared to delayed conversion after an LVAD.[25-27] If there is any question of the need for long term right ventricular support in the acute setting we advocate Thoratec BVADs which obviates the need for a second sternotomy.   In our experience we have found a cardiac index, right ventricular stroke work, preoperative RV dysfunction, creatinine, systemic blood pressure and prior cardiac surgery to be predictors of RVAD need.   Elevated CVP with a low pulmonary artery and systemic blood pressures has been a fairly reliable predictor of severe RV dysfunction and the need for RVAD.

CLINICAL EXPERIENCE

The clinical experience for the PVAD has occurred in over 260 hospitals worldwide for both BTT and postcardiotomy recovery. From March 30, 1982 to January 6, 2010, the Thoratec voluntary registry received reports of 4477 patients implanted with the PVAD. The mean age was 50 years (range, 6-77), median BSA was 1.91 mm² (minimum, 0.73 m²), with a median weight of 76 kg (minimum, 16.3 kg). Disease etiology was primarily ischemic (29%) and idiopathic (30%) cardiomyopathies, with various etiologies (acute myocardial infarction [AMI], myocarditis, viral and postpartum cardiomyopathies, failed transplants, etc) comprising the remainder.

Among 2928 BTT patients, biventricular assistance was used in 62% of patients, isolated LVADs in 31%, RVADs in 6%. For all patients receiving PVAD assistance, the mean period of support was 33 days, and the longest patient received paracorporeal BiVADs without any device exchanges for 3.3 years.

Current results with the PVAD are best described by several single-center reports recently published. The Pittsburgh group reported strategically using BiVADs as well as implantable LVADs for different clinical scenarios, with biventricular usage in 73 (32%) of 228 VAD patients, and encouraging results in morbid congestive heart failure.[6] The University of Pennsylvania group published a series of 99 (37%) BiVAD patients out of 266 VAD patients between 1995 and 2007 and achieved success (survived to transplant or were weaned) in 73% of patients who they preoperatively identified as BiVAD recipients, which compared favorably to a success rate of 79% for their LVAD

patients.[7] In contrast, of patients who later received an RVAD following LVAD implantation, only 45% survived to transplant or weaning. This study highlighted their success in preoperatively identifying BiVAD recipients and achieving outcomes that were comparable to LVAD-only recipients, resulting in dramatic improvements in survival when compared to the use of RVADs following LVAD implantation. The group at the University of California, Los Angeles, have also reported their single-center experience in 67 critically ill patients who received BiVAD support, of whom 47 patients (70.1%) were successfully bridged to transplant. Among patients who were bridged, the 1-year posttransplant survival rate was 89.4%.[28] A similar presentation by the group in Prague, Czech Republic, reported that of 49 patients implanted with BiVADs, 73.5% were successfully bridged to transplant with 1-year posttransplant survival of 89%.[29]

Kirsch et al from Henri Mondor Hospital in Paris, France, reported on 84 patients who were implanted with PVADs, with 62 patients (74%) receiving BiVADs.[8] Sixty-three percent of BiVAD patients were successfully bridged to transplant or recovered. Their success validated their belief in the use of PVAD as a primary device to support patients with cardiogenic shock and that the use of BiVADs prevents the risk of right ventricular dysfunction, and allowed rapid weaning of inotropic drugs. Compared to short-term devices, they concluded that the PVAD is capable of providing immediate ventricular unloading and adequate organ perfusion in patients with end-organ dysfunction.

Although most patients are implanted for BTT, the PVAD system is a very good option for recovery of ventricular function in postcardiotomy settings and for patients with fulminant myocarditis and acute onset cardiomyopathies.[30-32] A series of 22 young patients (average age 32) with myocarditis, postpartum and viral cardiomyopathies, were weaned from VAD support (13 BiVAD, 9 LVAD) after an average duration of 57 days before return of ventricular function and removal of the devices. The transplant-free post-VAD survival was 86% at 1 year and 77% at 5 years.[30]

■ PEDIATRIC EXPERIENCE

Though primarily designed for adults, PVADs have been implanted in over 250 pediatric and adolescent patients.[33-35] The patients' mean age was 14.5 years (range, 5-18 years), mean weight was 57 kg (range, 17-118 kg), mean BSA was 1.6 m² (range, 0.7-2.3 m²), and 65% were male patients. Most patients had cardiomyopathies (55.0%) or acute myocarditis (25.4%). Only 5.8% of patients had congenital heart disease. Average duration of support was 44.1 days (range, 0-434 days). BiVADs were used in 53.1% of patients and LVADs in 42.1%.

Overall survival (68%) was summarized by Reinhartz et al and was similar to results seen for adult patients who underwent VAD support as a BTT.[33,34] Subgroup analysis based on etiology found superior survival with Thoratec VAD support for patients with acute myocarditis (86%) and cardiomyopathies (74%), compared to patients having congenital heart disease (27%). The most important adverse events were thromboembolism and hemorrhage, which were higher than in the adult population. Size tends not to influence most outcomes as the success rate in patients less than 1.3 m² BSA with cardiomyopathies and acute myocarditis was the same, though it was worse (20%)

for patients with congenital heart disease. Successful use of the PVAD as a BTT for failure of a Fontan revision has also been reported in a 25-year-old patient who had the original procedure when he was 11 years old.[36]

CONCLUSIONS

First introduced over 20 years ago, the Thoratec PVAD remains an important therapeutic option in selected patients with left, right, or biventricular failure. With a clinical experience that involves more than 4400 patients, this device provides maximum versatility for physicians in meeting the left, right, or biventricular support needs of advanced heart failure patients requiring acute (weeks) or intermediate (months) support with the opportunity for home discharge. The device is approved in the United States for BTT and postcardiotomy recovery from open-heart surgery.

REFERENCES

1. Hill JD, Farrar DJ, Hershon JJ, et al. Use of a prosthetic ventricle as a bridge to cardiac transplantation for postinfarction cardiogenic shock. *N Engl J Med.* 1986 Mar 6;314(10):626-628.
2. Farrar DJ, Hill JD, Gray LA, Jr, et al. Heterotopic prosthetic ventricles as a bridge to cardiac transplantation: multicenter clinical study in twenty-nine patients. *N Engl J Med.* 1988;318:333-340.
3. McBride LR, Naunheim KS, Fiore AC, et al. Clinical experience with 111 Thoratec ventricular assist devices. *Ann Thorac Surg.* 1999;67:1233-1239.
4. Koerfer R, El-Banayosy A, Arusoglu L, et al. Single-center experience with the Thoratec ventricular assist device. *J Thorac Cardiovasc Surg.* 2000;119:596-600.
5. Farrar DJ, Hill JD, Pennington DG, et al. Preoperative and postoperative comparison of patients with univentricular and biventricular support with the Thoratec ventricular assist device as a bridge to cardiac transplantation. *J Thorac Cardiovasc Surg.* 1997;113(1):202-209.
6. Tsukui H, Teuteberg JT, McNamara DM, et al. Biventricular assist device utilization for patients with morbid congestive heart failure: a justifiable strategy. *Circulation.* 2005;112(9 Suppl):I65-I72.
7. Fitzpatrick JR, Frederick JR, Hiesinger W, et al. Early planned institution of biventricular mechanical circulatory support results in improved outcomes compared with delayed conversion of a left ventricular assist device to a biventricular assist device. *J Thorac Cardiovasc Surg.* 2009;137:971-977.
8. Kirsch M, Vermes E, Damy T, et al. Single-centre experience with the Thoratec paracorporeal ventricular assist device for patients with primary cardiac failure. *Arch Cardiovasc Dis.* 2009;102:509-518.
9. Slaughter MS, Tsui SS, El-Banayosy A, et al. Results of a multicenter clinical trial with the Thoratec ventricular assist device. *J Thorac Cardiovasc Surg.* 2007;133:1573-1580; Erratum: 2007;34A, Sep 2007.
10. Slaughter MS, Sobieski MA, Martin M, et al. Home discharge experience with the Thoratec TLC-II portable driver. *ASAIO J.* 2007;53(2):132-135.
11. Babu R, Gill R, Farrar D. Biostability of Thoralon left ventricular assist device blood pumping sacs after long-term clinical use. *ASAIO J.* 2004 Sep-Oct;50(5):479-484.
12. Sobieski MA, George TA, Slaughter MS. The Thoratec mobile computer: initial in-hospital and outpatient experience. *ASAIO J.* 2004 Jul-Aug;50(4):373-375.
13. Arabia FA, Paramesh V, Toporoff B. Biventricular cannulation for the Thoratec ventricular assist device. *Ann Thorac surg.* 1998;66:2119-2120.
14. Hill JD, Avery GJ, Egrie G, Turley K, Reichenbach S. Less invasive Thoratec LVAD insertion: a surgical technique. *Heart Surg Forum.* 2000;3(3):218-223.
15. Farrar DJ. Ventricular interactions during mechanical circulatory support. *Semin Thorac Cardiovasc Surg.* 1994 Jul;6(3):163-168.
16. Fukamachi K, McCarthy PM, Smedira NG, Vargo RL, Starling RC, Young JB. Preoperative risk factors for right ventricular failure after implantable left ventricular assist device insertion. *Ann Thorac Surg.* Dec 1999;68(6):2181-2184.

17. Ochiai Y, McCarthy PM, Smedira NG, et al. Predictors of severe right ventricular failure after implantable left ventricular assist device insertion: analysis of 245 patients. *Circulation.* 2002 Sep 24;106(12 Suppl 1):I198-I202.
18. Kormos RL, Teuteberg JJ, Pagani FD, et al. Right ventricular failure in patients with the HeartMate II continuous-flow left ventricular assist device: incidence, risk factors, and effect on outcomes. *J Thorac Cardiovasc Surg.* 2010;139:1316-1324.
19. Fitzpatrick JR, Frederick JR, Hsu V, et al. Risk score derived from preoperative data analysis predicts the need for biventricular mechanical circulatory support. *J Heart Lung Transplant.* 2008;1286-1292.
20. Matthews JC, Koelling TM, Pagani FD, Aaronson KD. The right ventricular failure risk score: a pre-operative tool for assessing the risk of right ventricular failure in left ventricular assist device candidates. *J Am Coll Cardiol.* 2008;51:2163-2172.
21. Drakos SG, Janicki L, Horne BD, et al. Risk factors predictive of right ventricular failure after left ventricular assist device implantation. *Am J Cardiol.* 2010;105(7):1030-1035.
22. Kormos RL, Gasior TA, Kawai A, et al. Transplant candidate's clinical status rather than right ventricular function defines need for univentricular versus biventricular support. *J Thorac Cardiovasc Surg.* 1996;111(4):773-782; discussion 782-773.
23. Morris RJ, Pochettino A, O'Hara M, Gardner TJ, Acker MA. Emergent mechanical support in the community: improvement with early transplant center referral. *J Heart Lung Transplant.* 2005;24(6):764-768.
24. Kavarana MN, Pessin-Minsley MS, Urtecho J, et al. Right ventricular dysfunction and organ failure in left ventricular assist device recipients: a continuing problem. *Ann Thorac Surg.* 2002;73(3):745-750.
25. Fitzpatrick JR, 3rd, Frederick JR, Hiesinger W, et al. Early planned institution of biventricular mechanical circulatory support results in improved outcomes compared with delayed conversion of a left ventricular assist device to a biventricular assist device. *J Thorac Cardiovas Surg.* Apr 2009;137(4):971-977.
26. Morgan JA, John R, Lee BJ, Oz MC, Naka Y. Is severe right ventricular failure in left ventricular assist device recipients a risk factor for unsuccessful bridging to transplant and post-transplant mortality. *Annals of Thorac Surg.* Mar 2004;77(3):859-863.
27. Deng MC, Edwards LB, Hertz MI, et al. Mechanical circulatory support device database of the International Society for Heart and Lung Transplantation: third annual report--2005. *J Heart Lung Transplant.* Sep 2005;24(9):1182-1187.
28. Moriguchi J, Kwon M, Plunkett M, et al. Improved clinical outcomes using biventricular assist devices as bridges to transplant in critically ill patients. *J Heart Lung Transplant.* 2008;27:S164. Poster presented at: International Society for Heart and Lung Transplantation 28th Annual Meeting and Scientific Sessions; 2008 Apr 9-12; Boston.
29. Netuka J, Pirk J, Szarszol O. Successful clinical outcomes following implantation of biventricular assist devices in patients at risk of right heart failure. Presented at 4th European Mechanical Circulatory Support Summit, 2009 Dec 2-5; Paris.
30. Farrar DJ, Holman WR, McBride LR, et al. Long-term follow-up of Thoratec ventricular assist device bridge-to-recovery patients successfully removed from support after recovery of ventricular function. *J Heart Lung Transplant.* 2002;21(5):516-521.
31. Slaughter MS, Silver MA, Farrar DJ, Tatooles AJ, Pappas PS: A new method of monitoring recovery and weaning the Thoratec left ventricular assist device. *Ann Thorac Surg.* 2001;71:215-218.
32. Zimmerman H, Coelho-Anderson R, Smith R, et al. Bridge to recovery with a Thoratec biventricular assist device for postpartum cardiomyopathy. *ASAIO J.* 2010 Sep-Oct;56(5):479-480.
33. Reinhartz O, Keith FM, El-Banayosy A, et al. Multicenter experience with the Thoratec ventricular assist device in children and adolescents. *J Heart Lung Transplant.* 2001;20(4):439-448.
34. Reinhartz O, Stiller B, Eilers R, Farrar DJ. Current clinical status of pulsatile pediatric circulatory support. *ASAIO J.* 2002 Sep-Oct;48(5):455-459.
35. Copeland JG, Arabia FA, Smith RG. Bridge to transplantation with a Thoratec left ventricular assist device in a 17-kg child. *Ann Thorac Surg.* 2001;71:1003-1004.
36. Newcomb AE, Negri JC, Brizard CP, et al. Successful left ventricular assist device bridge to transplantation after failure of a Fontan revision. *J Heart Lung Transplant.* 2006;25:365-367.

CHAPTER 28

THE SYNCARDIA TOTAL ARTIFICIAL HEART

Steven Langford

BACKGROUND AND HISTORY

The pneumatically actuated total artificial heart (TAH) is currently available through SynCardia Systems Inc (Syncardia Systems, Inc. Tucson, AZ). The SynCardia total artificial heart (Fig. 28–1) is the latest design that is descended from the original research done by William Kolff at the University of Utah and was formerly known as the Jarvik–7-70 total artificial heart. The original research and implantation techniques were pioneered by such luminaries as Robert Jarvik, Clifford Kwan-Gett, William Devries, Lyle Joyce, and Don Olsen. The first implantation of the original 100-cc Jarvik-7 TAH was performed at the University of Utah in 1982.

DESCRIPTION, DIMENSIONS, AND FEATURES

The SynCardia TAH is the modern version of CardioWest artificial heart produced in the 1990s. The 70-cc SynCardia artificial heart is a pneumatic diaphragm pump that is implanted orthotopically in the chest (Fig. 28–2). Diseased ventricles are completely removed along with the valves and replaced by right and left artificial ventricles. Right and left ventricles have a total displacement volume of approximately 400 cm^3 and weigh approximately 160 g. The heart is constructed of a biocompatible polyurethane. Ventricular cannulae are tunneled subcutaneously and are connected to a paratubal driveline that attaches to an external drive system. The SynCardia TAH is unique to other mechanical assist devices in that diseased ventricles are completely excised. Inflow cuffs are sewn directly to the remnant right and left atria. Outflow vascular grafts are joined by an end-to-end anastomosis to the pulmonary artery and aorta.

The currently available 70-cc-size device is generally used in patients who have a body surface area (BSA) of at least 1.6 m^2. Proper fit prediction may also be assessed by measuring a left ventricular end-diastolic diameter (LVEDD) of 70 mm or greater. Smaller artificial heart models are actively under development. Drivelines from the implanted artificial heart attach to an external drive system. Hospital-based drive systems provide operators an opportunity to optimize drive parameters to meet every patient's needs. Portable drive systems are designed to allow stable patients to be released from the hospital while awaiting heart transplant.

BENEFITS OF THE TOTAL ARTIFICIAL HEART

Total artificial heart (TAH) technology is the most aggressive of all mechanical circulatory support devices in that the diseased ventricles are completely removed from the patient. Removal of the diseased heart provides an immediate end to the underlying cardiac dysfunction. Clinicians can then regain total control over a failing circulatory system. Physiologic pressures and cardiac output are quickly restored to normal levels. The absence of inflow and outflow cannulae enhances filling and ejection of the blood allowing for high cardiac output with low inflow pressures. Inotropic support is not required and there is no more threat of arrhythmia. Cardiac output may be greater than 9 L/min with normal right and left atrial pressures. Lower central venous pressure (CVP) with normal systemic pressure provides greater perfusion differential pressure across the end organs. Cardiac dysfunction is completely eliminated. Support is immediate, and control and management of the device is simple and requires very little time. The artificial heart can provide long-term support with documented support times of around 3 years as a bridge device. Improved plastic technology, currently under development, is intended to allow even longer duration of support.

DRIVE SYSTEMS

The drivelines from the implanted artificial heart attach to an external drive system. There are two types of drive systems currently available: mobile hospital-based drive systems and portable drive systems. Hospital-based drive systems are mobile in the hospital and allow operators to have control of the operating parameters to optimize performance. Smaller portable drive systems are used to allow patients to leave the hospital and optimize patient mobility. Currently, there are two hospital drive systems and two portable drive systems. Older models are being phased out over the next few years in favor of newer drive systems.

■ HOSPITAL-BASED DRIVE SYSTEMS

Circulatory Support System (Big Blue)

The circulatory support system (CSS) (Fig. 28–3) is the original drive system designed in the 1980s and has been the work horse for the majority of more than 850 implants. This large console weighs about 440 lb (200 kg). A computer on top of the large metal frame allows operators to monitor device performance. Changes to drive pressures, rate, and vacuum are made by turning regulator knobs and dials. Within the drive system is an independent backup driver. Operators manually change to the backup driver if a problem is suspected with the driver. A panel of lights and audible alarms are activated when system performance is out of specified limits. Hospital compressed air provides the primary air pressure source, and internal regulators adjust the pressure to the appropriate levels used to control the heart. For patient transportation, two internal self-contained

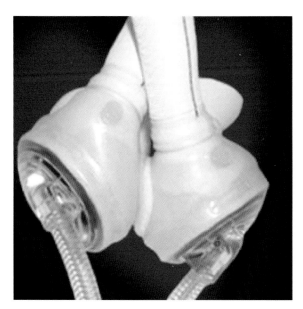

FIGURE 28–1. The SynCardia total artificial heart. (Courtesy of syncardia. com. www.syncardia.com.)

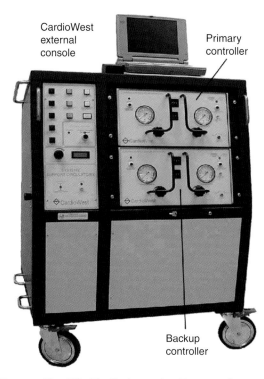

FIGURE 28–3. The CSS (Big Blue) console. (Courtesy of syncardia.com. www.syncardia.com.)

underwater breathing apparatus (SCUBA) air tanks provide about 2 hours of pneumatic backup air pressure. Internal batteries provide about 4 hours of electric backup power.

The Companion Drive System

The Companion drive system (Fig. 28–4) is intended to ultimately replace the CSS drive system. Like the CSS console, the drivers are leased to implanting hospitals and maintenance is

performed periodically by SynCardia. Redundant internal air compressors provide the regulated pulses of air to the ventricles. A touch screen interface allows the operator to control drive variables to optimize device management. Redundant compressors provide internal backup for compressed air. The system continually monitors its performance and alerts the operator if the system goes out of specified limits. The driver may be docked into a hospital cart or into a small caddy. The hospital cart docking configuration provides a larger screen on the top of

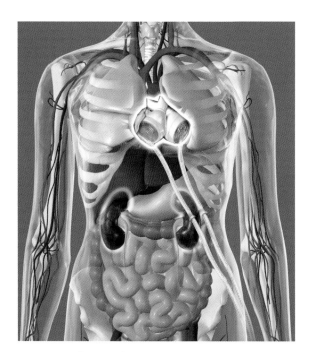

FIGURE 28–2. Orthotopic placement of the artificial heart. (Courtesy of syncardia.com. www.syncardia.com.)

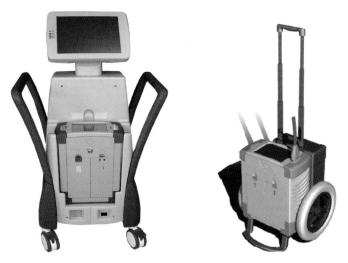

FIGURE 28–4. The Companion driver. Hospital cart and caddy docking configurations. (Courtesy of syncardia.com. www.syncardia.com.)

the cart. The touch screen display allows for driver management and system performance evaluation. The caddy docking configuration provides greater mobility within the hospital. While in the caddy, complete system management is by a touch screen on top of the driver. Operators may assess the waveforms and make driver changes from either of the touch screens.

■ PORTABLE DRIVE SYSTEMS

When a patient is stable, the hospital drive system may be switched to a portable external driver that allows the patient greater mobility. The two portable drive systems are the EXCOR TAH drive system and the Freedom drive system. These drive systems are intended to allow the patient to be released to home care while awaiting future heart transplant. The EXCOR drive system is currently available only in Europe and is being phased out by the Freedom driver. The EXCOR drive system is not discussed here.

Freedom Portable Driver

The Freedom drive system (Fig. 28–5) was introduced in 2010 in the United States and in Europe and offers the most lightweight drive system currently available. It is intended to be used on stable patients. This system provides maximum portability and minimum input requirements from the patient. Drive pressure and vacuum are preset. The clinician has the ability to vary the device rate to adjust for various patient needs. Depressing a button on the top of the driver allows visualization of the rate and the calculated fill volume and cardiac output of the left ventricle. The Freedom portable driver weighs about 13.5 lb (6.12 kg), including the two batteries. Replaceable external batteries provide approximately 3 hours of battery operation. The batteries may be exchanged by the patient or caregiver, or the driver can be plugged into wall power to recharge the batteries. A car charger is also provided to run the driver and recharge the

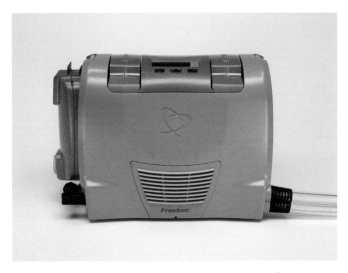

FIGURE 28–5. The Freedom driver. (Courtesy of syncardia.com. www. syncardia.com.)

batteries while in a car. The driver can be worn in a specialized back pack or shoulder bag. These bags may also be placed on a wheeled cart.

■ DRIVER MANAGEMENT

Control and management of the drive system is based on two principles. First, the pressures are adjusted to provide for complete emptying of the ventricle on each cycle. This is known as full eject or complete eject. Second, the rate is adjusted to provide filling of 50 to 60 mL of volume on each cycle. This is known as partial fill. Following these two principles of operation optimizes device performance. There are no electronics or sensors in the artificial ventricles. Management of the device is performed by assessing the pneumatic drive pressure waveforms and the flow volume of air through the driveline. Optimizing the performance of the artificial heart produces a Frank-Starling effect allowing increased cardiac output during periods of increased activity.

Full Ejection

Full ejection of the ventricle is assessed by observing the shape of the air pressure waveform. At the start of systole, air pressure is sent through the driveline to the ventricle and the pressure in the driveline increases rapidly until the pressure opens the outflow valve. When the outflow valve opens, the diaphragms begin to move forward. As the blood moves out of the device, the diaphragms move into the ventricle. The air pressure waveform flattens out as the diaphragm moves in the ventricle. When the diaphragm reaches the full extent of travel, the pressure increases rapidly to the operator set pressure. This second rapid rise in the pressure is known as the full eject flag of the pressure waveform and indicates that the ventricle has fully ejected all of the blood from the device. Figure 28–6 shows a typical full eject pressure waveform.

Partial Fill

Operator-made adjustments control the device to provide typical active filling volumes between 50 and 60 mL per beat. Filling volume characteristic is assessed using the attached external drive system. The attached drive system calculates the filling volume by measuring the volume of air exhausted during device diastole. Partial filling of the device is assessed by observing the air flow that is exhausted from the ventricle during diastole (Fig. 28–7). At the end of systole the diaphragms in the ventricles are in the fully distended position. The external driver opens a valve and releases the air pressure in the drivelines. As the air pressure decreases, the outflow valve in the ventricle closes and the inflow valve opens and atrial pressure begins to push the diaphragm into the ventricle. The air is pushed out of the driveline as the blood enters into the ventricle. Flow transducers in the external drive system measure the flow of air and calculate a volume of air that has exited the ventricle. The volume of air that is forced out of the ventricle is roughly equal to that of blood that entered into the ventricle. This volume is the filling volume of the ventricle and can be seen on the display of

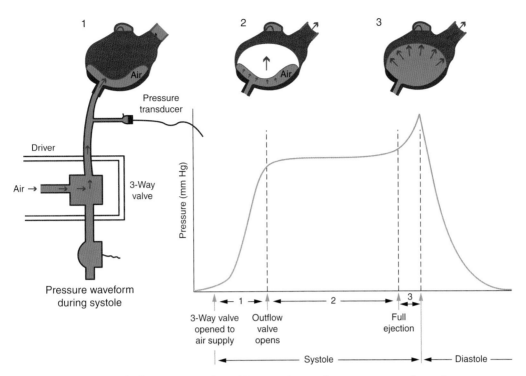

FIGURE 28–6. Full eject indicated by second rise in pressure waveform. (Courtesy of syncardia.com. www.syncardia.com.)

the external driver. The rate of the device is adjusted to allow the ventricle to fill about 80% of its full capacity. The target for the 70-mL ventricle is 50 to 60 mL per beat. Each cardiac filling cycle will vary depending on the inflow pressure to the ventricle. Having a variable stroke volume allows variable cardiac output

that provides a Frank-Starling–type effect on cardiac output. With proper adjustment of the rate and pressure, the ventricle will fully empty each cycle and will fill to 50 to 60 mL volume each cardiac cycle. Typical device rate for the 70-mL artificial heart is 125 beats/min, yielding a cardiac output of 6.3 to 7.5 L/min.

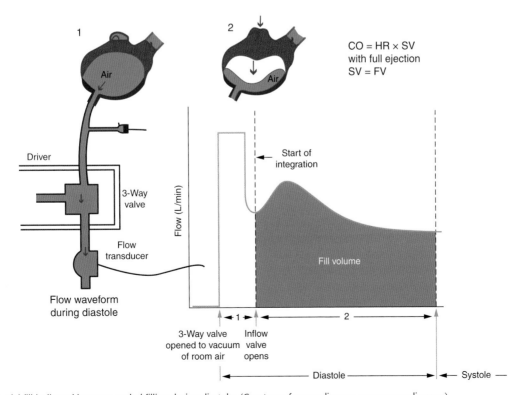

FIGURE 28–7. Partial fill indicated by open-ended filling during diastole. (Courtesy of syncardia.com. www.syncardia.com.)

REGULATORY APPROVALS

Use of the SynCardia temporary TAH (TAH-t) is currently Food and Drug Administration (FDA) approved for use in transplant-eligible patients suffering from biventricular failure who are at imminent risk of death. It is also authorized for use in the European Union with the CE mark and is also registered for use in Russia, Canada, and Australia. In the United States, the Freedom drive system is currently approved for use as part of an investigational device exemption (IDE) study. The study is intended to show the ability of the artificial heart patients to be managed outside of the hospital environment. In Europe the Freedom drive system has the CE mark approval for out-of-hospital use and is also approved for use in Russia. The Companion driver is approved for use in Europe and Russia and is intended to be introduced into the United States after final approval by the US FDA regulatory agency.

CLINICAL DATA

The August 2004 issue of the *New England Journal of Medicine* published clinical data collected as part of the clinical trial to support the premarket approval (PMA) application to the FDA.[1] In the clinical trial, 79% survival to transplantation was achieved in patients who received a TAH according to protocol. The overall survival rate of these patients at 1 year was 70%. The mean time of support in the clinical trail was reported to be 79 days. The maximum reported support time on an artificial heart to date is 971 days. Worldwide shortage of donor hearts will likely increase the importance of long-term support with the TAH. Since 1983, there have been over 860 implants of this artificial heart throughout the world. About half of these were in North America and the other half in Europe. Scarcity of external drive systems has limited wider use of the artificial heart, but new drive systems now offer an opportunity to expand the availability for use.

REFERENCE

1. Copeland JG, Smith RG, Arabia FA, et al. Cardiac replacement with a total artificial heart as a bridge to transplantation. *N Engl J Med.* 2004;351(9): 859-867.

CHAPTER 29

THE ABIOCOR TOTAL ARTIFICIAL HEART

Daniel H. Raess

The AbioCor implantable heart is the first available totally implantable artificial heart and has been designed as an alternative to transplantation. This device has been under development since the early 1980s by Abiomed Inc, (Danvers, MA).[1] The initial preclinical trials were conducted at the Texas Heart Institute and the University of Louisville.[2,3] In February 2001, permission to perform clinical trials was granted by the Food and Drug Administration (FDA). The first implantation was initiated on July 2, 2001 at the University of Louisville.

The AbioCor is a pulsatile electrohydraulic implantable replacement heart capable of delivering up to 8 L/min pump output over a broad range of physiologic pressures. System control is achieved on a beat-by-beat basis targeting a constant stroke volume to ensure repeated full filling and full ejection. Except for the inflow cuffs and the outflow graft connectors, which are constructed from standard medical grade velour patches and grafts, the blood-contacting components of the AbioCor are made from Angioflex, a polyether urethane. Titanium is used as the casing material to avoid corrosion. Medical grade epoxy is used to provide rigidity to nonmoving portions of the blood pumps. The flow paths through the pumps are designed to avoid creating regions of stasis. The inflow and outflow valves are designed to maintain proper washout of the leaflets. With the use of polyurethane valves, the AbioCor ventricles operate quietly.

The hydraulic system that powers the device consists of a miniature centrifugal pump and a reciprocating switching valve that reverses the direction of the fluid flow on every beat. The hydraulic fluid actuates the flexing membranes, which keep the hydraulic fluid separate from the blood, resulting in the simultaneous filling of blood on one side and ejecting of blood on the other side. Systole on the left side occurs synchronously with diastole on the right side and vice versa. The AbioCor System can accommodate the difference in cardiac outputs required between the left and right ventricles. In the normal anatomy, physiologic shunts exist to allow higher cardiac outputs on the left side of the heart than on the right side. In the AbioCor, a hydraulic balance chamber shunts the right chamber volume (also known as shunt flow), thus reducing cardiac output on the right side relative to the left side. This feature allows the maintenance of physiologic left atrial pressure.

The AbioCor System is implanted while the patient is on cardiopulmonary bypass (CPB).[4] The diseased ventricles are excised and cuffs are sewn to the two atrial remnants (Fig. 29–1A). Aortic and pulmonary grafts are sewn in place (Fig. 29–1B). The cuffs

and grafts have mating connectors to the inflow and outflow ports of the device to facilitate snap-on coupling (Fig. 29–1C). De-airing must occur before transition from CPB to the AbioCor System (Fig. 29–1D).

The AbioCor System can be divided into three subsystems:

- Implantable AbioCor System components
- External AbioCor System components
- Patient-carried electronics (PCE)

The following sections describe the functions of each of these subsystems.

IMPLANTABLE ABIOCOR SYSTEM COMPONENTS

The Implantable AbioCor System consists of all of the implantable components required for normal operation of the AbioCor System. The main components of this subsystem are described in the following text.

■ IMPLANTED COMPONENTS

Thoracic Unit

The Thoracic unit converts electric power into blood flow to support the circulatory system of the patient. It is implanted in the space vacated after excising the native diseased ventricles. It alternately ejects blood into the systemic and pulmonary circulations.

Implanted Controller

The Implanted controller is the "brain" of the entire system. It is microprocessor based and provides control and monitoring of the Thoracic unit. It also has the capability to receive and transmit information to the external systems via a radio frequency (RF) communication link.

Implanted Battery

The implanted battery is a rechargeable, lithium ion–based power source that can maintain normal operation of the implantable system in the absence of an external power source for approximately 45 minutes.

Implanted Transcutaneous Energy Transmission Coil

The implanted transcutaneous energy transmission (TET) coil receives power in the form of radio waves from an external power source (the external TET) and converts it into direct current (DC) to power the implantable AbioCor System.

Implanted Cable

The implanted cable provides electrical connections between the internal components of the AbioCor System. The implanted cable also has an integral RF antenna that is used for the RF communications.

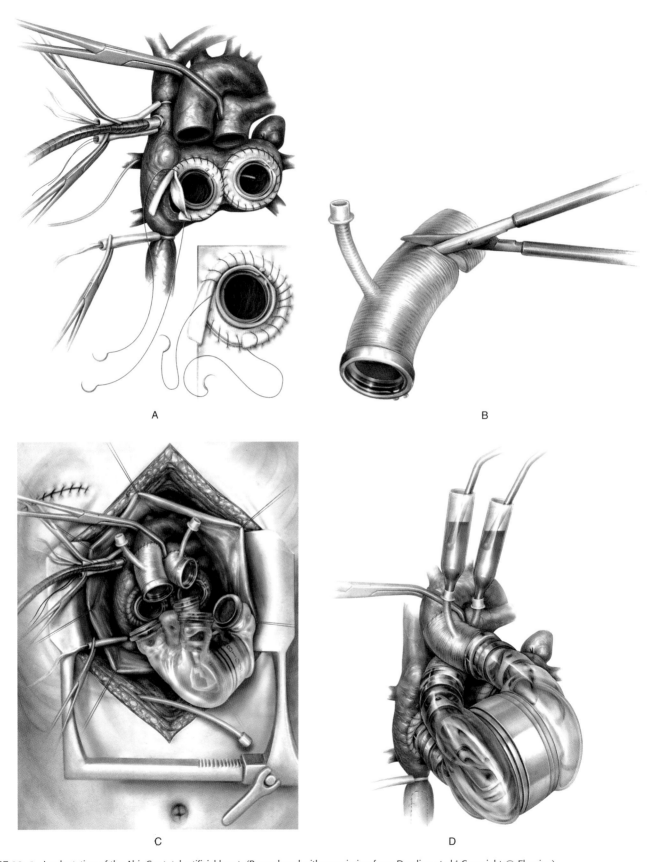

A

B

C

D

FIGURE 29–1. Implantation of the AbioCor total artificial heart. (Reproduced with permission from Dowling et al.[4] Copyright © Elsevier.)

EXTERNAL ABIOCOR SYSTEM COMPONENTS

The external subsystem consists of all of the components that are required to support normal operation of the AbioCor for implantation, intensive care unit (ICU) recovery, patient ambulation, and out-of-hospital use. The main components of this subsystem are described in the following text. Figure 29–2 illustrates the external components and their functional relationship with the implanted system.

■ CONSOLE

The AbioCor console is the primary interface and power source for the implanted AbioCor System components. The console is used to monitor AbioCor System parameters and alarms as well as make changes in system run conditions. Several modes of access help ensure safe system operation. For example, a user can use the console to stop operation of the Thoracic unit only during implantation. This function, essential during intraoperative de-airing of the Thoracic unit, is not accessible in any other functional mode. In the home mode, the display is significantly simplified to avoid information overload or potentially harmful actions by the user. Drive circuitry in the console powers the external TET coil.

■ EXTERNAL TRANSCUTANEOUS ENERGY TRANSMISSION COIL

The external TET allows delivery of electromagnetic energy to the implanted TET. There are two different TET cable lengths to accommodate various use environments. A DuoDERM-based Velcro patch is used to anchor the external TET at the skin region overlying the implanted TET.

■ RADIO FREQUENCY COMMUNICATION MODULE

The RF communication module uses bidirectional wireless radio communication to send data between the implanted controller and the console or PCE.

PATIENT-CARRIED ELECTRONICS

The Patient-carried electronics (PCE) consists of all of the components that are required to support normal operation of the AbioCor System when the patient is away from the AbioCor console (Fig. 29–3). It supplies battery power to the implanted AbioCor System through the external TET. The portable PCE system allows patients to be in different environments, such as

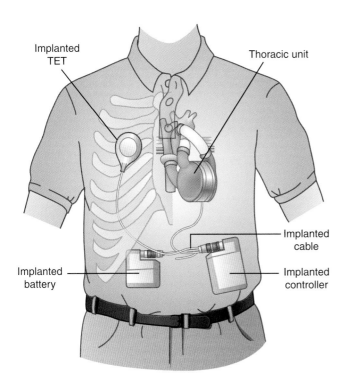

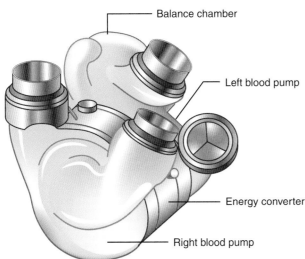

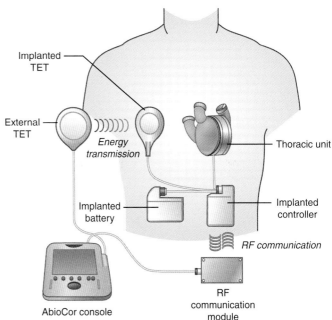

FIGURE 29–2. External components and their functional relationship with the implanted parts. (Reproduced with permission from Abiomed, Inc.)

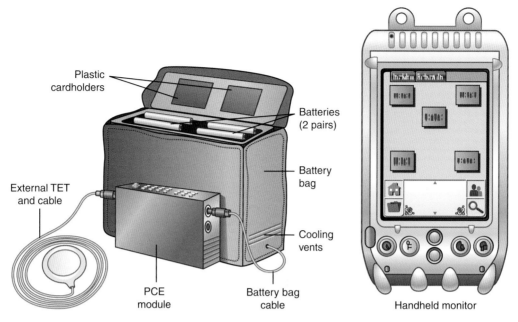

FIGURE 29-3. The patient-carried electronics (PCE) system and handheld monitor. (Reproduced with permission from Abiomed, Inc.)

restaurants, office buildings, vehicles, home, or outdoors, for extended periods of time. The main components of this subsystem are described in the following text.

■ PCE CONTROL MODULE

The lightweight PCE control module contains the circuitry to drive the TET and to produce simple alarms such as low battery, TET misalignment, high PCE temperature, and a general AbioCor System alarm.

■ EXTERNAL TRANSCUTANEOUS ENERGY TRANSMISSION COIL

The PCE uses the same TET coils that are used for the AbioCor Console.

■ PCE POWER AND BAG

The PCE batteries are the primary power source for the PCE control module. The PCE holds two pairs of batteries to allow for appropriate backup. The four batteries and the TET are housed in a nylon PCE bag specifically designed for portability.

■ HANDHELD MONITOR

The handheld monitor allows the user to view specific information about AbioCor System operation and alarms, and clear the alarm when the condition has resolved. This relieves the patient from needing to be near the console to have full diagnostic capability. The handheld monitor does not, however, provide control of the internal system. The console is needed to make changes to beat rate, motor speed, or balance settings.

■ ALTERNATING CURRENT POWER ADAPTER

The alternating current (AC) power adapter is an alternate power source for the PCE control module. It permits a patient, while stationary, to connect the PCE control module to standard AC power, ensuring a steady source of power to the PCE without using the PCE batteries.

■ PCE BATTERY CHARGER

The PCE battery charger is a 10-bay charger that allows the patient to charge up to five sets of PCE batteries. It also provides diagnostic information on the state of charge of the PCE batteries.

CLINICAL TRIAL RESULTS

The FDA approved an IDE clinical trial (IDE no. G000329) in January, 2001. The goal of this trial was to assess the safety and potential effectiveness of the fully implantable AbioCor replacement heart as a potential therapy for those cardiac patients whose therapeutic options have been exhausted. Candidate selection proceeded in two stages: a screening stage and an implant consent stage. During the screening stage, a comprehensive medical assessment was performed. This assessment included determining the severity of a candidate's heart failure and the potential fit of the device in the patient's thoracic cavity.

Candidates eligible for the trial were not eligible for heart transplant based on the center's criteria at the time of screening, were in biventricular failure not treatable with implantable left ventricular assist device a (LVAD), and were under optimal medical management, yet were unlikely to survive for a month based on the clinical judgment of the treating physicians. Patients with irreversible end-organ failure or inadequate psychosocial support were excluded from the trial.

Fourteen subjects were enrolled in the trial at four centers. Twelve of the 14 subjects were enrolled at two centers. All candidates were males, due primarily to size constraints. The mean age of this initial cohort was 67 ± 7.9 years, ranging between 51 and 79 years old. The percentage of subjects excluded from transplant was 43% (6/14) due to age; 29% (4/14) due to irreversible pulmonary hypertension; 14% (2/14) due to malignancy; and 14% (2/14) due to multiple comorbidities, including diabetes, neuropathy, renal dysfunction, and hepatic dysfunction.

Two centers performed 12 of the 14 AbioCor System implant procedures and each of the remaining two centers performed one implant procedure. Twelve subjects survived the implant surgery while two did not. All four centers were successful in their first implant. The 12 subjects were supported by the AbioCor for cumulative support duration of 5.2 years. The mean individual survival time for all 14 subjects was 4.5 months, ranging from 0 to 512 days. The median survival time was 3.6 months. Two patients did not survive the operative procedure. The remaining 12 AbioCor subjects in the trial lived out the remaining portions of their lives on the device. Support to six of the 12 subjects was withdrawn secondary to cerebrovascular accidents (CVAs). There were two device failures. Four subjects died of multiorgan failure or sepsis. One of the two operative deaths was caused by uncontrollable bleeding and the other by pulmonary embolism, most likely due to the use of factor concentrates following protamine reversal. Three of the six CVA-related deaths were due to inflow structure thrombosis, while the remaining three were due to factors preventing adequate anticoagulation of the subjects. One device failure was due to membrane wear and the other due to motor stoppage. The causes of multiorgan failure or sepsis in the remaining four patients were the result of (1) a vein puncture from a dialysis catheter leading to abdominal bleeding, aspiration, and subsequent sepsis, (2) unhealed suture wound, and (3) two cases of preexisting hepatic dysfunction that failed to reverse.

The results of the initial study of the AbioCor System provided the following safety data in subjects with severe end-stage heart failure facing imminent risk of death. Two device failures occurred, one anticipated and one unexpected, representing about 83% (10/12) failure-free device operation clinically consistent with the demonstrated 1-year bench operation. The observed stroke rate was 0.29 per subject-month. No device-related infection problems were observed in AbioCor subjects. Safety features for power management have been built into the system to avoid unintentional misuses that may result in hazards. The device restored normal hemodynamics and afforded dysfunctional end organs (eg, kidneys and liver), a chance of recovery. Although only two subjects were discharged from the hospital—one to home and the other to a hotel near the hospital—their experiences showed that the subjects and their caregivers were successful in managing the AbioCor System outside of the hospital environment, in their home and community settings.

Currently, the AbioCor has been granted Humanitarian Device Exemption (HDE) status and is available under this program in a very small number of centers under an FDA clinical trial. All patients are still required to be nontransplant candidates and to be in biventricular failure. If a patient should regain transplant status after AbioCor implantation, transplantation would be currently allowed pending acceptance of the transplant program.

REFERENCES

1. Dowling RD, Gray LA, Jr, Etoch SW, et al. The AbioCor implantable replacement heart. *Ann Thorac Surg.* 2003;75:S93-S99.
2. Dowling RD, Etoch SW, Stevens K, et al. Initial experience with the AbioCor implantable replacement heart at the University of Louisville. *ASAIO J.* 2000;46:579-581.
3. Dowling RD, Gray LA, Jr, Etoch SW, et al. Initial experience with the AbioCor implantable replacement heart system. *J Thorac Cardiovasc Surg.* 2004;127:131-141.
4. Dowling R, Etoch S, Gray L. Operative techniques for implantation of the AbioCor total artificial heart. *Op Tech Thorac Cardiovasc Surg.* 2002;7:139-151.

CHAPTER 30

THE BERLIN HEART EXCOR PEDIATRIC ASSIST DEVICE

Jennifer Rutledge, Christina VanderPluym,
Bob Kroslowitz, Ali Kilic, and Holger Buchholz

Mechanical circulatory support (MCS) with ventricular assist devices (VAD) has evolved in the pediatric population as an accepted modality for the failing heart refractory to maximal medical and surgical management.[1-3] Refinement of preimplantation planning and postimplantation management has resulted in survival rates to transplantation comparable to those without preceding VAD support. While there remains a more expansive armamentarium of VAD options for adult patients, the pediatric population has been limited to fewer devices with the EXCOR Pediatric gathering the most experience to date.

The EXCOR Pediatric was developed and approved for clinical use in Europe during the early 1990s and was granted CE mark approval in 1992. Worldwide acceptance of the EXCOR Pediatric grew over the first decade of use. Mounting experience began to clearly demonstrate its ability to provide stable circulatory support for children weighing as light as 2 kg for as long as 400 days. This device permitted physicians to be more aggressive in lifting sedation and paralysis, discontinuing ventilatory support, and promoting early ambulation and rehabilitation. These clinical benefits were widely considered infeasible with extracorporeal membrane oxygenation (ECMO) and while providing the necessary hemodynamic stability, EXCOR also allowed for child social interaction and development while awaiting cardiac transplantation or ventricular recovery.

In August 2000, the EXCOR Pediatric emerged in North America as an alternative for children requiring MCS. The use of the EXCOR Pediatric grew in North America under Humanitarian Use regulated by the Food and Drug Administration (FDA) Office of Orphan Products in the United States and the Special Access Regulations by Health Canada. By 2007, over 80 children in North America had been implanted, with each approved on a case-by-case basis after completing the process for emergency use or special access by the respective regulatory authorities. Because of the increasing demand for the device and need created by the North American pediatric medical community, the use of the EXCOR Pediatric had grown to a level where FDA, Health Canada, and Berlin Heart recognized the need for a formal clinical trial for potential approval of the device.

Approved in May 2007, the clinical trial is centered on assessing reasonable safety and probable benefit. The primary population for the EXCOR Pediatric was chosen to capture children at eminent risk of death from heart failure and listed for cardiac transplantation. In January 2009, Health Canada issued a Medical Device License and approved the device for use in Canada. However, the device has not yet been approved by the FDA, as the investigational device exemption (IDE) study is ongoing. As of May 2010, more than 300 pediatric patients have been supported in North America with the EXCOR Pediatric, while worldwide use of the device continues to grow. Berlin Heart hopes to complete the IDE study in 2010 and gain FDA approval soon thereafter.

DEVICE DISCRIPTION

The Berlin Heart EXCOR Pediatric is an extracorporeal, pulsatile, pneumatically driven VAD for children and infants over 2 kg.[4] It can be utilized for the left heart alone (LVAD), or as combination left and right heart for biventricular (BiVAD) support. Rarely, it has been used for right ventricular support alone (RVAD). The pump chamber is available as 10, 25, 30, 50, 60, or 80 mL sizes (Fig. 30–1).

■ BLOOD PUMPS

EXCOR blood pumps have transparent polyurethane housing which is divided into an air chamber and a blood chamber by a triple-layer membrane. The blood chamber has an inflow and an outflow stubs to which the inflow and outflow cannulae, respectively, are connected. The pump stubs themselves are made of polyurethane; the end of each stub is fitted with a titanium connector to which the cannula will be connected. The valves located in the pump stubs keep the blood flowing in one direction. The valves are trileaflet in the smaller pumps with the option of mechanical valves in the 50- to 80-mL chambers. The blood pump is equipped with a de-airing nipple which is used for de-airing the blood chamber when the pump is initially implanted. All blood-containing surfaces inside the pump, including the polyurethane valves, consist of the same material and are coated with heparin by the Carmeda process (Carmeda, Upplands Väsby, Sweden). The air chamber of the pump is equipped with a driving tube connector. This connector is used to connect the blood pump to the driving tube through which air is pumped from the driving unit (Ikus). The Ikus generates the suction and driving pressures required to move the blood pump's triple-layer membrane. A graphite powder layer is located between the membrane layers in order to minimize friction.

■ CANNULAE

Three different types of cannulae are available in varying configurations and sizes that are designed to ensure sufficient blood flow between the appropriate anatomical connection site and the blood pump, and that allow for anatomical and blood pump size variations. The three types of cannulae are atrial cannulae (inflow cannulae), ventricular apical cannulae (inflow cannulae), and arterial cannulae (outflow cannulae). Inflow cannulae deliver blood from the heart to the blood pump. Outflow cannulae deliver blood from the pump to the great vessels. For pediatric patients, internal diameters of 5, 6, 9, and 12 mm are available. The cannulae are constructed of silicone, and each cannula has a Dacron velour suture ring at the contact site with the

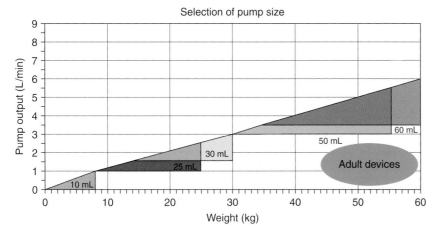

FIGURE 30-1. Selection of pump sizes. (Reproduced with permission from Berlin Heart, Inc.)

The arterial or outflow cannula is supplied with an angle and a Dacron velour–covered sewing rim at one end allowing for end-to-side anastomosis to either the aorta or the pulmonary artery. Like the arterial cannula, the atrial cannula incorporates an angle at their tissue-contacting end. The atrial cannulae are designed with various head lengths, all of which terminate in a basket that protrudes into the atrium after placement. The apical or inflow cannula also serves for inflow of blood into the pump from the heart. Unlike the arterial and atrial cannula designs, the apical cannula configuration *does not* incorporate an angled head at its tissue-contacting end.

abdominal wall which promotes tissue ingrowth. This provides a potential barrier to infection and migration along the skin tunnel. Some vascular cannulae have a shaping wire which allows the cannulae to be adapted to each individual patient's anatomic conditions. All cannulae are made to exit the body through the upper abdominal wall.

■ EXCOR STATIONARY DRIVING UNIT

The electropneumatic stationary driving unit (Ikus) generates the suction and driving pressure required to drive the blood pump (Fig. 30–2). Compressed air moves the pump membrane into its end-systolic position, which thereby ejects blood into the arterial circulation. Negative pressure is then created in pump

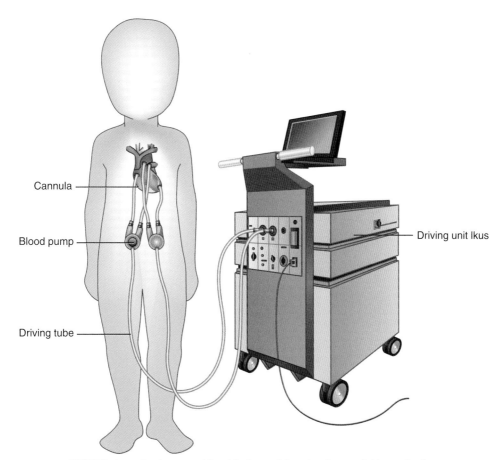

EXCOR shown in place as a biventricular assist system in a pediatric application

FIGURE 30-2. EXCOR biventricular assist configuration in pediatric patient. (Reproduced with permission from Berlin Heart, Inc.)

diastole to assist in filling of the pump. The casing of the driving unit contains the pneumatic/compressor and electronic components as well as a laptop computer that serves as an interface to the operator. The Ikus has three separate compressor systems that operate independently of each other. One pneumatic system is required for each blood pump (right or left heart), with the third serving as an emergency backup. In the case of malfunction of one unit, the backup will take over automatically without delay. If the two units fail simultaneously, the third unit will take over and can operate both pumps with a pump rate of 90 beats/min.

The compressor and pressure/vacuum cylinders are controlled by two redundant internal computers. The internal battery can provide power for up to 1 hour. In emergency situations, or if there is no working Ikus available, the system is equipped with a manual pump (mounted on the Ikus) which can be used to temporarily drive the blood pump(s).

The maximum positive driving pressure of the system is 350 mm Hg with a maximum negative driving pressure of −100 mm Hg. High pressures are needed to overcome the resistance of the smaller pediatric cannulae. The pump rate can be adjusted between 30 and 150 beats/min and the relative systolic duration from 20% to 70%. The system may be operated in uni- or biventricular modes. Additionally, the biventricular mode can be set for "synchronous" mode in which both pumps fill and eject simultaneously, "asynchronous" in which the right and left pumps alternate, or "separate" for completely independent pump function. Patients supported with the EXCOR stationary driving unit must remain as inpatients within a hospital setting. Suggested settings for initiation of the pump for LVAD and RVAD are systole 120 mm Hg, diastole −2.5 mm Hg, rate 30 beats/min, percentage of systole 40% parameters. Weaning from cardiopulmonary bypass settings is adjusted while monitoring pump membrane movement. The suggested settings for LVAD are systole 180 to 240 mm Hg, diastole −30 to −50 mm Hg, rate (dependent on patient weight and pump size), percentage of systole 35% to 50%; and for RVAD are systole 120 to 160 mm Hg, diastole −30 to −50 mm Hg, rate (dependent on patient weight and pump size), percentage of systole 35% to 50%.

The movement of the membrane in the blood chamber as well as the patient's clinical and hemodynamic status dictates any adjustment of the operating parameters. It is paramount to adequately assess the membrane ensuring that it is smooth with both filling and ejection. A membrane that appears wrinkled during filling is likely due to hypovolemia; fluid replacement should be the primary treatment prior to adjusting settings. Other causes for a wrinkled membrane in filling include inflow cannula obstruction, cardiac tamponade, or severe RV failure with LVAD support only. A wrinkled membrane during ejection requires prompt attention as incomplete ejection results in blood stasis and thrombus formation. Causes include high distal pressures (systemic hypertension for LVAD), outflow cannula obstruction, or insufficient pump systolic pressures.

The *Ikus* unit is constantly monitoring the internal drivers, computer, power supply, and battery. Dysfunction with any of these systems will result in an auditory alarm as well as a message on the laptop computer. The *Ikus* monitors the pump membrane movement indirectly through air movement in the driveline. As such, only acute changes will result in an alarm (eg, kinking of cannula), rather than slow gradual changes that may not be detected by the system (eg, cardiac tamponade). With major system failure, the Ikus will automatically switch to backup systems.

■ EXCOR MOBILE DRIVING SYSTEM

The EXCOR mobile driving system allows for stable adolescent and adult patients to be managed in an outpatient setting, following a period of stabilization in the hospital. This allows stable patients treated with the EXCOR pump as either a bridge-to-transplant, bridge-to-recovery, or destination therapy to achieve a more normal quality of life, attend school, or obtain employment while still being supported with the mobile driver. The mobile driver may only be used to drive EXCOR blood pumps of the 60 and 80 mL size. The mobile driver is intended exclusively for supporting mobile patients with stable hemodynamic parameters following a suitable period of support by the EXCOR stationary driving unit (Ikus). The mobile driver cannot be used for initiating therapy with the EXCOR blood pumps either during surgery or in the initial postoperative period. The mobile driver, with its piston pump, is designed to achieve a full stroke volume with the blood pumps for which it has been approved (60- and 80-mL pump), provided that the inflow and outflow conditions permit this. In general, criteria for outpatient care include underlying cardiac function that would support perfusion and blood pressure for at least 10 minutes without external assistance if the EXCOR mobile driver stops; the patient has received adequate training on the use of the mobile diver and is capable of carrying out the operating functions, and the patient is able to maintain adequate hydration.

UNIVENTRICULAR VERSUS BIVENTRICULAR SUPPORT

Consideration for a BiVAD versus an LVAD should be initiated prior to entering the operating room. Preimplantation assessment of right ventricle (RV) function can be done qualitatively with transthoracic and transesophageal echocardiography and quantitatively with cardiac magnetic resonance imaging (MRI). Clinical manifestations of systemic venous congestion with ascites and hepatic failure are also taken into the decision-making paradigm. If RV function is normal with no evidence of systemic venous congestion, LVAD alone is sufficient. In the event of severe ascites, hepatic dysfunction (three times the normal value for alanine transaminase and bilirubin), central venous pressure (CVP) greater than 20 mm Hg, and qualitative or quantitative RV dysfunction, BiVAD support is strongly recommended. Difficulty surrounds the scenario of unknown or moderate RV dysfunction with no clinical stigmata. In this event, intraoperative testing can be completed once the LVAD is implanted with a left atrial pressure of less than 10 mm Hg. If medical management is optimized and the cardiac index remains 2 to 2.5 L/min/m^2 or CVP 15 to 19 mm Hg, it is at the surgeon's discretion to implant an RVAD based on the complete clinical history.

POSTIMPLANTATION CONSIDERATIONS

◼ ANTICOAGULATION

Clinically significant thromboembolic events continue to be a devastating complication during VAD support (Fig. 30–3). The incidence of serious neurological events (thromboembolic or hemorrhagic) has been estimated at 7% to 8%.[4] Despite monumental advances in cardiac assist device technology, the monitoring and management of this hypercoagulable state, secondary to the presence of foreign material, altered rheological state, and peculiarities of pediatric hemostasis, remains a challenge. In addition, sepsis and other inflammatory states can greatly affect coagulation profiles, necessitating vigilant monitoring and adjustments of anticoagulation/antiplatelet (AC/AP) regimens. Current monitoring of AC/AP therapy has expanded past activated clotting time (ACT) traditionally used for ECMO, to include anti–factor Xa for unfractionated heparin level, international normalized ratio (INR), thromboelastograph (TEG), and Platelet Mapping. These tests provide valuable information required to monitor and adjust unfractionated heparin, low-molecular-weight heparin, and AP therapy. Monitoring of renal and hepatic function is also pivotal, as preexisting multiorgan dysfunction can further affect metabolism and excretion of these medications.

The Edmonton Anticoagulation and Platelet Inhibition Protocol guidelines for EXCOR Pediatric VADs have been applied to Berlin Heart EXCOR Pediatric with success. The guideline suggests no anticoagulation for the first 24 hours postimplantation, followed by the initiation of age-appropriate dosing of intravenous unfractionated heparin at 24 to 48 hours (Table 30–1). At 48 hours following surgery, a hemostatically and hemodynamically stable patient may be transitioned from unfractionated heparin to low-molecular-weight heparin (enox-

aparin) (Table 30–2). In patients older than 12 months, oral AC therapy with a vitamin K antagonist can be initiated (target INR 2.7-3.5) once they are hemodynamically stable and receiving adequate enteral feeds. Patients younger than 12 months are unstable on oral AC regimens due to difficulties monitoring the warfarin effect secondary to multiple drug and diet interactions. Based on results of TEG and Platelet Mapping, acetylsalicylic acid may be started at 48 hours and dipyridamole at 4 days postimplantation if the patient is hemodynamically stable, with no bleeding and a platelet count greater than 40000/μL (Table 30–3). Despite adherence to these guidelines, there remains a risk of thromboembolic or hemorrhagic events necessitating strict monitoring of coagulation profiles as well as vigilant surveillance of the pump and cannulae. In the initiation and transition stages of AC/AP therapy, frequent inspection of the pump with a flashlight for any fibrin or clot formation must be done every few hours. Once the patient has stabilized, pump and cannula inspection can be completed twice daily. In the event of significant fibrin or clot formation, additional AC dosing may be given and consideration must be given to changing the pump, depending on the location and size of the clot. Fibrin

TABLE 30–1. UFH Dosing at 24 to 48 Hours Post-VAD Surgery

	≤ 12 mo	≥ 12 mo
Initial dose[a]	15 IU/kg/h	10 IU/kg/h
After 6 h[b]	28 IU/kg/h	20 IU/kg/h

[a]Criteria for UFH initiation:
- Platelet count > 20,000/μL.
- Normal function on Platelet Mapping studies.
- Minimal bleeding (< 2 mL/kg/d).

[b] Six hours after increase to therapeutic dose, obtain a PTT and anti–factor Xa level (desired range 0.35-0.5 U/mL).

UFH, unfractionated heparin; VAD, ventricular assist device.

TABLE 30–2. LMWH at 48 Hours Post-VAD Surgery

	≤ 3 mo	≥ 3 mo	> 1 y
LMWH dosing[a,b]	1.8 mg/kg sc	1.5 mg/kg sc	1.3 mg/kg sc

[a] Criteria for LMWH initiation:
- No bleeding.
- Patient is hemodynamically stable.
- Normal renal function (normal creatinine and urea).

[b] Stop unfractionated heparin (UFH) and administer subcutaneous (sc) LMWH with anti–factor Xa 4 hours after second dose (therapeutic range 0.8-1.1 U/mL).

LMWH, low-molecular-weight heparin; VAD, ventricular assist device.

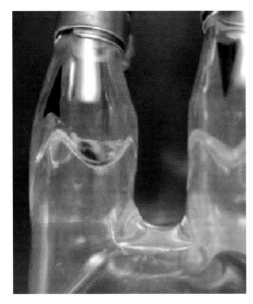

FIGURE 30–3. Polyurethane valve in pediatric pump with clot. (Reproduced with permission from Berlin Heart, Inc.)

TABLE 30-3. Antiplatelet Therapy Post-VAD Surgery

	Acetylsalicylic acid	Dipyridamole
First dose timing	> 48 h	> 4 d
Dosing	1 mg/kg/d divided into two doses[a]	4 mg/kg/d divided into four doses[b]

[a]Criteria for acetylsalicylic acid initiation:
- No bleeding.
- Patient is hemodynamically stable.
- Platelet Mapping does not show significantly decreased platelet function: net ADP G ≥ 4 and AA inhibition >70%.
- Platelet count > 40,000/μL.
- TEG MA > 56 from a CKH sample.

[b]Criteria for dipyridamole initiation:

Platelet Mapping shows platelet inhibition in the presence of net ADP G > 4.

TEG MA ≥ 72 mm from a CKH sample.

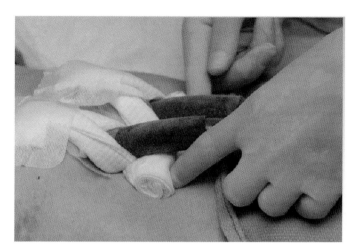

FIGURE 30-4. Pediatric dressing change. (Reproduced with permission from Berlin Heart, Inc.)

and clot formation tends to occur in areas of blood stasis and as such the valve leaflets are a nidus for growth. For LVADs, the presence of a clot in the pump dictates frequent neurological monitoring and decreases the threshold for a pump change. Pump changes can be done quickly with relatively low risk in the intensive care unit (ICU) under sedation, without the need for ventilatory support

■ INFECTION

VAD-related infections are a common complication and result in increased risk of thromboembolic events, multiorgan failure, need for VAD revision, and death. In addition, the presence of infection may adversely affect cardiac transplantation survival. The true incidence of VAD-related infection is difficult to discern, and published data range from 13% to 80% of cases in the adult population with implantable VADs.[5-9] However, the lack of a universal definition for device-related infections and the use of a multitude of different VADs make it difficult to extrapolate these data to the Berlin Heart EXCOR.

Infections with the Berlin Heart EXCOR can involve any aspect of the device with the surgical site and cannula acting as the origin in the majority of cases. The most common pathogens are gram-positive organisms; however, gram-negative species have also been described. As with all chronically hospitalized patients, infection with antibiotic-resistant organisms (methicillin-resistant *Staphylococcus aureus*, vancomycin-resistant enterococci, and *Pseudomonas*) can occur, along with the need for a broader armamentarium of antibiotic regimens.[10] This can then lead to a risk of *Clostridium difficile* enteritis and fungal infections. A high index of suspicion is required for fungal infections, as this patient population can be relatively asymptomatic until fulminant illness occurs. Fungaemia is associated with high mortality and is difficult to clear despite aggressive therapy.[11,12] Gordon and colleagues reported fungal infections during VAD

support to have the highest hazard ratio for death, followed by gram-negative and then gram-positive organisms.[13] *Candida* species are most commonly implicated in VAD-associated fungal infections.

Empiric treatment of VAD-associated infections will be dependent on the site, extent, and pathogen. Additional imaging may be necessary such as computer tomography (CT) to rule out infected collections deep to the cannula. Transthoracic and transesophageal echocardiography is also valuable in identifying vegetations suggestive of endocarditis. Pediatric patients pose an additional challenge due to the often subtle signs and symptoms and, sometimes, rapid clinical progression. Empiric broad-spectrum antibiotics should be initiated at the first clinical suspicion of infection. The addition of empiric antifungal therapy may depend on the degree of illness. Consideration for antibiotic choice must take into account the patient's previous infectious disease history and the institution's microbial resistance patterns. Once the organism is identified, the antibiotic regimen can be narrowed for optimal coverage.

Infection prevention is one of the most important management strategies. Prophylactic intravenous cefazolin is given to all patients for the first week postimplantation. Sterile dressing changes are necessary in monitoring the cannulae-skin interface for erythema, purulent drainage, and skin breakdown (Fig. 30–4). For the first 10 days postsurgery, dressing changes are completed once daily. If the patient is ambulating and the site appears to be healing well, then dressing changes can be extended to twice weekly with a concomitant shower. Even in very young patients, these dressing changes can be completed quickly without the need for analgesia or sedation.

CLINICAL EXPERIENCE

In 1988, the Berlin Heart EXCOR was first implanted in humans[14] with the first pediatric implant in 1990.[15] Clinical experience has shown that use of the EXCOR allows for long-term circulatory support, thereby allowing for restoration of end-organ function,

TABLE 30–4. Primary Diagnosis at Time of EXCOR Pediatric Implant

Idiopathic cardiomyopathy	371 (49.3%)
Congenital heart disease	155 (20.5%)
Myocarditis	97 (12.9%)
Restrictive cardiomyopathy	26 (3.5%)
Postcardiotomy	17 (2.3%)
Toxic cardiomyopathy	13 (1.7%)
Posttransplant	12 (1.6%)
Ischemic cardiomyopathy	7 (0.9%)
Postmyocarditis cardiomyopathy	6 (0.8%)
Acute myocardial infarct	2 (0.3%)
Other	36 (11%)
Unknown	11 (1.5%)

patient extubation and mobilization, enteral feeding, neurologic assessment, physiotherapy, and, ultimately, improved candidacy for transplantation or explantation of the device. Worldwide, 116 sites are currently implanting the EXCOR Pediatric. From 1990 to February 2010, a total of 753 pediatric implants have been performed (48% female/52% male) in children ranging in age from 2 days to 17 years (median 2 years, mean 5 years) (Berlin Heart Registry). Duration of support ranged from 0 to 902 days (mean 72 days). Primary diagnosis at the time of implant is included in Table 30–4, and current patient status is shown in Fig. 30–5.

Hetzer and colleagues reviewed the largest single-center pediatric experience and compared the outcome of children who were supported by the Berlin Heart EXCOR according to

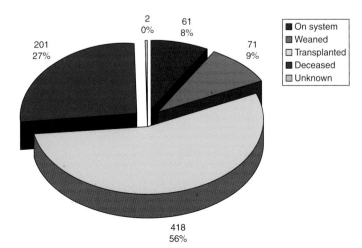

FIGURE 30-5. Berlin Heart Registry–current patient status. (Reproduced with permission from Berlin Heart, Inc.)

the period of treatment.[16] Period 1 consisted of 34 patients supported between 1991 and 1998; period 2 consisted of 28 children supported between 1999 and 2004. The primary outcomes were survival (defined as 30-day survival, heart transplantation, or myocardial recovery) and hospital discharge (discharge home or a rehabilitation center). Comparison of the two treatment periods demonstrated a significant improvement in survival and hospital discharge over time. Discharge from hospital after either device explant or heart transplantation was possible in 35% of patients in period 1 compared to 68% in period 2 ($P = .011$). In period 1, there were no survivors in the group of children younger than 1 year; during period 2, survival in this age group was similar to that of the groups of older children (Fig. 30–6A). Regarding indication for VAD support and ultimate discharge, there was an improvement in the discharge rate over time with 76% of cardiomyopathy patients being discharged in the most recent era compared to 43% in the earlier experience. Similarly, in those with postcardiotomy heart failure, 57% of patients were discharged in period 2 compared to 0% in period 1 (Fig. 30–6B). Reoperation for bleeding was similar in both time periods (eight patients in period 1, seven in period 2). The pump exchange rate per month for thrombus formation was 1.0, 0.3, and 0.4 in period 1, and 0.36, 1.1, and 0.27 in period 2 in the age groups younger than 1 year, 1 to 8 years, and older than 8 years, respectively. Neurologic complications were noted at a similar frequency in both periods: there were two cerebral strokes in the survivors of the group of children older than 8 years in period 1 and one stroke in the survivors of each age group (1-8 years and > 8 years) in period 2. All patients, except one, recovered without neurologic impairment. Cause of death for nonsurvivors during both time periods was not reported. The authors credit modifications to the device system itself, changes in AC protocols, and, importantly, clinical decision making and patent care to have contributed to improvements in clinical outcome. In the earlier experience, the majority of children younger than 1 year were placed on support in an advanced state of circulatory failure, resulting in no hospital survival in this group of children. Subsequently, an institutional policy of earlier VAD support resulted in nearly 75% hospital survival in this group of children in the latter period. Criteria for implant included rapid deterioration of the circulation, critical peripheral perfusion, metabolic acidosis, cardiac index less than 2.0 L/min/m², mixed venous saturation less than 40%; signs of renal and hepatic failure, patient on ventilator with rising Fio_2, and massively impaired cardiac function defined by echocardiography. Similarly, in the postcardiotomy population there was a gradual change in policy for VAD implantation. During period 1, the decision for VAD support was often delayed, following a protracted ICU course with no long-term survivors. The authors subsequently recommended implantation as early as during the initial operation when it became apparent that the cardiac function could not be stabilized postoperatively.

Recent comparisons of outcome of children bridged to transplant with Berlin Heart EXCOR Pediatric versus ECMO show that EXCOR Pediatric provides substantially longer support times without significant increase in the rates of stroke or multisystem organ failure, improved survival to transplant as well

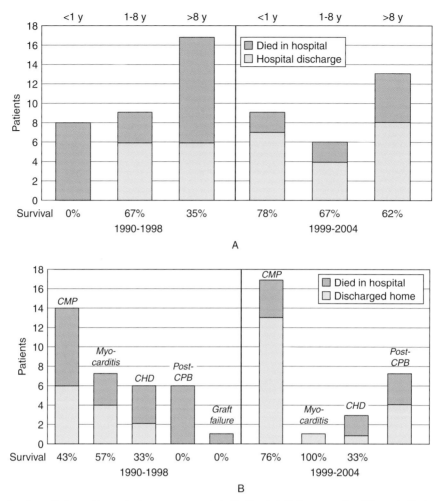

FIGURE 30–6. A. Number of patients discharged home in the treatment periods. **B.** Hospital discharge rate for different indications for ventricular assist device support in the two treatment periods. CHD, congenital heart disease; CMP, cardiomyopathy; post-CPB, postcardiotomy heart failure. (Reproduced with permission from Hetzer R, Potapov EJ, Stiller B. et al. Improvement in survival after mechanical circulatory support with pneumatic pulsatile ventricular assist devices in pediatric patients. Ann Thorac Surg 2006;82:917-925.)

as posttransplant hospital discharge, and long-term survival.[17,18] Experience in the single ventricle population is limited; however, patients following the bidirectional Glenn and Fontan have successfully been supported with EXCOR to transplantation or decannulation.[19-22] Results of the North American FDA trial are expected by the completion of 2010.

REFERENCES

1. Hetzer R, Ptoapov EV, Stiller B, et al Improvement in survival after mechanical circulatory support with pneumatic pulsatile ventricular assist devices in pediatric patients. *Ann Thorac Surg.* 2006;82:917-924.
2. Hetzer R, Alexi-Meskishvilli V, Weng Y, et al. Mechanical cardiac support in the young with the Berlin Heart EXCOR pulsatile ventricular assist device: 15 years' experience. *Semin Thorac Cardiovasc Surg Pediatr Card Surg Ann.* 2006;9:99-108.
3. Stiller B, Weng Y, Huber M, et al. Pneumatic pulsatile ventricular assist devices in children under 1 year of age. *Eur J Cardiothorac Surg.* 2005;28: 234-239.
4. Kirklin J. Mechanical Circulatory support as a bridge to pediatric cardiac transplantation. *Semin Thorac Cardiovasc Surg Pediatr Card Surg Ann.* 2008; 11:80-85.
5. Gordon R, Quagliarello B, Lowy F. Ventricular assist device-related infections. *Lancet Infect Dis.* 2006;6:426-437.
6. Frazier OH, Rose EA, Oz MC, et al. Multicenter clinical evaluation of the HeartMate vented electric left ventricular assist system in patients awaiting heart transplantation. *J Heart Lung Transplant.* 2001;20:201-202.
7. Poston RS, Husain S, Sorce D et al. LVAD bloodstream infections: therapeutic rational for transplantation after LVAD infection. J Heart Lung Transplant.2003;22:914-21.
8. Simon D, Fischer S, Grossman A, et al. Left ventricular assist device-related infection: treatment and outcome. *Clin Infect Dis.* 2005;40:1108-1115.
9. Baddour LM, Bettmann MA, Bolger AF, et al. Nonvalvular cardiovascular device-related infections. *Circulation.* 2003;108:2015-2031.
10. Beiras-Fernandez, Kur A, Kiefer F, et al. Multidrug-resistant gram-positive infections in patients with ventricular assist devices: the role of daptomycin. *Transplant Proc.* 2009;41(6):2589-2591.
11. Aslam S, Hernandez M, Thornby J, Zeluff B, Darouiche RO. Risk factors and outcomes of fungal ventricular assist device infections. *Clin Infect Dis.* 2010.50(5):664-671.
12. Goldstein DJ, el-Amir NG, Ashton RC, Jr, et al. Fungal infections in left ventricular assist device recipients. Incidence, prophylaxis and treatment. *ASAIO J.* 1995;41:873-875.
13. Gordon SM, Schmitt SK, Jacobs M, et al. Nosocomial bloodstream infections in patients with implantable left ventricular assist devices. *Ann Thorac Surg.* 2001;72:725-730.
14. Hetzer R, Hennig E, Schiessler A, et al. Mechanical support and heart transplantation. *J Heart Lung Transplant.* 1992;11:175-181.

15. Warnecke H, Berdijs F, Hennig E, et al. Mechanical left ventricular support as bridge to cardiac transplantation in childhood. *Eur J Cardiothorac Surg.* 1991;5:330-333.

16. Hetzer R, Potapov EJ, Stiller B, et al. Improvement in survival after mechanical circulatory support with pneumatic pulsatile ventricular assist devices in pediatric patients. *Ann Thorac Surg.* 2006;82:917-925.

17. Imamura M, Dossey AM, Prodhan P, et al. Bridge to cardiac transplant in children: Berlin Heart versus extracorporeal membrane oxygenation. *Ann Thorac Surg.* 2009;87:1894-1901.

18. Jeewa A, Manlhiot C, McCrindle BW, et al. Outcomes with ventricular assist device versus extracorporeal membrane oxygenation as a bridge to pediatric heart transplantation. *Artif Organs.* 2010 Jun 10 [Epub ahead of print].

19. Irving CA, Cassidy JV, Kirk RC, et al. Successful bridge to transplant with the Berlin Heart after cavopulmonary shunt. *J Heart Lung Transplant.* 2009;28(4):399-401.

20. Calvaruso DF, Ocello S, Salviato N, et al. Implantation of a Berlin Heart as single ventricle by-pass on Fontan circulation in univentricular heart failure. *ASAIO J.* 2007;53(6):e1-e2.

21. Chu MW, Sharma K, Tchervenkov CI, et al. Berlin Heart ventricular assist device in a child with hypoplastic left heart syndrome. *Ann Thorac Surg.* 2007;83(3):1179-1181.

22. Cardarelli MG, Salim M, Love J, et al. Berlin heart as a bridge to recovery for a failing Fontan. *Ann Thorac Surg.* 2009;87(3):943-946.

CHAPTER 31

THE BERLIN HEART INCOR ASSIST DEVICE

Johannes Müller, Bob Kroslowitz,
Robert Halfmann, and Peter Göttel

With Appendix by Jennifer Rutledge, Christina
VanderPluym, Ali Kilic, and Holger Buchholz

INTRODUCTION

Cardiac assist devices are capable of supporting the hemodynamic conditions of patients with heart failure in order to overcome the compromised end-organ status. The indications for implantation of a system of this kind include cardiogenic shock, acute deterioration of chronic cardiac insufficiency, and heart failure following cardiac surgery. The device is implanted at a point when medication therapy no longer has any effect. Cardiac functions are usually being supported by intravenous administration of catecholamines; often an intra-aoratic balloon pump (IABP) has already been implanted and no donor organ is available.[1] This article describes the INCOR system (Berlin Heart, Berlin, Germany), a nonpulsatile axial-flow pump (Fig. 31–1, see Appendix).

TECHNICAL ATTRIBUTES

The principle of the axial pump is that a rotor (synonymous designations: spindle, impeller) which rotates within a tube creates a volume flow, comparable to the screw named after Archimedes and used for irrigation purposes in ancient cultures.[2] Four main aims were pursued when developing the INCOR system: (1) to keep the size of the pump as small as possible (< 100 cm^3), (2) to minimize hemolysis, (3) to keep energy consumption as low as possible (< 5 W), and (4) to achieve a long service life of the system (> 5 years). As shown in Fig. 31–2 (see Appendix), one must visualize the blood flowing into the pump from the right. There it first passes between the blades of an inducer (inlet guide vane) which is mounted stationarily in the pump tube. This inducer serves to align the flow and minimize the reflows occuring along the walls of the tube in pumps utilizing this principle. The blood then enters the impeller space. The impeller rotates at speeds of 5,000 to 10,000 rpm (revolutions per minute). The rotating motion of the impeller generates the required volume flow. Downstream of the impeller, there is a diffuser (outlet guide vane) which is also rigidly mounted in the tube and serves to stop rotation of the flow and build up the required blood pressure. The shape of the blades and the gap between the blades and the surrounding tube are responsible for the degree of blood trauma and the fluid dynamic performance of the pump. For this reason, the design of the blades has been optimized using computer simulation models with the aim of minimizing hemolysis and overall blood trauma.[2] The pump was optimized for a blood flow of 5 L/min against a pressure of 100 mm Hg. As the software tools for the design of the fluid dynamic performance underlay a continuous process of improvement, it was verified at regular intervals whether the application of the always latest software version could lead to a further optimization of the blades. Furthermore, the application of the system in more than 250 patients revealed that in the vast majority of patients in the long-term use, the average blood flow was 4.5 L/min against a pressure of 80 mm Hg. Because of this and the progress in the software, the diffuser was redesigned with the goal to reduce the shear stress by application of the new software and to optimize the shape of the blades at a different but favorable working point. An examination of the new design showed no changes in the rate of hemolysis—which is already clinically not detectable—but a significant reduced influence on platelet activation.[3] The motor is located outside of the pump tube. It drives the rotary motion of the impeller, achieving an efficiency of more than 90%. This ensures that the pump does not heat up, this being an essential requirement for successful long-term applications. If the system gets too warm, this can lead to denaturation of proteins which, in unfavorable cases, leads to deposits in the pump and may even cause a pump stoppage.

In order to fulfill the requirement of a long service life of the system, magnetic bearings have been designed for the impeller instead of the commonly used mechanical bearings. The magnetic bearings keep the impeller suspended in the blood without touching the surrounding tube or the ends of the inducer and diffuser hubs. In this way, absolute wear-free and totally silent operation of the system can be achieved (see Fig. 31–2). The magnetic levitation stabilizes the rotor in the axial direction actively and in the radial direction passively. As the rotor is always kept in the position of minimum power consumption, the active stabilization is in the range of 0.4 W. Regarding the gaps between the floating rotor and the inducer and the diffuser, because of reciprocation of the impeller in the axial direction induced by the pulsatility of the beating heart, the gaps are perfectly washed out. Therefore, thrombus formation or deposits could never be detected inside the gaps.

All pump parts are made of medical-grade titanium alloy. Titanium parts which come in contact with blood have a heparin coating. The shape of both cannulae has been optimized according to fluid dynamic principles, the cannulae being made of silicone with a special inside coating. The material enures a flexibility of the inflow and outflow cannulae (Fig. 31–3, see Appendix). Therefore the movement of the cannulae reflects the movement of the heart. Thus, a dislocation of the pump after placement that could be seen in pumps with a stiff inflow cannula can not happen as the cannulae are able to absorb forces from the contracting heart. The sensors in the pump which control the magnetic bearings are also used for measuring the pressure head across the pump and the flow through the pump.[4] A comparison of the measured flow with that measured with ultrasound transducers revealed that the accuracy of this method is at least as high as the one with the ultrasound sensors. To get the information on the flow and the pressure head, the knowledge of the actual blood viscosity is not necessary. Both parameters are displayed on the screen of a laptop PC and can be used to optimize therapy (Fig. 31–4, see Appendix). So opening of the aortic valve can be derived from these curves which is valuable information for the optimal adjustment of the rotor speed. The system is controlled and powered via a transcutaneous cable leading to an external control unit and two accumulator batteries (see Fig. 31–4).

INDICATIONS (TABLE 31-1)

At present, the implantation of a ventricular assist system is considered as last-resort therapy for cardiac failure which can no longer be treated with probable success by other means.[5] It is therefore indicated when conservative measures such as optimum medication or implantation of an electrical resynchronization system have been exhausted or no longer show promise of success. This includes both the situation of chronic cardiac failure and cardiogenic shock. To date, these systems have been used with the objective of bridging the time up to heart transplant. Because of the former large, unwieldy drive systems and the resulting impaired quality of life for patients, applications in destination therapy were inconceivable until recently. Because of a reduction in the number of donor hearts, the waiting times up to transplant have increased considerably with the result that the periods in which ventricular assist devices (VADs) have to be used for support have also extended.

The demand for considerably smaller and lighter systems which has emerged as a result of this problem has led to the development of small, mobile drive systems which make it possible for patients to spend the waiting time at home. At the same

TABLE 31-1. Use of the System

Indications

The INCOR is an implantable LAVD that is indicated for use for as BTT, BTR, or DT in patients with end-stage left ventricular failure (NYHA class IV or INTERMACS levels 1-5) of different etiologies including:
- Dilatative cardiomyopathy
- Ischemic cardiomyopathy
- Myocarditis
- Congenital HD
- Peripartal cardiomyopathy
- Toxic cardiomyopathy
- Restrictive cardiomyopathy

Contraindications
- Predominantly right ventricular heart failure
- Biventricular heart failure
- Signs of infection which do not correspond to a *sepsis-like syndrome*
- Sepsis
- Progressive multiorgan failure

Relative contraindications
- Coagulation system disorder

Considerations for patient selection
- Carefully assess patient's RV function and pulmonary vascular resistance
- Failure of RV to deliver sufficient volume will result in low pump flow with increased risk of thrombus formation and suction phenomenon

Consider BiVAD support (Berlin Heart EXCOR) in patients with sustained RV dysfunction. Indications of RV dysfunction include elevated CVP, low PAP, and signs of liver dysfunction (elevated bilirubin).
- LVAD implantation in patients with preserved end-organ function leads to improved outcomes

BiVAD, biventricular assist device; BTR, bridge-to-recovery; BTT, bridge-to-transplantation; CVP, central venous pressure; DT, destination therapy; HD, heart disease; INTERMACS, Interagency Registry for Mechanically Assisted Circulatory Systems; LAVD, left ventricular assist device; NYHA, New York Heart Association; PAP, pulmonary arterial pressure; RV right ventricular/right ventricle.

time, this has paved the way for long-term applications in which the patient is supported by this kind of device when there is no suitable indication for a subsequent transplant.

Regarding the comparable *performance* of the systems, there is no fundamental difference between the indications for implanting an INCOR system and those for other implantable VADs.[6,7] In other words, the INCOR system is suitable for supporting patients with left ventricular insufficiency of New York Heart Association (NYHA) class III or IV, irrespective of the cause of the heart failure. However, it is important to make sure that the reduced function of the right ventricle and the increased pulmonary flow resistance can be reversed by reducing the load on the left ventricle and the corresponding filling pressure. Further aspects to be taken into account when assessing the indication are the time the patient is expected to remain under system support, in as far as this can be predicted and the patient's quality of life. Patients whose circulation needs to be assisted for a longer period benefit from a wear-free system, since the pump does not need to be replaced, even after years of use. In addition, noise reduction in the INCOR pump improves the patient's quality of life.

SURGICAL TECHNIQUES (FIG. 31–5, SEE APPENDIX)

Axial pumps can be implanted in two positions. In both positions, the inflow cannula leading to the pump is anastomosed to the apex of the left ventricle. When the pump is placed in the frontal position, the outflow cannula is anastomosed to the ascending aorta. When the pump is placed in the lateral intrapleural position, this cannula is anastomosed to the descending aorta. The lateral position is preferred for patients who have undergone prior cardiac surgery. However, the advantage of an uncomplicated placement may be countervailed by a nonphysiologic flow pattern in the aortic arch and ascending aorta with a subsequent higher complication rate.

First, cardiopulmonary bypass is initiated and preparations are made for anastomosis to the apex of the left ventricle. The anastomosis technique is similar to that used for other implantable pumps and is usually applied under induced fibrillation conditions.[8,9] The cannulae can be anastomosed without the pump being in place as the pump can easily be connected to the pump by the provided snap-in connectors. It must be ensured that the cannulae and pump are air free before the pump is started. The cable has to be tunneled transcutaneously to the contralateral exit side using a tunnelator. The intracorporeal distance between the pump and the transcutaneous exit is made as long as possible in order to prevent infections. Since anticoagulation therapy ought to be commenced soon after surgery, care must be taken to get the operated regions as dry as possible before closing the chest.

POSTSURGICAL TREATMENT AND DEVICE OPERATION

As opposed to the postoperative therapy of patients treated using other cardiothoracic procedures, there are three aspects which must be given special attention in the postoperative therapy management of patients with axial pumps: (1) right ventricular function, (2) hemodynamics, and (3) anticoagulation/platelet inhibition. Furthermore, antibiotic treatment of the location where the cable passes through the skin is needed.

Malfunctions of the right heart should always be expected after the implantation of a left ventricular assist device (LVAD). These are ideally treated using inotropic substances and, in order to reduce the afterload for the right ventricle, with an adequate dose of nitric oxide (NO).[10,11] Apart from excessive unloading of the left ventricle, the right ventricular functions may be impaired if the septum shift to the left side leads to enlargement of the right ventricle. Echocardiographic examination can be used to determine and control the optimum settings for left ventricular unloading, in this way avoiding *reshaping* of the right ventricle.

When treating patients with axial-flow pumps, care must be taken to maintain suitable hemodynamic conditions for ensuring optimum pump flows.[12] The physical principle on which axial pumps are based means that the flow through the pump depends on the pressure gradient across the pump. Thus, if the impeller rotates at a fixed speed of 7500 rpm, depending on the blood pressure, a flow of between 3.5 L/min (if the mean arterial pressure is 110 mm Hg) and 6 L/min (if the mean arterial pressure is 75 mm Hg) can be achieved. For this reason, it may be necessary to initiate antihypertensive therapy (eg, angiotensin-converting enzyme [ACE]–inhibitors) soon after surgery for maintaining blood pressure at arterial mean values between 70 and, at the most, 80 mm Hg. There is no benefit in raising the pump speed in an attempt to compensate a flow which is too low due to high blood pressure, since this would lead to a dramatic increase in energy losses in the system and the related hemolysis levels. However, a flow rate which is too low (< 2.5 L/min) will also lead to increased hemolysis, since the continuity of the flow pattern within the pump would then break down.

Because of the effect of shear forces on the cellular blood components inside the pump, axial pumps, at their present stage of development, subject the blood to stresses, leading to activation of the coagulation system and platelets.[13,14] In order to avoid thromboembolic complications resulting from activation, all patients must be given anticoagulation and platelet therapy. This is started roughly 12 to 24 hours after surgery using heparin if no noteworthy bleeding has occurred and the platelet count exceeds 50,000. The heparin dose is adjusted to achieve an initial partial thromboplastin time (PTT) of 60 to 70 seconds (later on this is raised to 80 seconds). Once the patient has recovered further, platelet-aggregation inhibitors (clopidogrel or/and acetyl-salicylic acid) are included in the anticoagulation therapy, the doses being adjusted in relation to the thromboelastogram and aggregometry results. The transition from heparin to oral administration of vitamin-K antagonists is made when all drainage and catheter accesses have been removed. The recommended international normalized ratio (INR) is in the range of 2.5 to 3. Clinical practice revealed that patients need an individually tailored anticoagulation and platelet inhibition. So, for example, the patient who was on support for more than 3 years was exclusively anticoagulated with vitamin-K antagonists targeting an INR of 2.8 to 3. There was no need for any platelet inhibitors. A summary of anticoagulation and antiplatelet management of the INCOR patient is given in Fig. 31–6 (see Appendix). Additional medication consists of heart failure therapy in accordance with the American Heart Association (AHA) guidelines.

The pump is easy to operate. The flow rate through the pump and the pressure head across the pump are displayed on the monitor of a laptop computer, both in numerical form and as a continuous graph (see Fig. 31–4). The pressure graph enables the viewer to estimate the patient's current blood pressure at the time of the cardiac diastole, as the pressure at the pump's inflow site can be assumed to be zero at that point (the intraventricular pressure during the diastole). This form of display permits permanent monitoring of the blood pressure management. If the flow rates are too high, venous return to the left ventricle may not be sufficient, in which case a suction effect may occur, causing the left ventricle to collapse. A straight line displayed in the pressure head graph is an early indication of this phenomenon. From a technical aspect, this can be counteracted by reducing the pump speed; from a medical aspect, the suction phenomena may also be the result of hypovolemia or right ventricular failure, which can be treated by volume substitution or other right heart failure therapy. Current INCOR software versions include an automatic control mechanism to reduce the pump speed automatically in such cases and then increase it, step by step, until the original set speed is reachieved.

RESULTS OF THE ANIMAL TRIALS AND CLINICAL OUTCOMES (FIG. 31–7, SEE APPENDIX)

Before the authorities granted Berlin Heart permission to conduct clinical trials, the INCOR system was tested exhaustively in animal trials with 22 bovine calves in 2002. The data obtained in the animal trials demonstrated that the magnetic-suspension bearings worked, not just in the laboratory, but also under realistic application conditions, that the pump was absolutely wear free, and that hemolysis, if it occurred at all, was below levels detectable by laboratory methods. The animal trials also showed that the software controlling the pump had some faults that needed to be eliminated and that some program enhancements were still necessary.

The first human implantation was performed in June 2002. At this time, an inflow cannula with a long tip (34 mm) that extended clearly into the left ventricular cavity was used in the first four patients. In the following 165 patients, an inflow cannula with a short tip (24 mm) was used which caused problems in some patients because the cannula did not always extend fully in the ventricle or was overgrown with tissue in long-term patients. After this problem had become evident, the primary version of the inflow cannula was reinstated.

As of July 2010, the pump has been implanted in 546 patients (mean age, 52.9 years; range, 15-77 years; male, 478; female, 68) at 56 different hospitals in 18 different countries. At time of placement, all patients were in the terminal stages of congestive heart failure. The majority of patients suffered from ischemic cardiomyopathy (205 patients) and dilated cardiomyopathy (240 patients). The average observation period per patient is 256.3 days (ranging 0-2194 days). The accumulated observation period has exceeded 381.2 patient-years. The number of patients supported for more than 1 year is 135, with 58 more than 2 years, 16 more than 3 years, 3 more than 4 years, 2 more than 5 years, and 1 more than 6 years. A more detailed analysis of the data revealed some risk factors which influenced the overall outcome. Just as the use of an inflow cannula with a short tip had higher rates of cerebrovascular accident (CVA), placement of the device in the lateral intrapleural cavity adversely influenced this outcome. Implantation in a high-volume center improved outcomes.

PERSPECTIVE

Optimization of the devices regarding minimizing hemolysis—always a primary objective—has obviously been successful in the case of INCOR to such an extent that it is not possible to detect any hemolysis at all using routine laboratory/chemical methods. The challenge now confronting the developers of such devices is to take activation of the coagulation system into account when designing the axial pumps in order to achieve a considerable reduction in this activation potential and to allow a significant reduction in anticoagulation and/or platelet inhibition.

There is an ongoing discussion whether or not and on how to make blood pumps "intelligent." Intelligent blood pumps would optimize the benefit of the pump while simplifying management. By means of sensors, the blood flow can be automatically adapted to the patient's needs, blood temperature can be controlled, coagulative status of the blood can be screened, and the ventricular function can be verified. Rotary blood pumps in general and axial-flow pumps in particular are the ideal devices to introduce these kinds of features. Because of the sensitivity of rotary blood pumps to the pressure across the pump, there is some degree of self-control of the pump if the intraventricular pressure goes up during physiologic stress which is, however, not sufficient enough for an ideal adaptation of the flow to the need of the patient. Therefore for the INCOR system, several sensors have been developed which are already in the final testing phase. Sensors in the hub of the inflow inducer and the diffuser are able to measure the absolute pressure and the temperature of the blood. Tests on the long-term stability of the sensors revealed a deviation of less than 0.25 mm Hg per year. As the sensor in the inflow tract of the pump is very closely located to the left ventricle, the pressure in the ventricle can be given as a function over time. This information can be used to fully control the pump, with the intraventricular pressure as a control variable. As functional recovery of the heart depends, besides on other parameters, on the degree of unloading of the heart, the sensor can be used to adjust the pressure so optimal improvement can be achieved at any given time. Further, sensors can be applied to screen the blood temperature, which may be useful to detect infection that can influence platelet function and as a consequence anticoagulation parameters. With the Doppler signals of very little ultrasound parameters (3 mm diameter), the blood flow can be measured, but, additionally, by using the backscatter function of these sensors, the blood viscosity and the formation of even very little clots or fibrin fibers can be detected.

It is still a subject of much controversy as to whether pulsatile displacement pumps are the only means of conserving physiologic pressure pulsatility successfully over extended periods. A new component is to be integrated into INCOR which can vary the impeller speed within a single heartbeat cycle in relation to the rate in such a way that the flow through the pump will be pulsatile and independent of the pulsatile flow received from the left ventricle. The pulse amplitude achieved in this way will be roughly equal to 70% of the physiologic pulsatility.

Axial pumps have all the qualifications for full implantability in future. They are compact, do not need a compensation chamber, and consume little energy. This means that the dimensions of an implantable accumulator battery and the control electronics and the TET (transcutaneous energy transmission) system can be kept very compact too.[15] INCOR system development is to be continued to make it into a fully implantable system, the objective being to use only two additional components the size of an implantable defibrillator, whereby it may also be possible to implant these pectorally.

REFERENCES

1. Hetzer R, Jurmann MJ, Potapov EV, et al. Heart assist systems—current status. *Herz*. 2002 Aug;27(5):407-417.
2. Goldowsky M. Mini hemoreliable axial flow LVAD with magnetic bearings: historical overview and concept advantages. *ASAIO J*. 2002 Jan-Feb;48(1):96-98.
3. Mueller J, Brodde M, Nuesser P, et al. Hemolysis testing is not the adequate method to verify optimization of the flow profil of rotary blood pumps. *Int J Artif Organs*. 2006;29:504.
4. Goldowsky M. Mini hemoreliable axial flow LVAD with magnetic bearings: modeling of demo-magnetic bearing and verification. *ASAIO J*. 2002 Jan-Feb;48(1):101-105.
5. Pagani FD, Aaronson KD, Swaniker F, Bartlett RH. The use of extracorporeal life support in adult patients with primary cardiac failure as a bridge to implantable left ventricular assist device. *Ann Thorac Surg*. 2001 Mar;71 (3 Suppl):S77-S81.
6. Grinda JM, Latremouille CH, Chevalier P, et al. Bridge to transplantation with the DeBakey VAD axial pump: a single center report. *Circulation*. 2002 Jun 4;105(22):2588-2591.
7. Westaby S, Banning AP, Saito S, et al. Circulatory support for long-term treatment of heart failure: experience with an intraventricular continuous flow pump. *Circulation*. 2002 Jun 4;105(22):2588-2591.
8. MCCarthy PM, Sabik JE. Implantable circulatory support devices as a bridge to heart transplantation. *Semin Thorac Cardiovasc Surg*. 1994;6:174-180.
9. Frazier OH. The development of an implantable, portable, electrically powered left ventricular assist device. *Semin Thorac Cardiovasc Surg*. 1994;6:181-187.
10. Salamonsen RF, Kaye D, Esmore DS. Inhalation of nitric oxide provides selective pulmonary vasodilatation, aiding mechanical cardiac assist with Thoratec left ventricular assist device. *Anaesth Intensive Care*. 1994 Apr;22(2):209-210.
11. Wagner F, Dandel M, Gunther G, et al. Nitric oxide inhalation in the treatment of right ventricular dysfunction following left ventricular assist device implantation. *Circulation*. 1997 Nov 4;96(9 Suppl):II-291-296.
12. Wieselthaler GM, Schima H, Hiesmayr M, et al. First clinical experience with the DeBakey VAD continuous-axial-flow pump for bridge to transplantation. *Circulation*. 2000 Feb 1;101(4):356-359.
13. Apel J, Paul R, Klaus S, Siess T, Reul H. Assessment of hemolysis related quantities in a microaxial blood pump by computational fluid dynamics. *Artif Organs*. 2001;25(5):341-347.
14. Schlitt A, Hauroeder B, Buerke M, et al. Effects of combined therapy of clopidogrel and aspirin in preventing thrombus formation on mechanical heart valves in an ex vivo rabbit model.*Thromb Res*. 2002 Jul 15;107(1-2): 39-43.
15. Diegel PD, Mussivand T, Holfert JW, et al. Electrohydraulic ventricular assist device development. *ASAIO J*. 1992 Jul-Sep;38(3):M306-M310.

APPENDIX

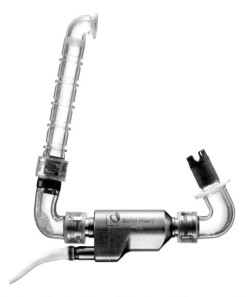

FIGURE 31–1. INCOR® left ventricular assist device. (Reproduced with permission from Berlin Heart, Inc.)

The INCOR® LVAD is a CE-certified axial-flow pump with a magnetically levitated impeller. The bearing system operates without any mechanical contact to ensure wear-free long-term support for patients with heart failure. The inner surface is composed of titanium with Carmeda® (heparin) coating. All implanted components are computational fluid dynamics (CFD) optimized for flow and blood trauma.

With an external diameter of just 30 mm, length of 120 mm, and a weight of approximately 200 g, the pump is able to provide a flow of 6 L/min against a pressure of 80 mm Hg. This is achieved at an impeller speed of 7500 rpm and a low power consumption of 4 W.

INCOR generates a constant mean flow. The difference between systolic and diastolic blood pressure arises exclusively as a result of the remaining pumping function of the heart and is superimposed by the pressure generated by the pump.

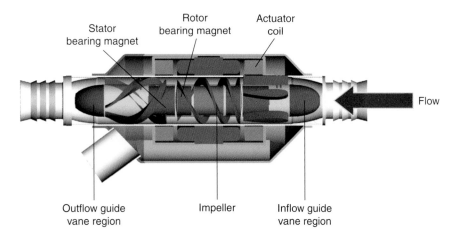

FIGURE 31–2. Longitudinal section. Magnetic suspension of the INCOR impeller. (Reproduced with permission from Berlin Heart, Inc.)

- Magnetically levitated impeller allows the following pump control algorithms:
  1. PC (Pulsatility Control)
  2. SP (Suction Protection)
  3. PFC (Periodically Flow Change)
- This design achieves the desired situation in nonpulsatile LVAD systems:
  1. Pulsatile arterial blood flow
  2. Optimal LV washout
  3. Aortic valve opening
  4. Low risk of ventricular collapse and suction
  5. No risk of pump thrombosis

■ SYSTEM COMPONENTS

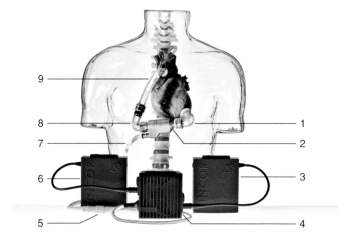

1. Inflow cannula
2. Axial pump
3. Backup battery
4. Control unit
5. Plug coupling
6. Main battery
7. Pump cable
8. Outflow angle section
9. Outflow cannula

FIGURE 31–3. INCOR in situ (configuration for medial access) with all permanently active components. (Reproduced with permission from Berlin Heart, Inc.)

INCOR Cannulae and Snap-in Connectors

All cannulae are made of medical grade silicone. They are strengthened with a plastic mesh and partially surrounded by polyester velour. The pump and the cannulae are connected to each other intraoperatively using snap-in connectors.

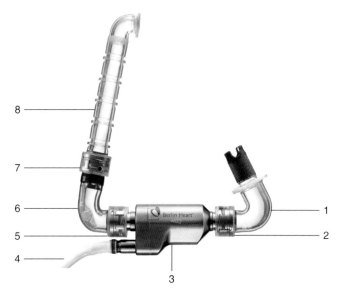

1. Inflow cannula
2. Snap-in connector
3. Pump
4. Pump cable
5. Snap-in connector
6. Outflow angle section
7. Snap-in connector
8. Outflow cannula

FIGURE 31–3A. Pump with cannulae, connected with snap-in connectors. (Reproduced with permission from Berlin Heart, Inc.)

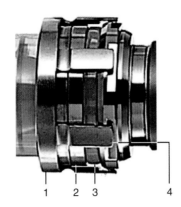

1. Guide ring
2. Stop ring
3. Detent ring
4. Snap-in position on detent ring

FIGURE 31–3B. Detailed view of snap-in connector: Guide ring snapped into detent ring (without protective cover). (Reproduced with permission from Berlin Heart, Inc.)

Inflow Cannula

All four jags are sealed with silicone. The complete crown area is dipped into silicone up to this mark. Outer surface of the titanium crown is made of sintered titanium.

On the inflow side of the inflow cannula, there is a titanium-reinforced head with a suture edge made from polyester velour.

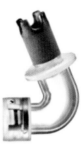

FIGURE 31–3C. Inflow cannula with textured titanium surface. (Reproduced with permission from Berlin Heart, Inc.)

Outflow Cannula

The inflow side of the outflow cannula has collars at which the cannula can be cut to the required length.

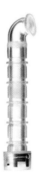

FIGURE 31–3D. Outflow cannula. (Reproduced with permission from Berlin Heart, Inc.)

■ INCOR CONTROL UNIT

INCOR is delivered with two identical control units. One control unit is active, while the second control unit serves as replacement.
Tasks of the control unit:

- The control unit controls the pumps motor, magnetic bearing, and power supply.
- Data concerning the status of the pump are stored in the control unit. These data can be requested via the laptop.
- In the event of malfunctions or empty batteries, the control unit generates messages.

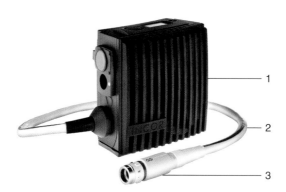

1. Control unit
2. Control unit cable
3. Control unit plug

FIGURE 31–4A.   Control unit with patient cable and patient plug. (Reproduced with permission from Berlin Heart, Inc.)

INCOR Batteries

Each INCOR includes two main batteries and two backup batteries with identical performance data. The run time of a battery is around 3.5 hours; the charging time is around 2 to 4 hours.

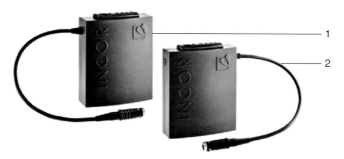

1. Mains battery
2. Backup battery

FIGURE 31–4B.   Mains and backup battery. (Reproduced with permission from Berlin Heart, Inc.)

INCOR Mains Power Supply Unit

The mains power supply unit is used for supplying power (mains power operation) and for charging the batteries. An indicator lamp on the On/Off toggle switch shows the operation of the mains power supply unit. On the top of the mains power supply unit, there is also an indicator LED. If the mains power supply unit is providing the correct output voltage, the indicator LED is green. If the charge status of one of the batteries connected to the control unit is less than 85%, the mains power supply unit recharges it. In doing so, its LEDs constantly show the charge status.

The time of mains power operation:

• Patient is sleeping.
• Patient is not mobile.
• The backup batteries are being changed because of two empty batteries (backup battery empty).

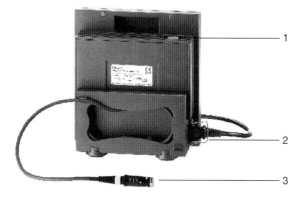

1. On/Off toggle switch
2. Mains power cable (secured in connector with safety bar)
3. Connection cable to control unit

FIGURE 31–4C.   Mains power supply unit, back view. (Reproduced with permission from Berlin Heart, Inc.)

INCOR Charging Unit

The charging unit provides two identical charging slots, each holding one battery. Above each charging slot, there is a connector for the battery plug. During the charging process, the battery LED shows the charge status of the battery. The charging time for an empty battery is around 2 hours. An indicator lamp on the toggle switch shows the operation of the charging unit.

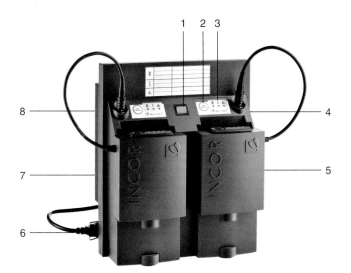

1. On/Off toggle switch
2. Button for calibration
3. LED
4. Plug socket for backup battery
5. Backup battery
6. Mains power cable (secured with safety bar)
7. Mains battery
8. Ventilation slot

FIGURE 31–4D. Charging unit with two batteries. (Reproduced with permission from Berlin Heart, Inc.)

Laptop With INCOR Monitoring Program

The pump is started, monitored, and configured using the laptop with the preinstalled monitoring program.

If the laptop is connected to the control unit, it provides the user with continuous data on the status and function of the implant as well as detailed information on all events and malfunctions. The data are simultaneously stored on the hard drive for later evaluation.

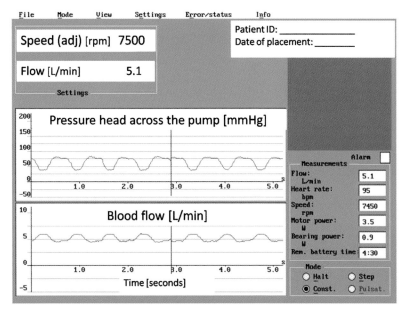

FIGURE 31–4E. Flow and pressure data are continuously displayed on the laptop computer's monitoring program. (Reproduced with permission from Berlin Heart, Inc.)

General surgical principles

- Standard cardiovascular techniques are used.
- Initiation of CPB with right atrial cannulation and aortic cannulation close to the aortic arch allowing proximal anastomosis of INCOR outflow cannula.
- INCOR implantation can be achieved on the beating or fibrillating heart.
- Snap-in connectors allow easy and fast connection between INCOR pump and its cannulae.

Surgical steps

- Step 1: LV apex hole is established by using the INCOR coring knife. All trabeculae next to the Inflow cannula must be excised to avoid thrombus formation and embolization. The suture ring holder should not be removed until all sutures are tied in order to maintain the round shape of ring (preserved shape of the suture ring provides blood impermeability between suture ring and inflow cannula).

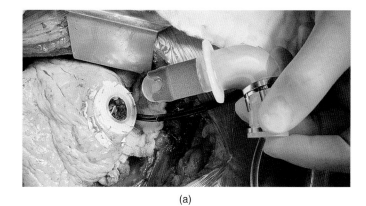

(a)

FIGURE 31–5. Surgical procedure. (Reproduced with permission from Berlin Heart, Inc.)

- Step 2: Connect inflow cannula with pump. Vent LV via outlet of pump (using the vent adapter supplied), thus de-airing the pump antegrade.

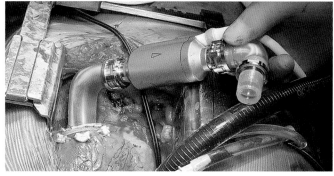

(b)

FIGURE 31–5. (Continued)

- Step 3: Aortic anastomosis with outflow cannula (end-to-side).
- Step 4: Trim outflow cannula to desired length, de-air retrograde, and connect to pump.

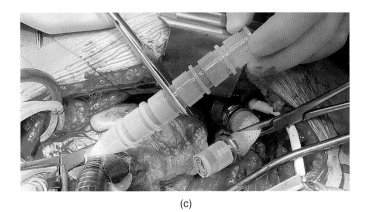

(c)

FIGURE 31-5. (*Continued*)

- Step 5: Tunnel driveline subcutaneously.
- Step 6: Start system, increase rpm as needed, and wean from cardiopulmonary bypass.

INCOR® — Anticoagulation Guideline Summary

Medications	Dosing Guidelines	Labs and Target Values

Unfractionated Heparin (UFH)
Start when:
   • 12 - 24 h post-op
   • No bleeding (<50 mL/h)
   • Platelet count (>50k/µl)
   • Normal coag. status (TEG)
	Start with:
	
	5-7 IU/kg/h (no bolus)
		- aPTT – check every 6 hours until aPTT stable, then every 24 h unless dose changes
		               Target aPTT Ratio
		POD 1 and normal plt. count: 50-60 s
		POD 2 and later:
		   - plt. count < 40 k/µl normal
		   - plt. count 50 – 100 k/µl 50-60 s 1.5 - 2.0
		   - plt. count > 100,000 60-80 s 2.0 - 2.5

Vitamin K Antagonist Start when: enteral feeding possible	**Dosing:** - Depends on liver function - Hold dose if INR >3.5	- Check INR daily - Target INR 2.5-3.0 - If low INR (<2.5), use LMWH guidelines
Platelet Inhibitors **Dipyridamole** – POD 2 and ADP >50% **Aspirin** – POD 4, drains out, and ARA >50% or POD 7 if drains still in **Clopidogrel** – if resistant to aspirin or if thrombotic complications	**Start with:** - 150 mg/d (up to 1 g/d) - 50 mg/d (increase if necessary) - 75 mg/d	**Targets: Platelet aggregation** - ADP <50% - ARA <30% - ADP <30% Collagen acts as a control and should not be suppressed. Epinephrine target 40%-50%

Low-Molecular-Weight Heparin (LMWH)
- Enoxaparin recommended
Start if suboptimal INR or if
   • Unable to tolerate PO
   • Unstable INR's
   • Frequent antibiotic changes
	Dosing (eg: Enoxaparin): - every 12 h
	INR = 2.0 to 2.4
	- Prophylactic dose (1 mg/kg/d)
	INR <2.0 (or use IV UFH)
	- Therapeutic dose (1 mg/kg 2x/d)
		Target: anti-factor Xa
		
		Therapeutic level 0.6 -1.0 U/mL for twice-daily dosing
		   - Draw blood 4 h after 2nd dose given
		   - Can check once a week when stable

Omega – 3 Fatty Acids (prescription strength) • EPA/DHA	**Dosing:** 1-3 g/d	

Source: INCOR Instructions for Clinical Use – Version 4.2   Version 3.0
* This is only a guideline and does not substitute clinical evaluation and judgment of each individual patient. This guideline does not factor in the usage of thromboelastography.

FIGURE 31-6 Anticoagulation/antiplatelet therapy. (Reproduced with permission from Berlin Heart, Inc.)

The INCOR® LVAD is the only CE-certified third-generation axial-flow pump. Its magnetically levitated impeller operates without any mechanical contact and ensures wear-free long-term support of patients with terminal heart failure. Since June 2002 INCOR® LVAD has been successfully used at 56 heart centers in 18 countries.

1. Demography

Implantations: 546

Female	Male
68	478
12%	88%

Mean age: 52.9 years
            (15 – 77 years)
Median age: 55 years

2. Indications

Dilative cardiomyopathy:	240	(44%)
Ischemic cardiomyopathy:	205	(37%)
Acute myocardial infarction:	43	(8%)
Myocarditis:	17	(3%)
Toxic cardiomyopathy:	7	(1%)
Postcardiotomy:	8	(2%)
Other:	26	(5%)

3. Results

Cumulative time on device: 381.2 years

Mean time on device:	256.3 days [0 – 2194]
	more than 1 year: 135
	more than 2 years: 58
	more than 3 years: 16
	more than 4 years: 3
	more than 5 years: 2
	more than 6 years: 1

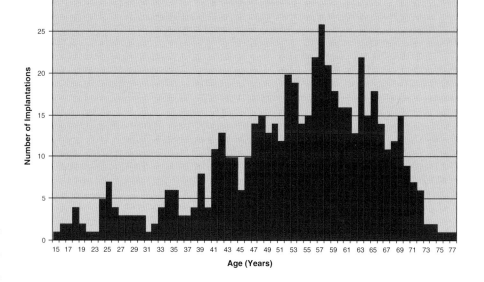

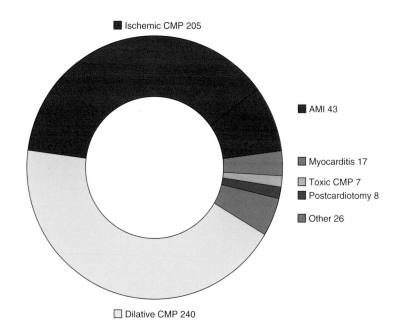

FIGURE 31–7. Clinical data. (Reproduced with permission from Berlin Heart, Inc.)

REFERENCES FOR APPENDIX 31–1

1. Hetzer R, Weng Y, Potapov EV, et al. First experiences with a novel magnetically suspended axial flow left ventricular assist device. *Eur J Cardiothorac Surg.* 2004;25:964-970.
2. Schmid C, Tjan TD, Etz C, et al. First clinical experience with the INCOR left ventricular assist device. *J Heart Lung Transplant.* 2005;24(9):1188-1194.
3. Garatti A, Bruschi G, Colombo T, et al. Clinical outcome and bridge to transplant rate of left ventricular assist device recipient patients: comparison between continuous-flow and pulsatile-flow devices. *Eur J Cardiothorac Surg.* 2008;34(2):275-280.
4. Welp H, Rukosujew A, Tjan TD, et al. Effect of pulsatile and non-pulsatile left ventricular assist devices on the renin-angiotensin system in patients with end-stage heart failure. *Thorac Cardiovasc Surg.* 2010;58(Suppl 2):S185-S188.
5. Schmid C, Jurmann M, Birnbaum D, et al. Influence of inflow cannula length in axial-flow pumps on neurologic adverse event rate: results from a multi-center analysis. *J Heart Lung Transplant.* 2008;27;3:253-260.
6. Schmid C, Etz C, Welp H, et al. Clinical situations demanding weaning from long-term ventricular assist devices. *Eur J Cardiothorac Surg.* 2004;26(4):730-735.
7. Komoda T, Komoda S, Dandel M, Weng Y, Hetzer R. Explantation of INCOR left ventricular assist device after myocardial recovery. *J Card Surg.* 2008;23(6):642-647.
8. Genta F, Colajanni E, Sbarra P, Tidu M, Rinaldi M, Bosimini E. Flow mediated dilation in patient with Berlin Heart INCOR left ventricle assist device. *Monaldi Arch Chest Dis.* 2008;70(1):38-40.
9. Tschirkov A, Nikolov D, Papantchev V, et al. New technique for implantation of the inflow cannula of Berlin Heart INCOR system. *Eur J Cardiothorac Surg.* 2006. 30(4):678-679.
10. Nakashima K, Kirsch ME, Vermes E, Rosanval O, Loisance D. Off-pump replacement of the INCOR implantable axial-flow pump. *J Heart Lung Transplant.* 2009. 28(2):199-201.

CHAPTER 32

HEARTMATE II CONTINUOUS-FLOW LEFT VENTRICULAR ASSIST SYSTEM

David J. Farrar

DEVICE DESCRIPTION

The HeartMate II Left Ventricular Assist System (LVAS) (Thoratec, Pleasanton, CA) consists of an implanted axial-flow blood pump (weight: 290 g; implant vol: 63 mL), a system controller and batteries worn by the patient, and external system components, including battery charger, power supply, and system monitor. The device has been well-described in the literature along with results from the clinical trials.[1-10] The left ventricular assist device (LVAD) blood pump is implanted just below the heart and has a flexible inflow conduit which is attached to the apex of the left ventricle, and an outflow graft is anastomosed to the ascending aorta with a polyester graft (Fig. 32–1). Blood is pumped continuously throughout systole and diastole from the conduit in the left ventricular apex, through the blood pump, and to the ascending aorta.

Control and power to the LVAD are through a percutaneous lead connected to the external controller and power source. The LVAD has only one moving part; the rotor. Vanes on the spinning rotor move blood through the pump, which is capable of providing flow from 3 to 10 L/min. There are no valves. Both the inflow conduit and outflow elbow feature textured titanium microsphere blood-contacting surfaces designed for thromboresistance. The pump's internal components that come in contact with the blood (pump rotor, stators, and pump chamber) have smooth, polished titanium surfaces. The HeartMate II rotor is suspended between the inlet and outlet stators with ball-and-cup bearings designed for long-term reliability and minimal blood damage. In clinical experience and in-vitro test results, there has been negligible bearing wear in explanted pumps, and the data suggest bearing life of well over 10 years.

The HeartMate II system components include the implantable LVAD with its percutaneous lead, as well as the external peripheral components, including the system controller, power module and cable, batteries and battery charger, and system monitor. The system controller is a small computer control package worn by the patient that regulates LVAD function and serves as the primary user interface. Batteries are used in pairs to power the LVAD during mobile operation. The power module provides alternating current (AC) electric power to the LVAD during tethered operation, for example at night. The battery charger charges, tests, and calibrates HeartMate 14-V Li-ion (lithium ion) or 12-V NiMH (nickel metal hydride) batteries. The system monitor functions as an enhanced display and control monitor when connected to the power module. It is used during LVAD implantation and during regular checkups, for changing settings and reviewing pump status.

MECHANISM OF ACTION

The HeartMate II LVAD is an axial-flow rotary pump connected in parallel to the native circulation. A rotor assembly inside the pump contains a magnet and is rotated by the electromotive force generated by the motor. Rotation of the rotor provides the driving force to propel the blood from the left ventricle through the pump out to the natural circulation. Pump output is dependent on the rotational speed of the rotor as well as the pressure difference between the inlet and outlet of the pump. The HeartMate II LVAD operates at a fixed rotational speed, which may be varied via commands from the system monitor under the control of qualified personnel. The patient does not have access to change the fixed speed set point.

Blood flow through the HeartMate II LVAD has reduced pulsatility compared to the native heart or to pulsatile LVADs, with a pattern following the native cardiac cycle and varying during diastole and systole. The amount of flow generated by the pump is determined by the pump speed and by the pressure gradient across the pump, which is the difference between the pressure at the pump outlet (connected to the aorta) and pump inlet (connected to the left ventricle). For a specified pump speed, flow varies inversely with pressure across the pump. Therefore, increasing pump pressure gradient decreases flow and decreasing pump pressure gradient increases flow.

SYSTEM CONTROLLER AND SYSTEM MONITOR IN THE POSTOPERATIVE SETTING

This section provides a brief overview of features in the system controller and system monitor for interacting with the HeartMate II LVAD. Always refer to the manufacturer's instructions for use and clinical operational guides for details concerning the proper use of the device.[11-14] Also, refer to the comprehensive clinical management guidelines for the HeartMate II continuous-flow LVAD.[15]

The HeartMate II system controller (Fig. 32–2A) controls LVAD operation and serves as the primary user interface of the HeartMate II LVAS. The system controller functions include the following: controls motor power and speed; monitors, interprets, and responds to system performance; performs diagnostic monitoring; provides hazard and advisory alarms; records and stores events in memory; and transfers system performance data to the system monitor.

The system controller has two power leads for connection to its power source. The white lead also contains a data link cable

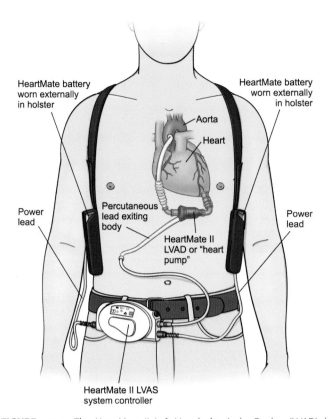

FIGURE 32–1. The HeartMate II Left Ventricular Assist Device (LVAD) is implanted below the heart and is connected by a percutaneous lead to a controller and batteries worn by the patients. Blood is pumped continuously throughout systole and diastole from a cannula inserted into the left ventricular apex with flow redirected to the ascending aorta. (Reproduced with permission from Thoratec Corporation, Pleasanton, CA.)

that transmits information from the system controller to the system monitor during tethered operation. A small battery—the controller—provides limited power to the system controller's audible alarms during situations when external power has been disrupted. The system controller alarm battery module does not provide backup power to the pump.

The system controller keypad (Fig. 32–2B) has buttons to interact with the system and displays and sounds for battery status, alarms, and warnings. A summary of the various warning lights and sounds on the system controller are presented in Fig. 32–3.[14]

The system controller is connected to the system monitor during start-up, for changing the pump speed settings and for diagnostics. The following pump parameter information is available on the system monitor when connected to the controller: speed, power, flow, and pulsatility index (PI) (Fig. 32–4). No single parameter can replace the importance of monitoring the clinical status of the patient, which should be the first priority.

Flow is directly related to speed and power. As the fixed speed is increased, flow will increase. Pump flow is not directly measured but is an estimated value based on pump power. Any increase in power will result in an increase in estimated flow. Any condition that causes an increase in pump power not related to increase flow, such as thrombus on the bearings or obstruction of the rotor, will display an erroneously high flow.

The amount of power used by the pump is determined by pump speed and blood flow through the pump. Under normal conditions, the power increases with either pump speed or flow. Gradual power increases (over hours or days) may signal a deposition of thrombus inside the pump.

The pulsatility index, or pulse index (PI) is a measure of the magnitude of the flow pulse through the pump during the cardiac cycle. It is measured and averaged over a 15-second interval and displayed on the monitor.

$$PI = \frac{(\text{max flow} - \text{min flow}) \times 10}{\text{average flow}}$$

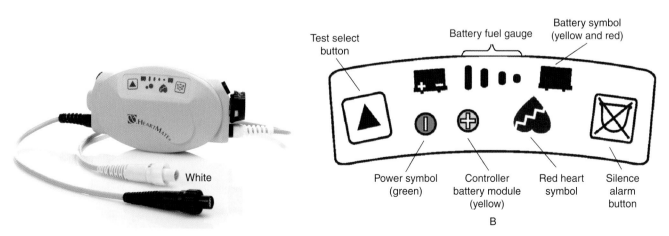

FIGURE 32–2 A. HeartMate II LVAD System Controller. (Reproduced with permission from Thoratec Corporation, Pleasanton, CA.) **B.** System controller keypad. (Reproduced with permission from Thoratec Corporation, Pleasanton, CA.)

System Controller Warning Lights and Sounds

Warning Lights	Audio Tone	Alarm Message	Meaning	Action
Red Heart	Steady Audio Tone	LOW FLOW HAZARD (on Display Module) LOW FLOW, PUMP OFF and/or PUMP DISCON-NECTED (on System Monitor)	Pump flow < 2.5 lpm, pump has stopped, perc lead is disconnected, or pump is not working properly.	1. Make sure System Controller is connected to the pump. 2. Make sure System Controller is connected to a power source (batteries, PBU/Power Module, or Emergency Power Pack [EPP]). 3. If alarm continues, immediately seek additional help.
NONE: No Warning Lights and No Green Power Symbol	Steady Audio Tone	NONE	System Controller is not receiving power.	1. Make sure System Controller is connected to a power source (batteries, PBU/Power Module, or EPP). 2. If connected and alarm continues, switch to alternate power source. 3. If alarm continues after switching power source, replace Controller (see otherside forinstructions.)
Red Battery	Steady Audio Tone	LOW VOLTAGE	Less than 5 minutes of battery power remain, voltage is too low, or the System Controller is not getting enough power from the PBU/Power Module.	Immediately replace depleted batteries with new, fully-charged set. Change batteries **one at a time**. If fully-charged batteries are not available, switch to PBU/PowerModule or EPP. **WARNING! Do NOT remove power from both power leads at the same time, or the pump will stop.** **Note**: Pump speed will gradually decrease to save power (i.e., "Power Saver Mode") until the condition is resolved and the alarm clears.
Yellow Battery	1 Beep Every 4 Seconds	Low Voltage Advisory	Less than 15 minutes of battery power remain, voltage is too low, or the System Controller is not getting enough power from the PBU/Power Module.	Immediately replace depleted batteries with new, fully-charged set. Change batteries **one at a time**. If fully-charged batteries are not available, switch to PBU/PowerModule or EPP. **WARNING! Do NOT remove power from both power leads at the same time, or the pump will stop.**
NONE: No Warning Light	Broken Audio Tone (repeating cycle: 1 beep per second for 2 seconds, followed by 2 seconds of silence)	REPLACE SYSTEM CONTROLLER (on System Monitor) REPLACE SYSTEM DRIVER (on Display Module)	System Controller is operating in back-up mode.	1. Replace the System Controller (see other side for instructions). 2. Notify the patient's physician. 3. Obtain a new backup System Controller. 4. Program the new backup Controller with settings prescribed for this patient.
Yellow ControllerCell	1 Beep Every 4 Seconds	SC CELL MODULE LOW (on System Monitor) Driver Cell Low (on Display Module)	The battery module that powers the System Controller audible alarm is depleted.	Replace the System Controller Battery Module.
Rapidly Flashing Green Power Symbol and 4 Green Battery Fuel Gauge Lights Flashing Once Per Second	1 Beep Every Second	POWER CABLE DISCONNECTED	One of the power leads is damaged or disconnected.	1. Reconnect or tighten disconnected/loose power lead. 2. If alarm continues, check System Controller power lead and PBU/Power Module patient cable for damage. 3. If System Controller power lead is damaged, replace the Controller. If PBU/Power Module patient cable is damaged, replace PBU/Power Module patient cable. 4. Obtain a new, backup System Controller for this patient, if necessary.
NONE: No Warning Light	NONE on PBU w/ System Monitor 1 Beep Every 4 Seconds when on Batteries or PBU (w/Display Module)	WARNING: Low Speed Operation	Pump is operating below low speed limit.	Connect System Controller to System Monitor (audio alarm will stop) and increase fixed speed setting or reduce low speed limit.

FIGURE 32–3. System Controller warning lights and sounds. (Reproduced with permission from Thoratec Corporation, Pleasanton, CA.)

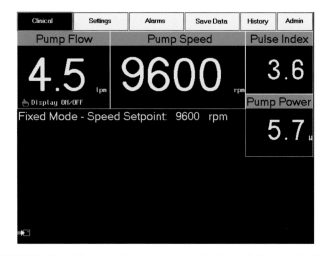

FIGURE 32–4. The clinical screen on the HeartMate II System Monitor. (Reproduced with permission from Thoratec Corporation, Pleasanton, CA.)

CURRENT APPROVAL STATUS

After completion of multicenter clinical trials for both indications, the HeartMate II LVAS was approved by the Food and Drug Administration (FDA) for bridge-to-transplantation (BTT) and for destination therapy (DT) in advanced heart failure patients. Approval for the BTT indication was obtained in April 2008 and for DT in nontransplant-eligible patients in January 2010.

■ INDICATIONS FOR USE

The HeartMate II LVAS is intended for use as a BTT in cardiac transplant candidates at risk of imminent death from nonreversible left ventricular failure. The HeartMate II LVAS is also

TABLE 32-1. Improvements in Outcomes With Bridge-to-Transplantation from Clinical Trial to Posttrial Postapproval Study

Reference	Study	Enrollment Period	n	30-Day Operative Mortality (%)	Transplantation, Recovery, or Ongoing Device Support at 180 Days (%)	Kaplan-Meier Survival at 1 Year (%)
Miller et al[1]	HM II pivotal trial	3/05-5/06	133	11	79	68
Pagani et al[2]	HM II pivotal trial	3/05-3/07	281	8	84	74
Starling et al[3]	Postapproval INTERMACS registry study	4/08-8/08	169	4	91	85

indicated for use in patients with New York Heart Association (NYHA) class IIIB or IV end-stage left ventricular failure who have received optimal medical therapy for at least 45 of the last 60 days and are not candidates for cardiac transplantation. The HeartMate II LVAS is also intended for use both inside and outside the hospital, or for transportation of ventricular assist device (VAD) patients via ground ambulance, fixed-wing aircraft, or helicopter.

SUMMARY OF CLINICAL RESULTS

Initial results of the BTT trial were published on 133 patients implanted from March 2005 through May 2006 by Miller et al,[1] followed by an updated report on 281 patients with enrollment extended through April 2008 with a continued access protocol by Pagani et al.[2] A postapproval study was also performed on the first 169 patients reported to Interagency Registry for Mechanically Assisted Circulatory Systems (INTERMACS) after FDA approval and reported by Starling et al.[3] This study showed improved survival in real-world settings compared to initial patients in the clinical trial (Table 32–1). The 30-day operative mortality has decreased from 11% to 4% since the initial clinical trial cohort. Similarly, 1-year Kaplan-Meier survival improved from 68% to 74% and now to 85% in the current report (Fig. 32–5). The percentage of patients reaching transplant, cardiac recovery, or ongoing LVAD support by 6 months was 91%. Results appear to be maintained in the next implanted patients in the INTERMACS registry, as 88% survival was reported in over 850 HeartMate II patients at 6 months in the annual report.[16]

The clinical trial for DT in nontransplant-eligible patients has also been completed and results published on the initial 200 patients, which were randomized 2:1 between the HeartMate II continuous-flow LVAD and the HeartMate XVE pulsatile-flow LVAD.[4] A comparison of results from this trial and the REMATCH (Randomized Evaluation of Mechanical Assistance for the Treatment of Congestive Heart Failure) trial was published by Fang,[17] (Fig. 32–6) which shows the improved survival

provided by the HeartMate II. Two-year survival was 58% compared to the pulsatile LVAD of 25%, significantly greater than for patients continuing on medical therapy in the REMATCH trial of 8% at 2 years.

Bleeding remains the most reported adverse event with the HeartMate II.[1-4] Anticoagulation strategies are still being refined, but the target international normalized ratio (INR) levels on long-term warfarin therapy for the HeartMate II has been reduced from 2.0 to 3.0 when the trial was started to 1.5 to 2.5 at the end of the trial due to a low incidence of pump thrombosis and ischemic stroke compared to a higher rate of hemorrhagic events.[6] Another analysis showed that intravenous heparin may

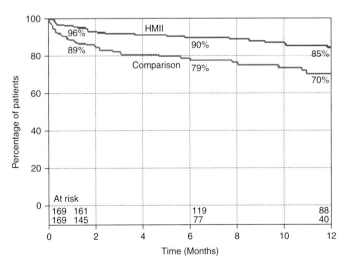

FIGURE 32–5. Kaplan-Meier survival for HeartMate II bridge-to-transplant patients in the post-FDA approval study conducted through the INTERMACS registry. The top line is the survival of HeartMate II (HMII) LVAD patients, and the bottom is the survival for patients receiving pulsatile VADs (comparison). (Reproduced with permission from Starling RC, Naka Y, Boyle AJ.[3])

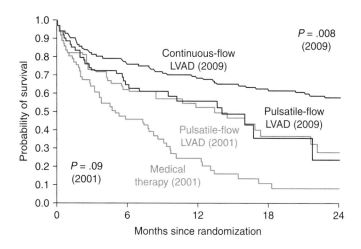

FIGURE 32–6. Kaplan-Meier survival for HeartMate II continuous-flow LVAD destination therapy trial results compared to pulsatile LVAD patients in the HeartMate II trial and in the REMATCH trial and patients receiving medical management in REMATCH. (Reproduced with permission from Fang JC.[17] Copyright © Massachusetts Medical Society.)

not be needed in the transition to warfarin therapy in the early postoperative period which was based on the observation of no increase in thrombotic events in patients who were managed without heparin and had less bleeding in the first 30 days.[7]

Right heart failure is another important adverse event. The incidence of the need for temporary RVAD support was 6% and an additional 7% required prolonged inotropic support as reported by Kormos et al along with an analysis of risk factors.[8] Russell et al[9] showed normalization of creatinine, blood urea nitrogen, and liver enzymes during continuous-flow LVAD support in BTT patients indicating improvements in renal and hepatic function over 6 months of support. Changes in neurocognitive function have also been evaluated for HeartMate II patients, with improvements seen in visual memory, executive functions, visual spatial perception, and processing speed from month 1 through 6, with stable function shown in other domains.[10]

Most importantly are significant improvements in functional capacity and quality of life which have been demonstrated in HeartMate II trial participants by Rogers et al.[5] Most patients had NYHA class IV symptoms at baseline. Following implantation, over 80% of patients had NYHA class symptoms class I or

II symptoms by 6 months, improvements that were sustained at 24 months.[5] Similar sustained improvements were seen with Minnesota Living With Heart Failure and the Kansas City Cardiomyopathy Questionnaires.

REFERENCES

1. Miller LW, Pagani FD, Russell SD, et al. Use of a continuous-flow device in patients awaiting heart transplantation. *N Engl J Med.* 2007;357:885-896.
2. Pagani FD, Miller LW, Russell SD, et al. Extended mechanical circulatory support with a continuous-flow rotary left ventricular assist device. *J Am Coll Cardiol.* 2009;54:312-321.
3. Starling RC, Naka Y, Boyle AJ. Results of the Post-FDA Approval Study with a continuous flow left ventricular assist device as a bridge to heart transplantation: a prospective study using the INTERMACS registry. *J Am Coll Cardiol.* 2011;57:1890-1898.
4. Slaughter MS, Rogers JG, Milano CA, et al. Advanced heart failure treated with continuous-flow left ventricular assist device. *N Engl J Med.* 2009;361:2241-2251.
5. Rogers JG, Aaronson KD, Boyle AJ, et al. Continuous flow left ventricular assist device improves functional capacity and quality of life of advanced heart failure patients. *J Am Coll Cardiol.* 2010;55:1826-1834.
6. Boyle AJ, Russell SD, Teuteberg JJ. Low thromboembolism and pump thrombosis with the HeartMate II left ventricular assist device: analysis of outpatient anti-coagulation. *J Heart Lung Transplant.* 2009;28:881-887.
7. Slaughter MS, Naka Y, John R. Post-operative heparin may not be required for transitioning patients with a HeartMate II left ventricular assist system to long-term warfarin therapy. *J Heart Lung Transplant.* 2010;29(6):616-624.
8. Kormos RL, Teuteberg JJ, Pagani FD. Right ventricular failure in patients with the HeartMate II continuous-flow left ventricular assist device: incidence, risk factors, and effect on outcomes. *J Thorac Cardiovasc Surg.* 2010;139(5):1316-1324.
9. Russell SD, Rogers JG, Milano CA. Renal and hepatic function improve in advanced heart failure patients during continuous-flow support with the HeartMate II left ventricular assist device. *Circulation.* 2009;120:2352-2357.
10. Petrucci RJ, Wright S, Naka Y. Neurocognitive assessments in advanced heart failure patients receiving continuous-flow left ventricular assist devices. *J Heart Lung Transplant.* 2009;28:542-549.
11. HeartMate II LVAS Instructions for Use. Document 103883. Thoratec Corporation, Pleasanton, CA.
12. HeartMate II LVAD Operating Manual, Document 103884, Thoratec Corporation, Pleasanton, CA.
13. HeartMate II LVAS Clinical Operation & Patient Management. Document 104181. Thoratec Corporation, Pleasanton, CA.
14. HeartMate II Alarm Guide for Clinicians. Document 103907. Thoratec Corporation, Pleasanton, CA.
15. Slaughter MS, Pagani FD, Rogers JG, et al. Clinical management of continuous-flow left ventricular assist devices in advanced heart failure. *J Heart Lung Transplant.* 2010;29:S1-S39.
16. Kirklin JK, Naftel DC, Kormos RL, et al. Second INTERMACS annual report: more than 1,000 primary left ventricular assist device implants. *J Heart Lung Transplant.* 2010;29:1-10.
17. Fang JC. Rise of the machines—left ventricular assist devices as permanent therapy for advanced heart failure. *N Engl J Med.* 2009;361:2282-2285.

CHAPTER 33
THE HEARTASSIST 5 VAD SYSTEM

Jay Kraemer

INTRODUCTION

Patients with end-stage heart failure have limited treatment options. Cardiac transplantation is an option for only a minority of these patients, who are found to be suitable candidates. Those patients awaiting cardiac transplantation whose condition deteriorates are placed on the highest priority UNOS (United Network of Organ Sharing) 1A or 1B list. Treatment options for this 1A or 1B subgroup include maximal continuous parenteral inotropic therapy (often requiring more than one inotropic medication) and intravenous vasodilators. For those patients who remain unstable despite maximal pharmacological therapy, mechanical support with a left ventricular assist device (LVAD) may be indicated.

The HeartAssist 5 VAD System (MicroMed Technology, Inc. Houston, TX) represents a new treatment option for patients with end-stage heart failure. This axial-flow pump was developed to provide a ventricular assist device (VAD) with adequate output that is small, lightweight, and mechanically simple. The potential benefits of this device include high reliability in light of a single moving part; a simple, short surgical implant procedure possibly limiting surgical morbidity and mortality; and a small flexible percutaneous cable that may result in fewer infections. Furthermore, the size of this VAD system may prove suitable for small patients who would otherwise not be candidates for implantable first-generation VAD support. In short, the HeartAssist 5 VAD System offers several benefits that may translate into better patient outcomes.

DEVICE DESCRIPTION

The HeartAssist 5 VAD is a miniaturized, auxiliary heart pump or VAD which was jointly developed by the famed heart surgeon Dr Michael E. DeBakey, Dr George P. Noon (Methodist Hospital, Houston, Texas), and the National Aeronautics and Space Administration (NASA). The HeartAssist 5 VAD is 30 mm × 76 mm, weighs 95 g (< 4 oz) and is designed to provide increased blood flow to patients who suffer from heart failure. MicroMed Cardiovascular, Inc. has exclusive rights to the technology.

The components of the HeartAssist 5 VAD System (Fig. 33–1) consist of the pump system (including the titanium pump and inlet cannula, the percutaneous cable, the flow probe and outflow graft), the controller (including batteries), VADPAK, ChargePAK, sterilizing tray and tools, and the HeartAttendant console. The individual components of the pump are illustrated

in Fig. 33–2. As can be seen in the illustration, the pump consists of a flow straightener, an inducer/ impeller, and a diffuser. These components are fully enclosed in a titanium flow tube that has been hermetically sealed. The pump is driven by a brushless, direct current (DC) motor stator that is contained in the stator housing. The inducer/impeller is the only moving part of the pump. It has six blades with eight magnets hermetically sealed in each blade. The inducer/impeller spins at 7500 to 12500 rpm (revolutions per minute) and is capable of generating flow in excess of 10 L/min.

The pump is attached to a titanium inlet cannula that is placed into the left ventricle of the heart. A graft is connected to the pump outlet and anastomosed to the aorta. A three-phase electric motor is an integral part of the pump and is driven by the controller. The pump is connected to the controller via a percutaneous cable that is passed through the skin. The percutaneous cable contains the pump power cable and the flow probe cable. The controller is designed to operate the pump (illustrated in Fig. 33–3). The controller's primary power is supplied by two external 12-V DC batteries, or by filtered DC power provided directly by the HeartAttendant or an independent power supply (both the HeartAttendant and the independent power supply are discussed below). The controller contains an internal 9-V battery that will not operate the pump, but will operate the controller alarms if both pump batteries are disconnected and direct power is not available. The controller displays pump-operating parameters such as speed, flow rate, power usage, and remaining battery life. The pump-operating parameters cannot be adjusted with the controller; they can only be adjusted using the HeartAttendant. After implantation of the HeartAssist 5 VAD, the patient will be able to carry the controller and batteries using the VADPAK, an ergonomically designed wearable pouch that enables the patient to be completely mobile.

The HeartAttendant (Fig. 33–4) is a portable console that supports the power and communication requirements for the HeartAssist 5 VAD by providing filtered DC power, charging and reconditioning batteries, and transmitting program data to the patient-worn controller. The software on the HeartAttendant allows real-time visualization of the pump performance and its interaction with the native heart via a flow waveform. Bar charts indicating battery charge levels, power usage, and mean flow are also displayed. Other screens allow technicians to program pump-operating parameters and alarm levels. In lieu of using the HeartAttendant for the sole purpose of supplying filtered power to the controller, an optional independent power supply (Fig. 33–5) is available, which is lightweight and easy to use. The independent power supply plugs directly into a wall outlet and then connects to the controller.

CURRENT APPROVAL STATUS

The HeartAssist 5 VAD received the CE mark in March, 2010 and the HeartAttendant was approved in April 2010.[1] Clinical experience has been gained on use of the device by individual centers in Europe. Clinical investigations in the United States are being orchestrated at the time of this writing, with comparison

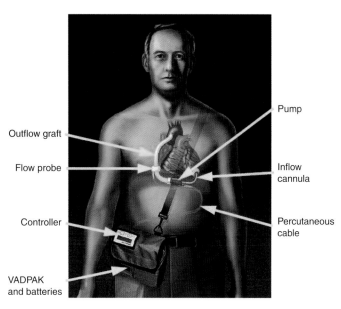

FIGURE 33-1. The HeartAssist 5 VAD System. (Courtesy of micromedcv.com.)

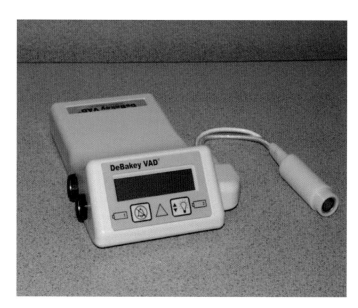

FIGURE 33-3. The controller. (Courtesy of micromedcv.com.)

to a concurrent control in order to establish safety and effectiveness of the device as a left ventricular support in patients awaiting cardiac transplantation. The study design is a multicenter, prospective, nonrandomized two-arm study using the INTERMACS (Interagency Registry for Mechanically Assisted Circulatory Systems) registry as a concurrent control. Up to 40 US centers will be participating in the study. A total of 105 patients will be enrolled over a period of 12 to 18 months, with the observation phase of the study being the first 180 postoperative days. The success of the device will be measured at the end of the observation phase and will include all patients

undergoing a heart transplant before 180 postoperative days, survival on the original device, or device removal due to recovery of heart function followed by a minimum of 60-day survival. Failure will include death before 180 postoperative days, device exchange due to failure of the original HeartAssist 5 VAD System before 180 postoperative days, and device removal for cardiac recovery without a minimum 60-day survival. Patients surviving beyond the observation phase, while implanted with the original device, will continue to be followed until death, cardiac transplant, device exchange, or device removal due to cardiac recovery.

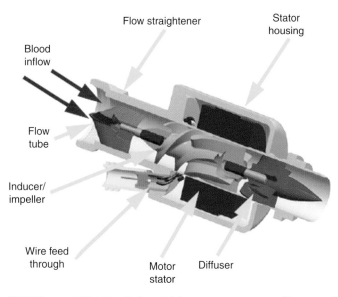

FIGURE 33-2. The HeartAssist 5 VAD pump components. (Courtesy of micromedcv.com.)

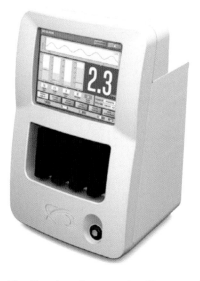

FIGURE 33-4. The HeartAttendant console. (Courtesy of micromedcv.com.)

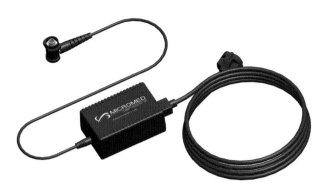

FIGURE 33-5. Optional independent power supply. (Courtesy of micromedcv.com.)

PATIENT SELECTION

Patients are considered eligible for support with the HeartAssist 5 VAD System if they meet the following criteria:

- Age > 18.
- Body surface area (BSA) > 1.2 m².
- Approved for cardiac transplant and LVAD by the institution's multidisciplinary transplant committee.
- Listed with UNOS for heart transplant.
- Patient is New York Heart Association (NYHA) class IV.
- Patient is able to return to the clinical site for all routine follow-up visits.

Patients are considered ineligible for support with the HeartAssist 5 VAD System if they meet the following criteria:

- Patient has undergone cardiothoracic surgery within 30 days.
- Patient had an acute myocardial infarction within 14 days with no signs of hemodynamic improvement.
- Patient has prior cardiac transplant, left ventricular reduction surgery, cardiomyoplasty, or LVAD.
- Patient has a mechanical, animal, or human tissue heart valve, or requires a valve or left ventricular aneurysm resection.
- Patient has history of untreated abdominal or thoracic aortic aneurysm > 5 cm.
- Patient on ventilator support for > 72 hours within 4 days immediately prior to enrollment.
- Patient has a proven history of pulmonary embolism within 6 months of enrollment.
- Patient has moderate to severe aortic insufficiency as determined by echocardiogram without plans for correction during pump implantation surgery.
- Patient has uncorrected thrombocytopenia or generalized coagulopathy (eg, platelets < 100,000, international normalized ratio (INR) > 1.6, or partial thromboplastin time (PTT) > 2.5 times control in the absence of anticoagulation therapy).
- Patient has severe right ventricular failure as defined by the anticipated need for right ventricular assist device (RVAD) support or extracorporeal membrane oxygenation (ECMO) at the time of implantation *or* right atrial pressure > 20 mm Hg while on multiple inotropes.
- Patient has fixed pulmonary vascular resistance which is unresponsive to pharmacologic manipulation as evidenced by a pulmonary artery systolic pressure exceeding 60 mm Hg *and* any one of the following three variables:
  - Pulmonary vascular resistance > 5 Wood units
  - Pulmonary vascular resistance index > 6 Wood units · m⁻²
  - Transpulmonary gradient exceeding 16 to 20 mm Hg
- Patient has significant renal dysfunction defined as serum creatinine > 3.0 (mg/dL) or requires hemo or peritoneal dialysis for renal failure (excluding ultrafiltration for fluid removal).
- Patient has evidence of intrinsic hepatic disease as defined as liver enzyme values (aspartate aminotransferase [AST] or alanine aminotransferase [ALT] that are > 3 times the upper limits of normal *or* a total bilirubin > 2.5 mg/dL *or* biopsy-proven liver cirrhosis or portal hypertension).
- Patient has serum albumin < 3.3 g/dL.
- Patient has positive serum pregnancy test.
- Patient has active systemic infection prior to study enrollment not yet resolved by treatment. Active systemic infection is defined by any one of the following in spite of antibiotic, antiviral, or antifungal treatment: two or more consecutive positive cultures; elevated temperature and white blood cell count; and hypotension, tachycardia, and generalized malaise.
- Patient has had a stroke within 90 days prior to enrollment *or* patient has a history of cerebral vascular disease, with > 80% extracranial stenosis documented by carotid Doppler study during transplant evaluation.
- Patient has significant lower extremity peripheral vascular disease accompanied by rest pain or leg ulceration.
- Patient has contraindication to the administration of heparin, warfarin, or antiplatelet agents.
- Patient is intolerant to any peri- or postoperative therapy that the investigator may administer based on the patient's health status.
- Patient has a history of psychiatric disease (including drug or alcohol abuse) that is likely to impair compliance with the treatment.
- Patient has a condition, other than heart failure, that may limit survival to < 2 years and/or would exclude cardiac transplantation.
- Patient has been diagnosed with cancer.

CONCLUSION

In the MicroMed experience using the earlier-generation DeBakey VAD design, over 440 implants were performed worldwide, accounting for more than 130 patient years of life. With CE approval of both the adult and pediatric versions of the device, this pump offers a new form of therapy for patients who require mechanical circulatory support. The HeartAssist 5 VAD System features several important modifications to the original design. The inflow cannula has been textured to promote better ingrowth inside the left ventricle to reduce blood activation as well as shortened to allow for implantation above the diaphragm in the pericardial space. A modified inlet flare serves to maximize smooth blood flow into the pump. The rear hub has been modified to provide smoother blood flow and improve washout, thereby improving physiologic response and widening the spectrum of cardiac support. These features, along with an improved interface with the portable console, have the potential to improve therapy for patients with end-stage heart failure.

REFERENCES

1. Noon GP, Loebe M. Current status of the MicroMed DeBakey Noon Ventricular Assist Device. *Tex Heart Inst J.* 2010;37(6):652-653.

CHAPTER 34

THE JARVIK-2000 FLOWMAKER

Robert K. Jarvik

The Jarvik-2000 (Jarvik Heart, Inc. New York, NY) mechanical circulatory support devices comprise a family of miniature axial-flow blood pumps configured for many applications, including left ventricular assist device (LVAD), right ventricular assist device (RVAD), total ventricular assist (tVA), pediatric applications, and regional perfusion.[1]

BACKGROUND

Dr Jarvik first developed miniature axial-flow pumps in 1976 to pump hydraulic fluid and provide a portable electrohydraulic heart to improve upon the bulky pneumatic power technology used at that time. Pumps only 1 in in diameter and 2 in long could provide over 30 L/min at 12000 rpm (revolutions per minute) and were reversed in under 20 milliseconds to alternately pump silicone hydraulic fluid from the right to the left ventricle, and vice versa. The hydraulic fluid was used to actuate the diaphragms of the Jarvik-7 heart. Such a high flow was needed to reach the peak ejection flow during pulsatility where the left percent systole was 33% and the cardiac output was 10 L/min.

In 1986 Dr Jarvik began development of miniature rotary blood pumps using rotors supported on a very fine wire held in tension to provide rigidity. Small axial-flow blood pumps using this bearing design avoided hemolysis and functioned well in animals for about a week. The wire in tension bearings failed because blood in the tiny gap between the stationary wire and elongated pyrolytic carbon rotating sleeve essentially glued the parts together and stopped the pump.

Development of small ceramic pin bearings overcame this problem, and during the 1990s the adult-size Jarvik-2000 blood pump was developed to the point of clinical readiness under a 5-year National Institute of Health (NIH) IVAS (Innovative Ventricular Assist System) contract. Transicoil, Inc, an aerospace manufacturer of motors and electromechanical assemblies, was the prime contractor with Dr Jarvik as principal investigator. In parallel with this work, Jarvik Heart, Inc developed the highly simplified analog control system intended for manual pump output adjustment directly by the patient.

When clinical implants were initiated in the year 2000, Dr Frazier implanted the first bridge-to-transplant (BTT) patient in the Jarvik-2000 Pilot Study.[2] That patient continues an active life as a transplant recipient after more than 10 years. Dr Westaby initiated long-term use with the postauricular connector. Dr Westaby's first long-term use patient lived for 7½ years supported by the Jarvik-2000 and was rehabilitated to New York Heart Association (NYHA) class I for most of that time.[3]

From 2004 to 2010 Jarvik Heart, Inc developed child- and infant-size models under the NIH pediatric contract program. During the first 3 years of this research, the small pin bearings used successfully in adult-size pumps proved unsuccessful in the child model because of excess thrombus formation that caused the pumps to bind. This problem was solved with the development of cone bearings that have subsequently been applied to the adult Jarvik-2000 and to all other configurations.

CLINICAL SUMMARY

By July 2010, the Jarvik-2000 had been implanted as BTT and for permanent use in more than 400 patients at over 50 hospitals in 10 countries. There is now more than 250 patient-years of experience with its use. Kaplan-Meyer 10-year survival of the bridge patients after transplant is 80%. The 5-year survival with pump support is over 40% which includes patients with earlier versions of the system prior to important improvements. With the present model having major improvements, including the microsphere surface, intermittent low speed (ILS) controller, cone bearings, and improved abdominal cables, 5-year survival results are expected to be similar to heart transplant.

INTRAVENTRICULAR PLACEMENT

The Jarvik-2000 is implanted in the left ventricular apex with the outflow graft to either the descending thoracic aorta when the left thoracotomy is used or to the ascending aorta with sternotomy (Fig. 34–1A). In most cases the pump is implanted without cardiopulmonary bypass. Two pumps may be used to support both the right and the left natural ventricles. This procedure, called total ventricular assist (tVA), is performed via left thoracotomy as shown in Fig. 34–1B.[4]

UNIQUE CHARACTERISTICS OF THE JARVIK-2000

1. The intraventricular placement of the blood pump avoids any pump pocket and contributes to the extraordinarily low pump infection rate.

2. The device is available with either a cable exiting the abdomen or a head-mounted cable, called the postauricular model (Fig. 34–3). Both cables have a very low infection rate of about 3%.

3. The postauricular connector, which has remained infection free over 7 years, is based on cochlear implant pedestals that have remained infection free for over 20 years.[5] The postauricular site is highly resistant to infection because of the high vascularity of the scalp and other tissue characteristics evolved to minimize wound infection and enhance wound healing around the head and neck.[6] There is practically no motion of the scalp tissue against the connector post. This reduces tissue trauma. No wound dressing is required, improving patient self-sufficiency and also permitting normal showering and bathing. The postauricular cable

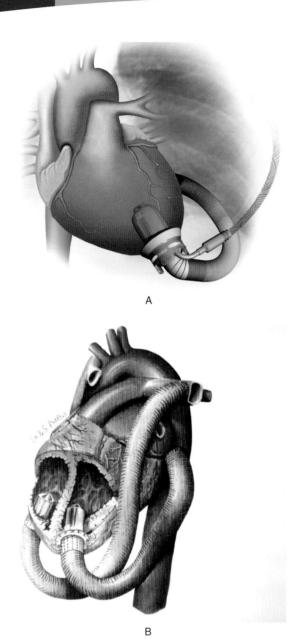

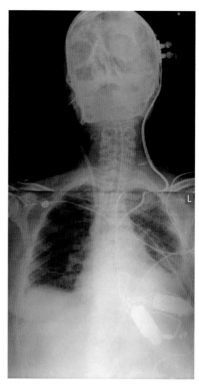

FIGURE 34–2. Total ventricular assist (tVA) may be performed via a left thoracotomy off bypass. Two Jarvik-2000 pumps are implanted in the apex of the right and left ventricles using a sewing cuff. The power cables are tunneled together to the postauricular pedestal, where they exit the skin. Right/left balance is easily achieved by running the left pump 1000 rpm faster than the right.

FIGURE 34–1. Position of the pump in (A) the left apex and (B) as biventricular support.

is comfortable and represents successful "human engineering." In our era of head-mounted communication devices the cable and connector are cosmetically acceptable.

4. The implanted cable uses a triple redundant cable. There have been no failures of the internal cable. A connector is located within the flange-mounted percutaneous post, which provides the ability to completely change the external cable and connector components in the event of damage or as a periodic routine maintenance procedure.

5. The Jarvik-2000 analog controller is manually adjustable by the patient, with no software or automatic speed control. This permits the patient to dial in a speed setting from numbers 1 to 5 which corresponds to motor speeds from 8000 to 12000 rpm. Since the patient has the controller with him or her at all times, speed adjustment related to the patient's exercise level is always available. This is advantageous compared to other control systems which require the patient to use a nonportable console to change pump speed, and therefore requires the patient to return home or to the hospital for speed changes.

6. The Jarvik-2000 may be safely turned off for a few minutes up to hours in most patients because the net regurgitant flow is relatively low due to the small area of the flow path through the device. The rotor spins in reverse (like a turbine) driven by the differential pressure gradient between the aortic pressure and intraventricular pressure during diastole, and is therefore well washed to avoid stagnant zones predisposed to thrombus formation. Other axial-flow pumps have a higher regurgitant flow, and many patients rapidly go into heart failure if the pump is turned off. Centrifugal pumps are unsafe to turn off because the rotors do not spin when stopped and reverse flow from the aorta into the ventricle through the pump takes the shortest path between the tangential pump outflow diffuser and the central inflow port. This leaves a large stagnant area in the pumping chamber opposite the outflow where thrombus forms.

7. The Jarvik-2000 system utilizes an ILS mode to ensure washing of the aortic valve each minute. The ILS mode lowers the pump speed to 7000 rpm for 8 seconds each minute. This

permits the natural ventricle to open the aortic valve for six or eight beats and thereby wash the aortic root. During the other 52 seconds of each minute the pump operates at the speed set on the dial.

8. The Jarvik-2000 requires no inlet cannula, reducing the risk of the inlet cannulae becoming displaced against the ventricular wall and partially occluded which may occur with extraventricular pumps if the position of a relatively heavy pump in the abdomen shifts or if the relative anatomy changes due to reverse remodeling of the left ventricle. Long inlet cannulae add resistance to the flow entering the pump, and increased fluid inertia within long inlet cannulae damps pump pulsatility in response to natural intraventricular pressure changes over the cardiac cycle. The intraventricular impeller of the Jarvik-2000 combined with the lack of an inlet cannula favorably affects pulsatility. In most patients a pulse can be palpated by the time of hospital discharge, and blood pressure can often be measured with a cuff.

9. The Jarvik-2000 does not require pump removal in recovery patients. In patients who have recovered sufficient ventricular function to no longer need the device, the Jarvik-2000 was left in the apex, the outflow graft was ligated, and the power cable was cut and removed. Patients have survived for years after the pump was stopped, without infections of the pump or thromboembolic events.

10. The adult-size Jarvik-2000 is small (30 cc) and lightweight (90 g) and the Jarvik-2000 infant ventricular assist device (VAD) is only 4 cc weighing 11 g. A catheter-mounted 21-Fr permanent partial support pump (2 L/min) that is only 2 cc and weighs only 6 g is under development.

These characteristics provide many quality-of-life benefits to patients. Additionally, other characteristics of the system include simplicity of the user interface, small lightweight long life batteries, silent operation, and exceptionally high durability and reliability of the implant.

■ THE CONTROLLER AND BATTERIES

The Jarvik-2000 uses a small portable controller and lithium ion (Li-ion) battery pack to provide 10 to 12 hours of use when the battery is new and over 7 hours of use with a battery pack that has been recharged 500 times. The system also includes a larger reserve battery weighing 12 lb that is used by the patient's bedside for nighttime power. These batteries provide more than 24 hours of use when fully charged. Figure 34–3 shows the controller (black) and Li-ion pack (grey) in the palm of a patient's hand.

Patients must keep a charged spare battery with them at all times. The system provided to each patient at hospital discharge includes two controllers, two reserve batteries (with built-in chargers), three Li-ion portable battery packs, two Li-ion battery chargers, and backups for all cables.

The controller and batteries are designed with clips to be worn on the belt (Fig. 34–4). Alternatively, patients may carry the external components in a "camera bag" or wear them in a strap-on carrying bag such as a "fanny pack" (Fig. 34–5).

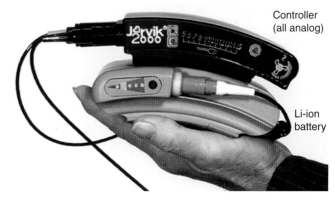

FIGURE 34–3. The controller and portable battery pack.

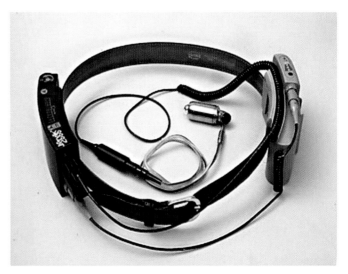

FIGURE 34–4. The controller and battery shown mounted on a belt with the cables to the Jarvik-2000 blood pump shown at the center.

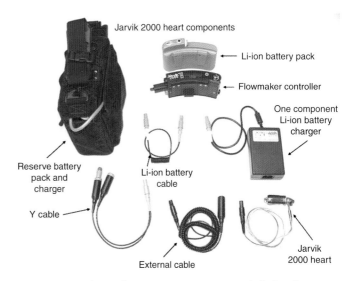

FIGURE 34–5. The Jarvik-2000 system components, including the reserve battery (red), cables, and chargers.

FlowMaker controller

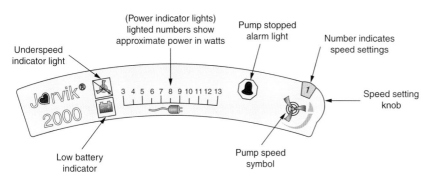

FIGURE 34–6. The speed is set using the dial at the right. The controller includes alarms for low battery, low pump speed, and pump stopped. A wattmeter continuously indicates the power used.

■ SETTING THE PROPER SPEED

The controller speed is initially adjusted by the physician, VAD specialists, and nursing staff. The principle is to keep the speed as low as possible while achieving sufficient flow augmentation (Fig. 34–6). This is judged by clinical information in the immediate postoperative period, including blood pressure, lung function and blood gasses, renal function, and flow data from a cardiac output–monitoring catheter if one is in place. Using transthoracic echo, the pump speed can be set low enough that the aortic valve opens on some beats and usually will open on all beats during the ILS portion of the cycle.

■ PATIENT ADJUSTMENT OF THE CONTROLLER

By the time patients have recovered sufficiently to go home and before they may be discharged, they are trained in the use of the equipment and changing batteries and cables. A normal pump speed for rest and mild exercise is determined; usually setting 2 or 3 is used most of the day (Fig. 34–7). To match the speed

to exercise level, patients make adjustments to the speed control dial. They are able to judge whether their controller is running the pump optimally or if it is too fast or too slow. When patients exercise strenuously enough to become short of breath, they turn the pump speed up for more flow. Then, when they cut back their exercise level, they have a sense that the flow is too high, which reminds them to turn the speed back down. Some patients must turn the speed to a lower value in order to sleep and will get insomnia if the speed is too fast.

SUMMARY

The Jarvik-2000 technology provides a family of small axial-flow blood pumps for a variety of clinical applications. The adult model is in wide use around the world, the child and infant sizes are beginning clinical use, and new applications such as the catheter-mounted model (Fig. 34–8) are under development.

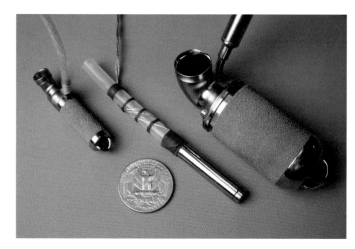

FIGURE 34–8. The infant- and adult-size Jarvik-2000 hearts are shown with a research prototype of the 7-mm-diameter catheter-mounted pump, under development for long-term support with insertion in the cath lab.

FlowMaker controller
Blood flow, power indicator

- Actual blood flow not measured
- Flow through the Jarvik-2000 based on data from animal studies

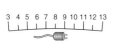

	Speed rpm	Flow L/min	Power W
1	8,000	1-2	3-4
2	9,000	2-4	4-5
3	10,000	3-5	5-6-7
4	11,000	4-6	7-8-9
5	12,000	5-7	8-9-10

- Power indicator: lights may change with heartbeat, indicating pulsatile flow
- All lights are green except 13 which is yellow:
  – 13 indicates 13 W or more
  – 3 indicates 3 W or less

FIGURE 34–7. The approximate flow and power that are usual for each speed setting.

REFERENCES

1. Macris MP, Parnis SM, Frazier OH, Fuqua JM Jr, Jarvik RK. Development of an implantable ventricular assist system. *Ann Thorac Surg.* 1997;63(2):367-70.
2. Westaby S, Frazier OH, Beyersdorf F, et al. The Jarvik 2000 Heart. Clinical validation of the intraventricular position. Eur J Cardiothorac Surg. 2002;22(2):228-32.
3. Westaby S, Siegenthaler M, Beyersdorf F, et al. Destination therapy with a rotary blood pump and novel power delivery. *Eur J Cardiothorac Surg.* 2010;37(2):350-6.
4. Siegenthaler MP, Martin J, Gutwald R, et al. Anterior approach to implant the Jarvik 2000 with retroauricular power supply. *Ann Thorac Surg.* 2005;80(2):745-7.
5. Westaby S, Frazier OH, Banning A. Six years of continuous mechanical circulatory support. *N Engl J Med.* 2006;355(3):325-7.
6. Jarvik R, Westaby S, Katsumata T, Pigott D, Evans RD. LVAD power delivery: a percutaneous approach to avoid infection. *Ann Thorac Surg.* 1998;65(2):470-473.

CHAPTER 35

CIRCULITE SYNERGY PARTIAL CIRCULATORY SUPPORT SYSTEM

Arielle Drummond, Robert Farnan, Gail Farnan, Daniel Burkhoff, Carol Krieger, and John Burdis

INTRODUCTION

Implantation of left ventricular assist devices (LVADs) for the treatment of end-stage heart failure is becoming progressively more accepted within the heart failure community worldwide. These devices are designed to provide full hemodynamic support in New York Heart Association (NYHA) class IV or cardiogenic shock patients, with typical flow capacities of 5 to 10 L/min, providing complete left ventricular unloading, and with prolonged use, result in structural and functional reverse remodeling.[1,2] These devices are typically large, requiring a major surgical procedure (sternotomy and cardiopulmonary bypass [CPB] support), thus increasing the risk of adverse events and impacting the speed of patient recovery and lengthening hospitalization. Because of the size of these devices and associated major surgery, LVADs are still generally restricted to the most critically ill patients with a short life expectancy. A smaller device under development called the Synergy Pocket Micro-pump (CircuLite, Inc, Saddle Brook, NJ) was designed to provide partial hemodynamic support in a slightly "less sick" patient population (class IIIb and early class IV). The concept of the Synergy Micro-pump includes a less invasive off-pump surgery, in principle reducing the incidence of adverse events as compared to the major surgery associated with LVADs, thus justifying the use of the device in patients who are less sick than those currently receiving LVADs.

DEVICE DESCRIPTION

The Synergy Micro-pump (Fig. 35–1) is the size of an AA battery and weighs approximately 25 g with an outer body diameter of 14 mm and a length of 53 mm. The system includes a silicone nitinol-reinforced inflow cannula at 20.5 cm in length. The inner diameter of the inflow cannula is 6 mm and has a titanium tip with a Dacron cuff, allowing for enhanced healing. The outflow graft is a 1-mm-thick expanded polytetrafluoroethylene (ePTFE) prosthesis with an inner diameter of 8 mm. The system also incorporates a percutaneous lead connecting the micro-pump to two rechargeable batteries to a controller (Fig. 35–2).

This mixed-flow micro-pump has a rotor that is hydrodynamically levitated and magnetically stabilized. The micro-pump operates in a range from 20,000 to 28,000 rpm and provides partial support of between 2.5 and 3.5 L/min. The micro-pump draws blood from the left atrium via an inflow cannula into the pump inlet and then propels the blood out at a 90-degree angle via the outflow graft that is anastomosed to the subclavian artery (Fig. 35–3). The micro-pump is implanted without CPB or sternotomy which is unique to this device. The implant procedure is completed with two incisions: a right anterolateral mini-thoracotomy for placement of the inflow cannula into the left atrium via Waterston's groove and a right subclavicular incision to isolate the subclavian artery for the outflow graft anastomosis. This incision site is also used to create a pump pocket anterior to the pectoralis major muscle (Fig. 35–4). Clinically, the micro-pump has been implanted in an off-pump procedure as short as 90 minutes and on average an approximately 150-minute procedure.

Once the micro-pump is implanted, the device is powered by the patient controller connected to two battery modules or an alternating current (AC) power supply. The patient controller stores all the micro-pump parameters, such as pump current and alarms, and displays the pump speed, remaining battery charge, and controller error codes on an LCD (liquid crystal display) screen. In order to change the settings of the micro-pump, the physician or hospital staff connect the physician programmer to the controller and make adjustments accordingly. The controller is connected directly to the micro-pump via the percutaneous lead.

The controller incorporates various alarm algorithms that indicate any abnormal events experienced by the micro-pump such as a battery disconnect. The micro-pump status indicator on the controller has three LED (light-emitting diode) lights: green, amber, and red to assist the patient and physician in assessing the functioning of the pump. The green light indicates that the micro-pump is operating normally. The amber light is a nonemergent alarm, but a physician should be notified in order to assess the patient status and determine the action required. The red light is an urgent alarm with immediate action required. The controller also has an audible alarm.

CLINICAL EXPERIENCE

CircuLite is currently enrolling patients in a 50-patient clinical trial in Europe at up to 10 sites in support of a CE mark and European commercialization. Patients are eligible for inclusion in this study if they are between 18 and 75 years of age; have NYHA functional class IIIb or early class IV symptoms despite appropriate treatment with diuretics, angiotensin-converting

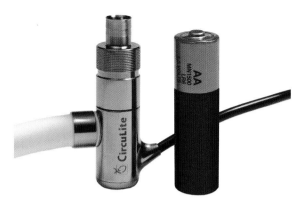

FIGURE 35-1. The CircuLite Synergy Pocket Micro-pump. (Reproduced with permission from CircuLite®, Inc.)

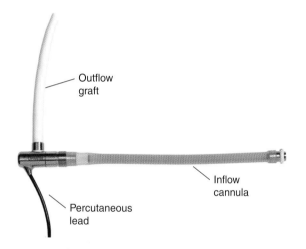

FIGURE 35-2. The CircuLite Synergy Pocket Micro-pump with inflow and outflow graft. (Reproduced with permission from CircuLite®, Inc.)

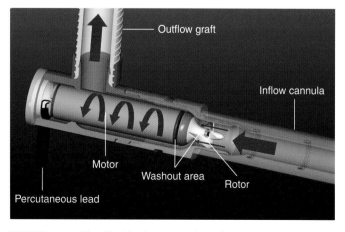

FIGURE 35-3. The CircuLite Synergy Pocket Micro-pump cross-section of the micro-pump (see text for details). (Reproduced with permission from CircuLite®, Inc.)

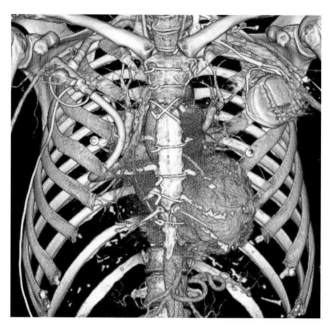

FIGURE 35-4. CT scan of implanted CircuLite Synergy Pocket Micro-pump. (Reproduced with permission from CircuLite®, Inc.)

enzyme inhibitor, angiotensin receptor blockade, and β-blocker (unless intolerant); are listed or eligible for heart transplant; and are ambulatory with a worsening clinically unstable condition (eg, frequent hospitalizations for heart failure or increasingly symptomatic). Exclusion criteria include the requirement for continuous inotropic support, isolated right heart failure, and previous surgery in the right chest that could obstruct access to the left atrium from the Waterston's groove for placement of the inflow cannula.

Enrollment for this clinical trial began in 2007, and, to date, 34 patients have been implanted with the Synergy device. Patient characteristics are summarized in Table 35–1. For comparison, similar data reported for the HeartMate II (Thoratec Corporation, Pleasanton, CA) bridge-to-transplant population are also provided.[3] The majority of the patients were male with ischemic cardiomyopathy. One-fourth of the patients had prior cardiac operations with sternotomy (eight coronary artery bypass grafting [CABG], including one CABG plus aortic valve replacement, one CABG plus mitral valve replacement, and one Dor procedure). Forty-four percent of the patients were in permanent atrial fibrillation and more than two-thirds had an implantable cardioverter defibrillator. Baseline hemodynamic and echocardiographic parameters confirmed an end-stage heart failure population with reasonably well-preserved end-organ function (Table 35–2) and were similar to those reported for the HeartMate II BTT population.[3]

Data from the initial 27 implants at 24 hours postsurgery estimated the nominal flow through the micro-pump to be 2.97 ± 0.39 L/min with actual flows ranging from 2.3 to 3.5 L/min. The hemodynamic improvements evaluated at 24 hours following the surgery included an increase in cardiac index (CI)

Table 35-1. Patient Demographic Data (n = 34) Compared to Those for HeartMate II (n = 133)

	CircuLite		HeartMate II[3]	
	Mean	SD	Mean	SD
Age (y)	56.2	9.8	50.1	13.1
BSA (m²)	1.9	0.2	2.0	0.3
BMI (kg/m²)	25.4	3.5	26.8	5.9
	n	%	n	%
Gender				
Male	29	85.3	105	79.0
Female	5	14.7	27	21.0
CHF etiology				
ICM	26	76.5	49	37.0
DCM	8	23.5	84	63.0
INTERMACS (n = 28)				
2	1	2.9		
3	1	2.9		
4	26	76.5		
Cardiovascular history				
Diabetes mellitus	10	29.4		
Atrial fibrillation	15	44.1		

BMI, body mass index; BSA, body surface area; CHF, congestive heart failure; DCM, dilated cardiomyopathy; ICM, ischemic cardiomyopathy; INTERMACS; Interagency Registry for Mechanically Assisted Circulatory Systems.

Table 35-2. Baseline Functional Data (n = 34) Compared to Those for HeartMate II (n = 133)

	CircuLite		HeartMate II[3]	
	Mean	SD	Mean	SD
Hemodynamics				
HR (beats/min)	77.2	15.8	91.8	18.5
SBP (mm Hg)	98.1	13.7	95.8	14.6
DBP (mm Hg)	64.3	10.0	61.7	11.3
MAP (mm Hg)	74.2	9.6	73.1[a]	12.4
CVP (mm Hg)	12.7	4.9	13.5	7.8
PAP (S, mm Hg)	55.0	15.8	53.0	14.1
PAP (D, mm Hg)	27.0	9.1	28.2	8.8
PAP (M, mm Hg)	37.6	9.9	36.5	9.7
PCWP (mm Hg)	27.0	8.2	26.1	7.9
CO (L/min)	3.9	1.0	4.0[a]	1.2
CI (L/min/m²)	2.0	0.5	2.0	0.6
SVR (Wood unit)	16.1	6.0	14.9[a]	3.8
Echocardiography				
EF (%)	20.9	5.7	16.3	5.7
LVEDD (cm)	15.8	21.3	n/r	
MR (grade)	1.7	0.8	n/r	
AR (grade)	0.3	0.5	n/r	
Peak Vo₂ (mL/kg/min)	10.8	3.1	n/r	
Laboratory findings				
BNP (pg/mL)	6231.7	5151.5	n/r	
Sodium	136.4	4.7	132.9	5.1
Creatinine (mg/dL)	1.5	0.5	1.4	0.5
Estimated CrCl	66.0	23.9	75.1	36.8
Total bilirubin (mg/dL)	0.9	0.6	1.2	0.8
LDH (mg/dL)	345.2	162.8	376.0	371.0
AST (U/L)	27.7	12.9	104.0	287.0
ALT (U/L)	35.9	23.3	67.0	168.0

[a] Values estimated from reported cardiac output and pulmonary pressures.

ALT, alanine aminotransferase; AR, aortic regurgitation; AST, aspartate aminotransferase; BNP, brain natriuretic peptide; CI, cardiac index; CO, cardiac output; CrCl, creatinine clearance; CVP, central venous pressure; DBP, diastolic blood pressure; EF, ejection fraction; HR, heart rate; LDH, lactate dehydrogenase; LVEDD, left ventricular end-diastolic diameter; MAP, mean arterial pressure; MR, mitral regurgitation; n/r, not reported; PAP, pulmonary arterial pressure; PCWP, pulmonary capillary wedge pressure; PVR, pulmonary vascular resistance; SBP, systolic blood pressure; SVR, systemic vascular resistance.

(from 2.0 ± 0.4 to 3.3 ± 0.9 L/min/m², $P < .001$), decreases in pulmonary systolic pressure (from 55 ± 15 to 53 ± 14 mm Hg, $P = .34$), and pulmonary diastolic pressure (27 ± 9 to 21 ± 5 mm Hg, $P = .002$). The average follow-up time was 9.5 ± 5.5 weeks. Data available from 17 patients (Table 35–3) showed continuous improvements in all parameters that include clinically and statistically significant reductions in pulmonary and arterial resistances. The European CE mark clinical trial is expected to complete enrollment in 2010, and a US investigation device exemption (IDE) pilot trial is expected to begin enrollment in 2011.

FUTURE DEVELOPMENTS

CircuLite's next-generation platform involves the surgical placement of the Synergy Pocket Micro-pump system into an endovascular system that can be implanted by an interventional

Table 35–3. Comparison of Hemodynamic Parameters at Baseline and After an Average (±SD) of 16.7 ± 12.3 Weeks of Follow-up on 17 Patients[4]

| | Baseline | Follow-up | |
Parameter	Mean ± SD	Mean ± SD	P
Mean arterial pressure (mm Hg)	76.94 ± 11.2	73.6 ± 6.6	.143
Pulmonary wedge pressure (mm Hg)	26.67 ± 9.15	19.9 ± 7.8	.006
Cardiac index (L/min/m²)	2.1 ± 0.5	2.7 ± 0.4	.000
Pulmonary vascular resistance (Wood units)	2.9 ± 1.4	2.1 ± 0.9	.016
Systemic vascular resistance (Wood units)	17.0 ± 6.3	15.47 ± 3.7	.264

cardiologist in the catheterization laboratory or in a hybrid surgical suite. The endovascular system features an inflow cannula that will access the left atrium via transseptal percutaneous placement of the inflow cannula from the right subclavian vein. Access to the left atrium will utilize standard transseptal techniques, and a custom-designed delivery system will deploy the tip of the cannula onto the atrial septum. The placement of the micro-pump and outflow connection to the subclavian artery will initially require a surgeon to perform a traditional surgical incision and graft anastomosis. As with the inflow cannula, the outflow connection will also evolve to an endovascular procedure as connection tools become available. At the time of this writing, this system is in preclinical trials with the first clinical implant targeted for 2011.

In addition to the endovascular system, CircuLite is modifying the Synergy system for use in pediatric patients with acquired or congenital heart disease. This development work is funded by the National Institute of Health under SBIR Fast Track grant: 4R44HL096214-02. The goal of this grant is to complete the feasibility work, required to modify the system for use in a pediatric patient population. Clinical evaluations of the pediatric system are targeted to begin in 2013/2014.

CONCLUSIONS

The CircuLite Synergy system is designed to provide a smaller, less invasively implantable assist device to benefit patients with severe symptomatic heart failure but who are not yet sick enough to require or justify implantation of a full-support ventricular assist device. Results to date support the concept that partial mechanical support with the CircuLite Synergy Pocket Micro-pump interrupts the progressive hemodynamic deterioration typical of end-stage heart failure.[4] These data support the previous theoretical work that earlier intervention with a smaller, partial-support device implanted using a minimally invasive procedure can provide substantial clinical benefits to less sick patients (NYHA class IIIb) with severe symptomatic heart failure with no other treatment options.[5]

CAUTION: Investigation Device. Limited by Federal and Local Law to Investigation Use Only. CircuLite and Synergy are registered trademarks of CircuLite, Inc. Additional information about CircuLite, Inc and the Synergy Pocket Micro-pump are available at: www.CircuLite.net.

REFERENCES

1. Meyns B, Klotz S, Simon A, et al. Proof of concept: hemodynamic response to long-term partial ventricular support with the synergy pocket micro-pump. *J Am Coll Cardiol.* 2009;54:79-86.
2. Kirklin JK, Naftel DC, Stevenson LW, et al. INTERMACS database for durable devices for circulatory support: first annual report. *J Heart Lung Transplant.* 2008;27:1065-1072.
3. Miller LW, Pagani FD, Russell SD, et al. Use of a continuous-flow device in patients awaiting heart transplantation. *N Engl J Med.* 2007;357:885-896.
4. Meyns B, Simon A, Klotz S, et al. Clinical Benefits of Partial Circulatory Support in New York Heart Association Class IIIB and Early Class IV patients. *Eur J Cardio-Thoracic Surg.* 2011;39:693-698.
5. Morley D, Litwak K, Ferber P, et al. Hemodynamic effects of partial ventricular support in chronic heart failure: results of simulation validated with in vivo data. *J Thorac Cardiovasc Surg.* 2007;133:21-28.

CHAPTER 36

THE HEARTWARE VENTRICULAR ASSIST SYSTEM

Marc T. Swartz and David R. Hathaway

INTRODUCTION

According to the most recent statistics from the American Heart Association, congestive heart failure (CHF) affects approximately 7.5 million or 2.5% of the US population with approximately 670,000 new cases diagnosed each year.[1] Despite new medical treatments and electrophysiologic interventions, the number of patients who die or endure a greatly diminished quality of life from end-stage heart failure continues to grow. While cardiac transplantation has proven to be an effective treatment for advanced heart failure, its application is limited by a lack of available donor organs that shows no significant trend to meet the demand. Over the last 20 years, with improvements in technology, survival, and a reduction in morbidity, bridging to cardiac transplantation with left ventricular assist devices (LVADs) has gained wider clinical use.[2,3] More recently, LVADs have been used as an alternative to transplantation to extend the life expectancy of nontransplant candidates. Permanent use of such devices or "destination therapy" (DT) has been approved this decade.[4,5] A major limitation of earlier pump technology was the necessity for complex components and wear on moving parts that limited long-term use. The HeartWare Ventricular Assist System (VAS) is one of a new generation of devices that employs a proprietary continuous-flow blood pump, the HeartWare ventricular assist device (HVAD) pump. This centrifugal pump was designed to be small, reliable, and easy to insert and operate.[6] The potential benefits include improved reliability and durability due to a single moving part that does not make contact with other components during operation.

DEVICE DESCRIPTION

The HVAD pump consists of a small round titanium housing that displaces a volume of 50 mL and weighs 160 g. Incorporated into the pump housing is a short inflow cannula to allow for placement in the apex of the left ventricle (LV). The pump utilizes magnetic and hydrodynamic forces to elevate and rotate the impeller. There are three main parts that make up the pump: (1) a front housing with an integrated inflow cannula, (2) a rear housing with a magnetic center post, and (3) the

rotating impeller (Fig. 36–1A). The front and rear housings are hybrid titanium-ceramic assemblies that contain hermetically sealed dual-motor stators to improve system efficiency and provide power redundancy to rotate the impeller.

■ PATHS

The wide-bladed impeller is designed to house four large rare-earth motor magnets that allow for short axial height and high motor efficiency. The impeller also contains a stack of three rare-earth magnets with like poles that contribute to the impeller suspension system. Another set of magnets stacked within the center post provides repulsive magnetic forces that maintain radial support for the impeller. The vertical alignment of the magnets within the center post is shifted downward relative to the impeller magnetic stack to develop an axial magnetic force to "push" the impeller toward the front housing. When the pump is turned on, blood entering the pump via the inflow cannula is distributed to the flow channels on the impellar by the center post (Fig. 36–1B). As the impeller rotates, lift is created by the hydrodynamic thrust bearings (Fig. 36–2) that continuously push the impeller away from the front housing. A fluid (blood) barrier maintains the gap between the impeller and the front housing.

The impeller rotates between 1800 and 4000 rpm (revolutions per minute) and can produce a maximum flow rate of 10 L/min. The rotating impeller forces blood through the pump and uses hydrodynamic and centrifugal forces to increase blood pressure and blood flow from the inlet of the pump to the outlet of the pump. The inflow cannula is made of titanium and contains a silicone O-ring to ensure a seal with the sewing ring. Table 36–1 lists some of the HVAD pump specifications

HVAD PUMP IMPLANTATION

The HVAD pump was designed to be implanted entirely in the pericardial space above the diaphragm without the need for an abdominal pocket or subdiaphramatic dissection (Fig. 36–3A,B). It can be implanted via a median sternotomy or left thoracotomy, most often with cardiopulmonary bypass (CPB) support, although implants have been done successfully without CPB support. Once the heart and LV apex have been exposed, a sewing ring is attached to the LV apex and a plug of tissue is removed using a proprietary coring tool. It is critical that the inside of the LV is inspected for preexisting thrombi, debris from the coring, or any intraventricular structures that may affect inflow cannula placement or position, and that these be removed. Once the inflow cannula is in place, the sewing ring clamp is tightened, securing the pump to the heart. Next, the outflow graft is cut to length and anastomosed end to side to the ascending aorta. The HVAD pump outflow conduit is a 10-mm gel-impregnated graft surrounded by a rigid strain relief. The driveline (4.2 mm diameter) is tunneled subcutaneously to a percutaneous exit site in either the right or left upper abdominal quadrant. The driveline connects the pump to all the external components. After the driveline is connected to the

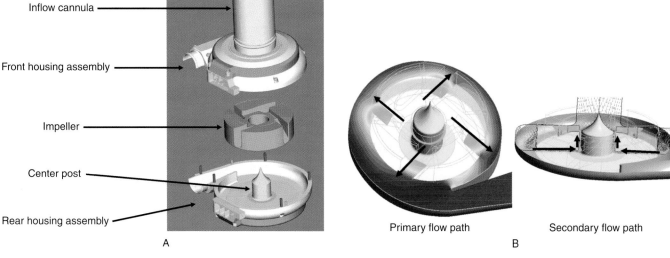

FIGURE 36–1. A. Exploded view of HVAD pump. (Reproduced with permission from HeartWare®, Inc.) **B.** Blood flow paths. (Reproduced with permission from HeartWare®, Inc.)

controller, the HVAD pump is started at 1800 rpm and run at lower speeds until all the air has been removed from the HVAD pump, cannulae, and native LV. Once deairing is complete, the HVAD pump speed is increased to an average of 2800 to 2900 rpm as CPB flow is decreased. When off CPB, drains are placed and the chest is closed in the usual manner.

EXTERNAL COMPONENTS

The HeartWare VAS includes the following external components:

- Controller
- Monitor

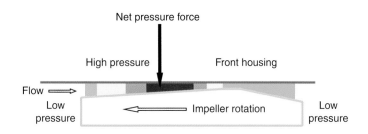

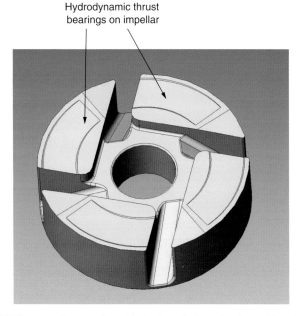

FIGURE 36–2. Cutaway view of hydrodynamic thrust bearing and location on impeller. (Reproduced with permission from HeartWare®, Inc.)

Table 36–1. Technical Features of the HVAD Pump

Pump technology	Centrifugal
Full output (up to 10 L/min)	Yes
Pump weight	160 g
Pump volume	50 cc
Wearless	Yes
Impeller suspension	Hydrodynamic, passive magnetic
Electric motor/driveline redundancy	Yes
Pump speed	1800-4000 rpm
Normal-operation pump power range	3.0-6.0 W
Inflow cannula length	25 mm
Inflow cannula OD	21 mm
Outflow graft ID	10 mm

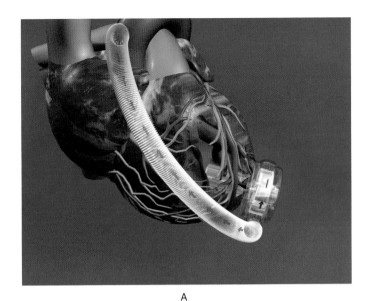

A

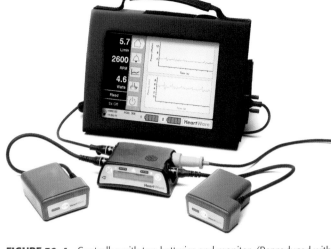

FIGURE 36–4. Controller with two batteries and monitor. (Reproduced with permission from HeartWare®, Inc.)

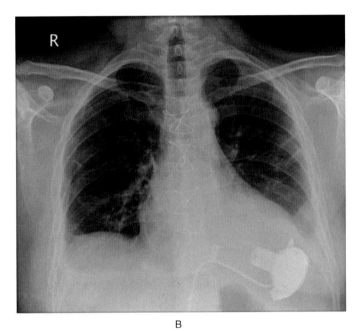

B

FIGURE 36–3. A. HVAD pump placement in the pericardium—LV apex to ascending aortic cannulation. (Reproduced with permission from HeartWare®, Inc.) **B.** Chest film showing HVAD pump placement. (Reproduced with permission from HeartWare®, Inc.)

- External power—battery, alternating current (AC) adapter, direct current (DC) adapter
- Battery charger

■ CONTROLLER

The controller (Fig. 36–4) is a microprocessor unit that controls and manages HVAD pump operation. The percutaneous driveline connects the pump to the controller. The controller sends and regulates power and operating signals to the pump and collects information from the pump. An LED (light-emitting

diode) screen displays real-time HVAD pump parameters, including power, speed, and flow estimation as well as alarm conditions. Alarms (low, medium, and high priority) are accompanied by specific LED colors or sequences and by audible sounds as well as a digital readout on the controller screen. The controller interfaces with the monitor through a data port to allow controller setup and permit changes in pump parameters. The controller has internal memory that stores pump- and battery-related data every 15 minutes for up to 1 month. This information can be downloaded to the monitor and then an external memory source. An example of the graphic created when charting controller log files is shown in Fig. 36–5. Flow is calculated by an algorithm that includes power output and a viscosity derived from the hematocrit. Log file graphics have been useful for detecting early stages of VAD thrombosis and for linking volume changes or arrhythmias to suction events. There are four connectors, two on either side of the controller. The power supply connections are identical and used to connect any of the power sources to the controller (batteries, AC adapter, or DC adapter). The controller should always be connected to two power sources for safety (two batteries or one battery and an AC adapter or DC adapter [car adapter]). If only connected to one power source, the controller will function but will alarm after 20 seconds. There is also a nonreplaceable rechargeable battery inside the controller that is used to power an audible "no power" alarm.

The batteries and controller are carried in proprietary belt or carry bag worn by the patient to provide mobility. The entire weight of this assembly is approximately 2.85 lb (see Fig. 36–5).

■ MONITOR

The monitor is a touch screen tablet PC computer (see Fig. 36–4) that uses proprietary software to display system performance information and permit adjustment of selected controller parameters. When connected to a controller, the monitor

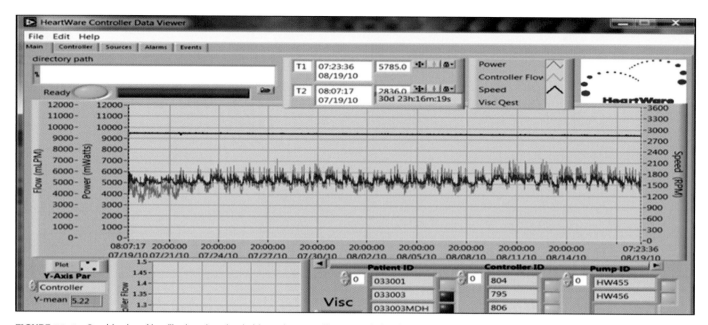

FIGURE 36–5. Graphic plot of log file data downloaded from the controller (green is flow in L/min; red is power in W; and black is speed in rpm). (Reproduced with permission from HeartWare®, Inc.)

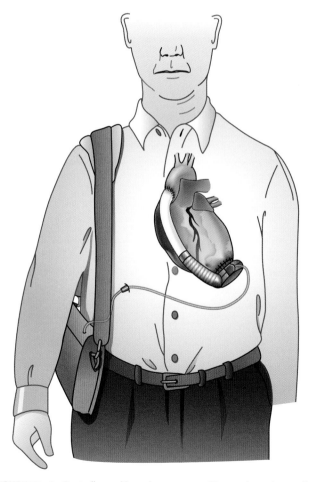

FIGURE 36–6. Controller and batteries are secured in carry bag when ambulatory. (Reproduced with permission from HeartWare®, Inc.)

receives continuous blood pump information from the controller and displays real-time and historical pump information. The monitor also displays alarm conditions and provides a means to download data collected from the controller.

■ EXTERNAL POWER SOURCES

The controller requires two power sources for safe operation: either two batteries (see Fig. 36–4) or one battery and an AC adapter or DC adapter. While active, patients will typically use two batteries which drain sequentially. Each battery provides approximately 5 to 6 hours of system power. While relaxing or sleeping, most patients use power from an electric outlet (AC adapter) because it provides power for an unlimited period of time. The batteries should be exchanged when their charge falls below 25% capacity.

■ BATTERY CHARGER

The battery charger (Fig. 36–7) is used to simultaneously recharge up to four batteries. It takes approximately 6 hours to charge all four batteries.

CLINICAL TRIALS

The HeartWare VAS received CE mark in Europe in January 2009 and is now commercially available for bridge-to-transplant (BTT). A pivotal trial for BBT in the United States (ADVANCE) completed enrollment in February 2010. One hundred forty subjects received the HVAD pump for a noninferiority comparison to a contemporaneous control group obtained from the Interagency Registry for Mechanically Assisted Circulatory

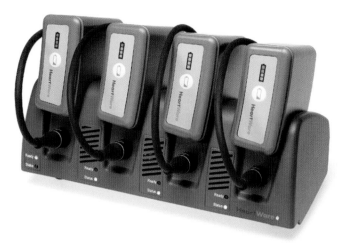

FIGURE 36–7. Battery charger. (Reproduced with permission from HeartWare®, Inc.)

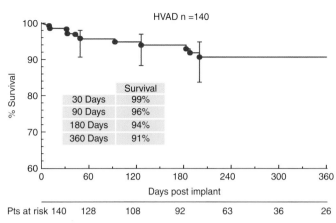

FIGURE 36–8. Kaplan-Meier plot of survival of 50 subjects enrolled in the International Clinical Trial (CE Mark trial).

Systems (INTERMACS). Submission of a premarketing application is planned for the end of 2010. A DT trial (ENDURANCE) was launched in July 2010 and will enroll 450 patients randomized 2:1 against a control LVAD. The trial was launched in August 2010 and has enrolled more than 100 subjects as of March 2011. The primary endpoint is survival on the originally implanted LVAD in the absence of any stroke with a Modified Rankin Score > 4.[7] A Kaplan-Meier plot of survival from the CE Mark trial is shown below in Fig. 36–8. Six-month survival was 90%.

SUMMARY

The HVAD pump is designed to fit into the pericardial space. Despite its small size, the HVAD pump can generate flows of up to 10 L/min. The only moving part, the impeller, makes no contact with the device housing because of a combination of magnetic and hydrodynamic forces. The first BTT clinical trial yielded a 6-month survival of 90%. A similar trial (ADVANCE) conducted in the United States was recently completed, and a destination trial (ENDURANCE) has been launched. The HeartWare VAS is an important advance in mechanical circulatory support for patients with end-stage heart failure.

Note: HeartWare and HVAD are registered trademarks of HeartWare, Inc.

REFERENCES

1. Jones DL, Adams R, Carnethon M, et al; American Heart Association Statistics Committee and Stroke Statistics Subcommittee. Heart disease and stroke statistics—2009 update: a report from the American Heart Association Statistics Committee and Stroke Statistics Subcommittee. *Circulation.* 2009;119(3):480-486. Published online Dec 15, 2008. DOI: 10.1161/CIRCULATIONAHA.108.191261.
2. Miller LW, Pagani FD, Russell SD, et al; HeartMate II Clinical Investigators. Use of a continuous-flow device in patients awaiting heart transplantation. *N Engl J Med.* 2007;357:885-896.
3. Pagani FD, Miller LW, Russell SD, et al; HeartMate II Investigators. Extended mechanical circulatory support with a continuous-flow rotary left ventricular assist device. *J Am Coll Cardiol.* 2009 Jul 21;54(4):312-321.
4. Rose EA, Gelijns AC, Moskowitz AJ, et al; Randomized Evaluation of Mechanical Assistance for Congestive Heart Failure (REMATCH) study group. Long term use of a ventricular assist device for end-stage heart failure. *N Engl J Med.* 2001;345:1435-1443.
5. Slaughter MS, Rogers JG, Milano CA, et al; HeartMate II Investigators. Advanced heart failure treated with continuous-flow left ventricular assist device. *N Engl J Med.* 2009 Dec 3;361(23):2241-2251.
6. Tuzun E, Roberts K, Cohn WE, et al. In vivo evaluation of the HeartWare centrifugal ventricular assist device. *Tex Heart Inst J.* 2007;34(4):406-411.
7. Strueber M, O'Driscoll G, Jansz P, Khaghani A, Levy WC, Wieselthaler GM and HeartWare Investigators. Multicenter Evaluation of an Intrapericardial Left Ventricular Assist System. *J Am Coll Cardiol.* 2011;57; 1375-1382.

CHAPTER 37

TERUMO DURAHEART MAGNETICALLY LEVITATED CENTRIFUGAL LEFT VENTRICULAR ASSIST SYSTEM

Thomas Gould

The Terumo DuraHeart (Terumo Heart, Inc. Ann Arbor, MI) is the world's first magnetically levitated centrifugal left ventricular assist system (LVAS) designed for long-term circulatory support in patients with late-stage heart failure. The system consists of the primary components listed in Fig. 37–1 (each primary component is discussed in detail later). The system also includes a battery charger, a hospital computer console (discussed below), and the following surgical instruments:

- Apical punch
- Wrench
- Tunneler
- Pump cable connector

COMPONENTS

This overview summarizes the features of the DuraHeart System's components. For a complete description of the system and its clinical operation, please refer to the *DuraHeart LVAS Hospital Guide.*

■ OUTFLOW CONDUIT

The outflow conduit measures 350 mm long, has a 14-mm outer diameter, and a 12-mm inner diameter. It incorporates a 12-mm Gelweave graft, a polyethylene reinforcement sleeve, and a titanium connector. During system implantation, the graft is anastomosed to the aorta and secured to the pump's outflow port using the DuraHeart wrench.

■ PUMP (FIG. 37–2)

Made of titanium, the DuraHeart centrifugal pump employs magnetic levitation to achieve friction-free blood propulsion. Through electromagnets and position sensors, the impeller is rigidly suspended within the blood chamber, leaving a 500-μm gap between the impeller and the device housing. Secondary blood flow around the impeller assists washout to eliminate areas of stasis that may lead to thrombus formation. All blood-contacting surfaces of the pump are prepared with a heparin coating. The DuraHeart pump is 73 mm in diameter, 46.2 mm thick, and weighs approximately 540 g.

■ INFLOW CONDUIT AND APICAL CUFF

The inflow conduit is a small titanium alloy tube that connects the left ventricle to the pump's inflow port. The conduit has a 60-degree angle and is available in three lengths to accommodate varying patient anatomies. The apical cuff is sewn onto the apex of the left ventricle and helps support the conduit. The cuff is constructed from a 16-mm Gelseal graft.

■ PUMP CABLE

The percutaneous pump cable is passed through the patient's abdominal wall and skin during implantation. It connects the implanted pump to the controller, providing the pathway through which the pump is powered and controlled.

■ CONTROLLER (FIG. 37–3)

The controller is an electronic device worn or carried by the patient. Outside the hospital, one of three external power sources can power the controller and pump:

- Two batteries
- Single battery and external battery backup
- Single battery and the battery charger

In the hospital, the console can power the system.

The controller coordinates pump functions and monitors system performance. As the system interface, it

- Displays system status including pump flow and rotational speed.
- Notifies patients of system alarms and alerts.
- Interfaces with external power sources.
- Communicates with the hospital console for system setup, monitoring, follow-up, and troubleshooting.

The face of the controller provides display information that enables the clinician to monitor the system and respond to alarms (Fig. 37–4):

- The **menu** button is used to monitor the system by scrolling through various functions shown on the controller screen. The menu button beeps each time it is pressed and glows green to indicate that the controller is powered.
- The **alarm and alert indicators** use lights and tones to alert the clinician to possible system emergencies. An emergency alarm (with a red light) sounds for serious problems indicating pump stoppage. A yellow caution indicator light illuminates when conditions may require immediate attention or monitoring.
- The **mute** button temporarily silences alarms. Any new alarm received while muting is active will re-sound the alarm.

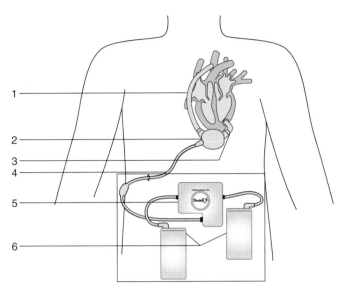

FIGURE 37–1. DuraHeart LVAS components (components in red border are not implanted). (Reproduced with permission from Terumo Heart, Inc.)

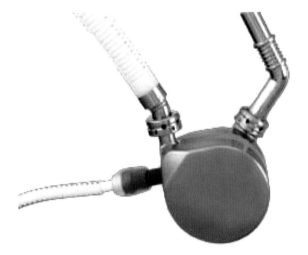

FIGURE 37–2. DuraHeart pump showing inflow and outflow conduits and controller cable attached. (Reproduced with permission from Terumo Heart, Inc.)

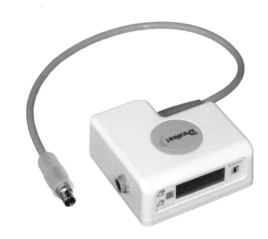

FIGURE 37–3. System controller. (Reproduced with permission from Terumo Heart, Inc.)

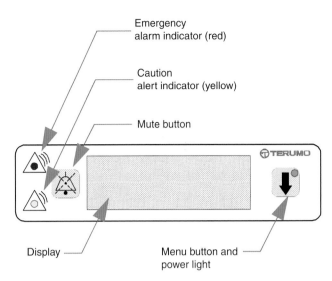

FIGURE 37–4. Display information on the controller face. (Reproduced with permission from Terumo Heart, Inc.)

Various system functions can be monitored through the controller's menu:

- Power supply status
- Flow rate in L/min (liters per minutes)
- Actual motor speed in rpm (revolutions per minutes)
- Motor current in A (amperes)
- Programmed motor speed in rpm

If the controller detects a serious problem with the pump or the controller itself, an emergency alarm (ie, a high-priority alarm) will sound and a red *emergency* triangle will illuminate. If a less serious condition is detected, a yellow caution symbol will light up and a caution alert will sound.

■ BATTERIES

The batteries power the system, allowing patients to go about their normal activities. Two batteries connect to the controller, one on each side. Together they provide up to 3½ hours of power. The exact amount of time each battery lasts varies depending on several factors, including how hard the pump is working. Each battery charges fully in 3 to 4 hours and can be recharged up to 200 times.

■ HOSPITAL CONSOLE (FIG. 37–5):

In the hospital setting, the DuraHeart controller connects to a special computer system called the hospital console. The console is used to set up, adjust, monitor, and troubleshoot the DuraHeart System, and can also be used to power the system. The console operates in two modes: Master and Safe (Fig. 37–6). The Master mode provides access to all system functions, including stopping and starting the pump and adjusting motor speed. The Safe mode is used for system monitoring and does not allow pump settings to be changed. The hospital console

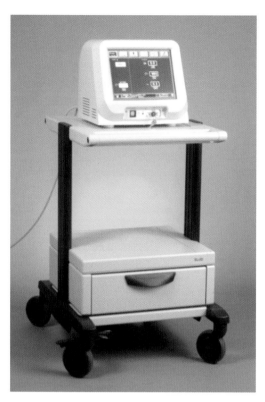

FIGURE 37–5. Hospital console. (Reproduced with permission from Terumo Heart, Inc.)

provides access to its primary functions through five buttons located at the top of the screen:

 Status: Shows the current state of the pump, including the flow rate, motor electric current, and rotational speed.

 Alarms: Flashes anytime there is a console or controller active alert or alarm.

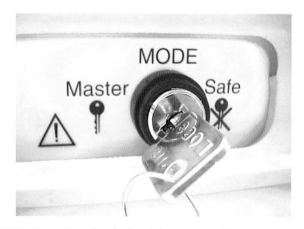

FIGURE 37–6. Operating the hospital console in either Master mode or Safe mode. (Reproduced with permission from Terumo Heart, Inc.)

 Patient: Displays patient information such as

- Patient name
- Identification
- Height
- Weight
- Hematocrit
- Implant date
- Birth date
- Gender

When the system is in Master mode, this information can be entered and changed.

 System: Provides system information including:

- Hospital name
- System date and time
- Pump and controller serial numbers

In Master mode, times and dates as well as language may be changed.

 Data: Displays real-time data, 1-hour and 30-day trend data in numeric or graphic format

An internal hospital console battery powers the controller and pump for approximately 1 hour, providing uninterrupted system operation while a patient is transported within the hospital. The internal battery recharges within 4 to 5 hours when the hospital console is connected to AC power.

PATIENT INDICATIONS

The DuraHeart LVAS is intended to provide mechanical circulatory support as a bridge-to-transplantation in patients at risk of death due to end-stage left ventricular failure. The DuraHeart System is suitable for use inside and outside of the hospital. The company had planned to begin a destination therapy trial during the summer of 2010.

CONTRAINDICATIONS

- Patients younger than 18 years.
- Patients ineligible for heart transplant.
- Patients ineligible for implantation of a left ventricular assist device (LVAD) based on surgical, physical, or psychological considerations; for example, primary right heart failure, noncorrectable aortic regurgitation, irreversible multiorgan failure, sepsis, primary coagulopathy, platelet disorder, allergies, or who are sensitive to materials in the device.
- Patients with a body surface area less than 1.1 m².
- Patients requiring magnetic resonance imaging.

MECHANISM OF ACTION

The DuraHeart System is a third-generation LVAD whose design eliminates all mechanical contacts inside the blood chamber through the use of magnetic levitation between the impeller and the pump housing (Fig. 37–7). This design offers several advantages[1]:

- More precise impeller control ensures consistent flow patterns and proper washing of blood-contacting surfaces inside the pump, reducing the potential for thrombus formation.

- Stable impeller position provides a gap between the impeller and pump housing (250 μm on both sides) that reduces shear stress, virtually eliminating hemolysis and improving washout to minimize thrombus formation.

- Friction-free operation minimizes heat production and reduces wear and tear on moving parts to extend device life.

In contrast to the DuraHeart System, some devices rely on hydrodynamic forces to suspend the impeller, requiring a tighter gap between impeller and blood chamber walls. The dimensional tolerances that this system entails are much more difficult to control in manufacturing. In addition, the hydrodynamic forces depend on rotational speed, blood properties, pump flow, and pressure changes, making the gap between the impeller and blood chamber wall critical. This may potentially vary the shear stress and secondary flow patterns.

Other systems rely on different design features, such as hydrodynamics or permanent magnets for stability in the radial plane, or magnetic levitation along one axis only (single degree of freedom (DOF) control), which may not prevent impeller wobble. This can potentially result in variations in secondary blood flow patterns and unpredictable shear stress. The DuraHeart System's closed-type impeller design incorporates straight rather than curved blades, creating a more stable flow pattern and minimizing turbulent flows.

APPROVAL STATUS

The device is currently undergoing multicenter prospective, nonrandomized pivotal trials in the United States, where it is limited by law to investigational use. The DuraHeart LVAS is commercialized in Europe with the CE mark. Now it is also commercially approved in Japan.

CLINICAL DATA

The DuraHeart LVAS is the only device of its kind that combines a centrifugal pump with magnetic impeller levitation. This configuration has proven reliable and effective at minimizing the potential for blood damage and development of thrombus. Results of the European clinical experiences as of July 31, 2009, show survival at 18 months to be 73% (Fig. 37–8).[2] Stroke-free survival at 1 and 2 years in the trial (33 patients) was 94% for the last 22 patients after implementing a less intensive anticoagulation/antiplatelet regimen. There was no pump mechanical failure, pump thrombosis, or hemolysis throughout the support duration.[1]

In 2010, Morshuis et al published results from two separate DuraHeart LVAS trials: the CE mark study referenced above and the postmarket study conducted in Europe. Data from 82 patients were reviewed from the two separate study groups at different points of follow-up[3]:

- Thirty-three patients from the CE mark study with data reported through to 13 weeks, including survival and adverse event rates.

- Forty-nine patients from the postmarket study with data reported through to 6 months, including survival, discharge rates, and freedom from device replacement events.

Overall outcomes of the study groups included

- Survival rates of 90% at 13 weeks, 85% at 6 months, 79% at 12 months, and 58% at 2 years.

Closed impeller design

Only one moving part

Wide gap (250 micron)

Low shear stress
Even flow of blood
Low hemolysis

Primary flow

Continuous, gentle pattern

Secondary flow/washout

Eliminates stagnation
No thrombus

FIGURE 37–7. DuraHeart LVAS magnetic levitation and active control. (Reproduced with permission from Terumo Heart, Inc.)

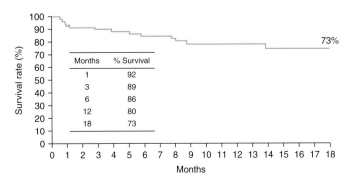

Months	% Survival
1	92
3	89
6	86
12	80
18	73

FIGURE 37–8. Kaplan-Meier survival data at 18 months. (Reproduced with permission from Terumo Heart, Inc.)

- Freedom from device replacement at 6 months was 96% with no additional replacement during 4 years of support.

- No clinically significant hemolysis observed in DuraHeart LVAS patients.

Adverse events reported in the DuraHeart CE mark study included[3]

- Lower event rate of bleeding (0.14% ppy) compared to first- and second-generation devices (1.47% and 0.78% ppy, respectively).

- Lower GI bleeds (0.105% ppy vs 0.63% ppy) compared to other rotary blood pumps.

- Reduced driveline or pocket infection rate (0.27% ppy vs 3.49%) compared to pulsatile pumps.

- Fifty percent improvement in cerebrovascular accident (CVA) rates over pulsatile pumps. The data demonstrated a significant reduction in rate of CVAs after optimization of anticoagulation and antiplatelet therapy regimen (mean international normalized ratio [INR] = 2.5; INR protocol was changed post first 11 patients).

- Rate of ventricular arrhythmia was 65% less than with axial-flow pumps.

REFERENCES

1. Morshuis M, El-Banayosy A, Arusoglu L, et al. European experience of DuraHeart magnetically levitated centrifugal left ventricular assist system. *Eur J Cardiothorac Surg.* 2009;35:1020-1028.
2. "Long Term Circulatory Support With the DuraHeart Mag-Lev Centrifugal LVAS for Advanced Heart Failure Patients Eligible for Transplantation: European Experience" Chisato Nojiri, MD, PhD, Chief Executive Officer for Terumo Heart, Inc, delivered the report at the meeting of the International Society for Heart and Lung Transplantation, Boston, 2008.
3. Morshuis M, Schoenbrodt M, Nojiri C, et al. DuraHeart magnetically levitated centrifugal left ventricular assist system for advanced heart failure patients. *Expert Rev Med Devices.* 2010;7(2):173-183.

CHAPTER 38
THE LEVACOR® VAD

Pratap S. Khanwilkar, Phillip J. Miller, Gill B. Bearnson, Gordon B. Jacobs, James Lee, Karl E. Nelson, Jal S. Jassawalla, and James W. Long

LEVACOR VAD OVERVIEW

The Levacor® (World Heart Corporation, Salt Lake City, Utah) VAD (ventricular assist device) is a next-generation rotary blood pump intended for adults with late-stage heart failure (Fig. 38–1). A unique, completely "bearing-less" pump was developed involving total magnetic levitation (MagLev) and rotation of the rotor.

Key design elements of the Levacor *blood pump* along with targeted clinical features include the following:

- Optimized *hemocompatability* and anticoagulation arising from unimpeded blood flow paths having wide gaps
- Extended *durability* resulting from a friction-free, "bearing-less" rotor suspension with integrated motor
- *Extended flow dynamics* afforded by a centrifugal pump with a multispeed controller
- Improved *anatomic fit* afforded by a flat, pancake design

The *peripheral components* of the Levacor VAD system were designed to deliver additional features, some also unique to the Levacor.

- *Safety* afforded by incorporating a backup battery into the controller mitigating the potential for serious errors of accidental battery disconnect
- The option of *replacement* of a modular percutaneous lead without having to replace the blood pump, adding to overall system longevity as well as adding a lead-only replacement option for managing infections
- The option of future *upgradeability* to a completely implantable system accommodated by a modular, removable percutaneous lead connector detachable at the blood pump
- Enhanced *usability* of the externals with a reduced weight, ergonomic controller design, and the option for single battery pack use

IMPLANTABLE COMPONENTS

The implantable components of the Levacor VAD are shown in Fig. 38–2. A compact, centrifugal blood pump (1) made from titanium with smooth blood-contacting surfaces receives blood from the left ventricle (LV) through an inflow cannula (2) that can be rotated around the pump inlet to adjust orientation of the cannula tip in relationship to the LV apex. The pump delivers blood to the ascending aorta via a polyester outflow conduit (3) reinforced with a kink-resistant tube. A modular, replaceable percutaneous cable (4) connects to an external, wearable controller and battery pack ([5,6] or electrically powered monitoring unit) via an inline connector and extension cable (7) beyond the exit site.

■ BLOOD PUMP CONFIGURATION

The pump's flat shape and placement location were selected to facilitate anatomic fit, especially in smaller patients. This was made possible by two approaches.

1. A flattened, low-profile pump inlet with a unique, redirecting blood flow pathway was designed to avoid the long perpendicular inflow conduit, usually used with centrifugal pumps. This allowed for improved anatomic fit markedly reducing anterior-posterior dimensions and offered greater flexibility with the orientation of the LV cannula avoiding inlet obstruction previously reported with the perpendicular inlet configuration.[1]

2. Pump thickness was further minimized by the use of an innovative flat, brushless direct current (DC) motor which operates without any stator iron. This motor is completely integrated within the body of the pump, unlike some other designs with MagLev of the rotor but requiring additional motor bearings or components.

■ LV INFLOW CANNULA

The hardware used for inserting and securing the Levacor's inflow cannula into the LV allows for an expedited approach with potentially less cardiopulmonary bypass (CPB) time. The sewing ring can be sutured to the LV apex before coring and CPB. A metallic ring in the center of the sewing cuff helps guide placement of the sutures, keeping them away from the region to be cored out. A coring knife with trocar is provided for removing the apical core following which the LV cannula is inserted and secured within the attached silicone rubber sleeve. An elongated version of the sleeve allows for the option of clamping it at the time of insertion (or removal with subsequent plug insertion during explantation) so as to minimize blood loss and time.

The smooth inlet tip of the titanium inflow cannula (see Fig. 38–2) projects well into the LV while the base of the inflow cannula, with a textured exterior (sintered titanium microspheres), is left in contact with the myocardium, allowing stable neointimal tissue formation and incorporation at its junction with the LV apical endocardium.[2] The base of the cannula, in contact with myocardial tissue, is about twice the diameter of the cannula tip, allowing for mechanical stenting of the LV walls and avoiding thrombus-promoting contact between the LV and the cannula tip.

■ OUTFLOW CONDUIT

The outflow pathway to the ascending aorta incorporates a 12-mm-diameter gelatin-impregnated woven polyester graft, with an external bend relief to resist kinking. The screw-ring

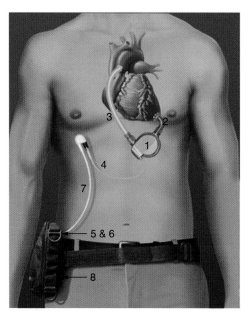

FIGURE 38–1. Levacor® VAD showing both implantable and wearable components. (Reproduced with permission from World Heart Corp.)

connector between the pump and the outflow conduit is designed to allow high-volume de-airing through the connector at time of implant by partially unscrewing the two-stage connector to its "loose-connection" first stage, allowing for a high-volume purge while still keeping the outflow graft loosely connected.

■ PERCUTANEOUS LEAD

The Levacor is the only implantable VAD having a modular percutaneous lead, detachable from the pump, permitting complete lead replacement without pump exchange (Item 4 in Fig. 38–2). The percutaneous cable terminates in an inline connector shortly after it exits the body (Item 4 in Fig. 38–1). The connector is

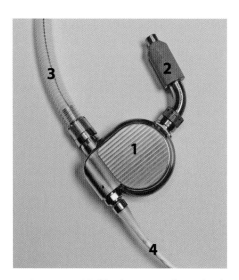

FIGURE 38–2. Levacor® VAD blood pump and associated components. (Reproduced with permission from World Heart Corp.)

only 12 mm in diameter, with a cable diameter of 6 mm, minimizing exit site trauma when exteriorized during implantation. One of optional length extension cables (10 ft for perioperative use, 3 ft for chronic use) connects the percutaneous lead to the controller and power supply. The extension segment is more susceptible to damage with mishandling and can be replaced rapidly without surgical intervention. Replacing the percutaneous lead connected to the pump requires a subxyphoid incision and surgical exposure to disconnect a damaged lead from the connector at the pump and replace it with a new lead, still avoiding pump replacement, something that is necessary with all other current VADs.

"BEARING-LESS" MAGNETIC LEVITATION

The magnetic levitation (MagLev) incorporated into the Levacor VAD employs a unique approach to suspending and stabilizing the rotor. All axes of potential rotor movement, except for one dimension, are passively controlled with permanent magnets. Movement in that one other axis is controlled by only one electromagnet and one sensor built into the pump housing (Fig. 38–3). This approach to MagLev allows for minimizing electronic complexity as no more than one electronic sensor and one active electromagnet is required to stabilize the rotor in all dimensions, achieving the least possible number as predicted by the laws of physics.

The overall design of the magnetics allows for enough stability to withstand 6 g of shock preventing the rotor from contacting the pump housing. This allows the recipient to be normally active and be able to tolerate moderately severe levels of trauma.

Some of the practical benefits of a MagLev design that have been considered include[3]:

- Improved gentleness with blood handling (hemocompatibility)
- Stable rotor suspension despite variations in rotor speed, flow, or changes in blood characteristics
- Friction-free operation reducing wear or localized heat generation

BLOOD PUMP DYNAMICS AND FLOW PATHWAY

■ BLOOD PUMP DYNAMICS

The pump can be operated between 800 and 3000 rpm, and can provide flows of greater than 9 L/min. This flow rate capacity makes it well suited to support larger patients.

A centrifugal pump such as that used in the Levacor VAD design has the potential for more physiological responsiveness as compared to an axial-flow pump. This offers some possible advantages:

- Provide a more Starling-like response,[4] that is, greater responsiveness of change in flow rate in response to changing preload.

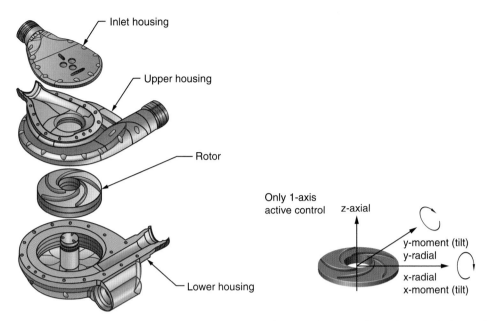

FIGURE 38–3. Simple complete MagLev used for the Levacor VAD rotor. Only one axis (z-axis shown) requires active control. The remaining four axes (x, y, two rotational) for positional control using MagLev are handled with permanent magnets. The remaining rotational axis (not shown about the z-axis) is controlled by motor action that causes the rotor to spin and pump blood. (Reproduced with permission from World Heart Corp.)

- Transmit greater pulsatility in the instantaneous flow to the systemic circulation.[5]

A centrifugal pump is a more hydraulically efficient pump than an axial-flow pump for adult blood flow rates.[6] This translates into less input power for the same cardiac output.

■ HEMOCOMPATIBILITY AND BLOOD FLOW PATHWAY

Unlike earlier generations of rotary pumps with mechanical or blood-lubricated bearings, the Levacor VAD is completely "bearing-less" with its rotor fully magnetically levitated.[7] Full MagLev has been successfully used for completely levitating much larger moving objects such as oil pumps, gas turbines, and even high-speed passenger trains.[8] When used for suspending the rotor of a blood pump, this approach allows for *wide gaps* and *unimpeded flow pathways* which offer potential advantages for blood handling.

The smallest gaps in the Levacor VAD are 180 μm wide and uniform across the secondary flow path. In comparison, the smallest blood flow gaps in pumps that depend on hydrodynamic, blood-lubricated bearings that suspend the rotor on thin fluid films, are a little more than 6 μm, about 30 times less than the Levacor gaps.[9] Further, in contrast to blood-lubricated bearing pumps, the impeller's position is independent of variations in volumetric and hemodynamic status of the patient, varying hematocrit (and resulting blood viscosity), or flow rate through the pump, factors which may affect fluid film thickness and performance.

With this distinctive feature, together with careful blood pump design, incorporating rigorous application of CFD (Fig. 38–4) and flow visualization,[10] targeting for a flow path with shortened

blood component transit times, minimal stagnation, and lowered shear stresses, the Levacor VAD was designed for improved *hemocompatibility*. In the current era of blood pumps, interest in the potential impact on blood extends beyond red blood cell hemolysis to consider effects on platelets, white cells, and even some larger subcellular components. Lower shear rates may impact on the challenge of acquired von Willebrands factor deficiency with *bleeding*, as observed with older-generation rotary VAD recipients.[11,12]

In addition to optimizing the geometry of the blood flow path, the blood-contacting smooth titanium surfaces of the Levacor VAD are coated with a phosphorylcholine (PC) coating. The PC

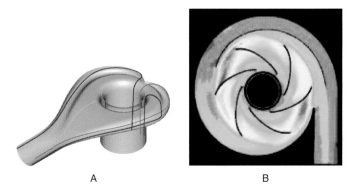

A   B

FIGURE 38–4. Levacor VAD-CFD models showing design for: **(A)** smooth flow via regular and smooth streamlines shown for particles entering pump into flat inlet, **(B)** uniform and reduced pressure distribution and gradients inside the pump. (Reproduced with permission from World Heart Corp.)

is a polymeric analog of the phospholipids that are naturally present in the lipid bilayer of the cell membrane. By mimicking cell membranes, the PC coating has the capacity to reduce the foreign body response. In addition, the hydrophilic PC head group acts as a barrier to protein and cell adhesion. PC coating has been shown to provide improved hemocompatibility, reduced inflammation and fibrosis, and reduced bacterial adhesion in other implantable blood-contacting applications.[13] A version has also been clinically used in another centrifugal blood pump.[14]

SYSTEM COMPONENTS

■ WEARABLE, EXTERNAL COMPONENTS

The Levacor VAD system (Fig. 38–5) was designed incorporating principles of flexibility, modularity, and user choice. The wearable controller (with integrated reserve battery) and separate battery pack(s) are external to, and designed to be worn by, the recipient. Nonwearable, stationary equipment includes the system monitor base unit and system monitor display, and the battery charger (see Fig. 38–5).

Batteries

External, rechargeable battery packs each provide power for about 4 hours and weigh less than 1 lb. These lithium-polymer packs are equipped with a remaining capacity indicator gauge. Patients have the option of one-battery operation (unique to the Levacor) for lighter-weight or two-battery operation for extended periods of use.

An integrated reserve battery within the wearable controller maintains system operation for a minimum of approximately 15 minutes. This feature, unique to the Levacor system, is what enables single external battery pack use since continuous power can still be assured during exchanges. The reserve battery also adds an important safety feature, reducing the potentially serious risk of accidental battery disconnects.

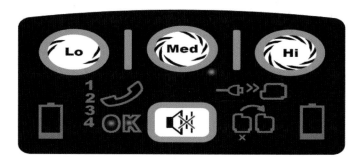

Wearable Controller

The external controller is the wearable, portable "brain" of the Levacor VAD system. A close-up of its display/interface panel appears in Fig. 38–6. Weight is only 1.5 lb.

Status indicators, *alerts*, and *alarms* provide information ensuring normal operation or denote recommended actions. Four possible responses may be indicated: (1) Change battery pack(s), (2) check the pump connection, and, if not resolved, replace the pump extension cable to the controller, (3) replace the controller, and (4) call the medical team.

Speed control buttons on the controller allow the user to choose among between pump speeds (low, medium, high) preset by the medical team, a feature not usually incorporated with blood pump systems.[15,16] This option extends the operating range to better match pump flow to a recipient's increased activity level (high) or a potentially lower flow state (low) caused by filling volume loss due to dehydration or arrhythmias, for example, adding an element of safety against LV suction.

■ STATIONARY COMPONENTS

Monitor and Power Unit

The monitor and the base unit are externals that can be connected to the wearable controller. This arrangement is always used periopeartively in the hospital. At home, the base unit provides power, as an alternative to wearable battery pack(s) in a "tethered" operating mode, for example, when sleeping.

The advanced system controller and monitor (see Fig. 38–5) is a PC-tablet computer displaying information and allowing parameter adjustments through its touch-screen display, when in the "Clinic" mode. It can also download and store system information from the wearable controller. A "Home" mode allows monitoring but locks out the user from making adjustments, except through the more user-friendly wearable controller interface.

CLINICAL EXPERIENCE

First clinical experience with the Levacor VAD was conducted outside the United States in an initial feasibility evaluation. This experience focused on the implantable components with

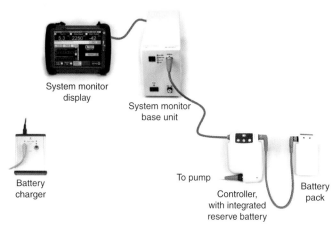

System monitor display

System monitor base unit

Battery charger

To pump

Controller, with integrated reserve battery

Battery pack

a hospital-only configuration of the external portable controller and battery unit.[17] This evaluation confirmed satisfactory performance of the blood pump and magnetic bearings as well as biocompatibility.

In that experience, the Levacor also demonstrated its potential to facilitate ventricular recovery following high-risk surgical repair of compromised hearts in patients with chronic advanced heart failure achieving sustainable recovery and explant by 3 months.[18]

After that, further development focused on the peripherals and system integration. The Levacor VAD system for out-of-hospital use was extensively tested in bench and animal studies.

In January 2010, the US Bridge-to-Transplantation trial began. It is expected to involve 160 subjects.

SUMMARY

A fully magnetically levitated centrifugal blood pump, the Levacor VAD was conceived and developed from principles of physics, physiology, and anatomy to meet projected clinical needs of late-stage heart failure patients. While early clinical results with the device appear promising, statistically significant clinical data will be derived from the clinical trial under way, with the expectation that this clinical study experience will lead to further enhancements.

ACKNOWLEDGEMENTS

The authors would like to acknowledge their colleagues at World Heart Corporation (Salt Lake City, Utah and Oakland, CA) and its predecessor, MedQuest Products Inc. Our development and commercialization associates and suppliers have included Dr James Antaki at the Carnegie-Mellon University (Pittsburgh, PA) and Dr Brad Paden and Dave Paden of LaunchPoint Technologies (Goleta, CA). We also appreciate the support of the State of Utah, the Heart and Lung Research Foundation, and the National Heart, Lung and Blood Institute. The authors appreciate the assistance with editing of Jeff Gibbs, John Kirk, and Dr John Woodard.

REFERENCES

1. Watterson PA, Woodard JC, Ramsden VS, Reizes JA. VentrAssist hydrodynamically suspended, open, centrifugal blood pump. *Artif Organs.* 2000; 24(6):475-477.

2. Houël R, Moczar M, Ginat M, Loisance D. Pseudointima in inflow and outflow conduits of a left ventricular assist system: possible role in clinical outcome. *ASAIO J.* 2001 May/June;(3):275-228.

3. Bearnson GB, Jacobs GB, Kirk J, Khanwilkar PS, Nelson KE, Long JW. HeartQuest ventricular assist device magnetically levitated centrifugal blood pump. *Artif Organs.* 2006;30(5):339-346.

4. Nojiri C, Harris GA, McCartney MH, et al. Terumo DuraHeart LVAS—inherent automaticity of a centrifugal flow pump. *ASAIO J.* 2003 Mar/Apr;49(2):164.

5. Ündar, A. Myths and truths of pulsatile and nonpulsatile perfusion during acute and chronic cardiac support. *Artif Organs.* 2004;28:439-443.

6. Maher TR, Butler KC, Poirier VL, Gernes DB. HeartMate left ventricular assist devices: a multigeneration of implanted blood pumps. *Artif Organs.* 2001;25:422-426.

7. Khanwilkar P, Olsen D, Bearnson G, et al. Using hybrid magnetic bearings to completely suspend the impeller of a ventricular assist device. *Artif Organs.* 1996;20(6):597-604.

8. Hyung-Woo L, Ki-Chan K, Ju L. Review of MagLev train technologies. *IEEE Transactions on Magnetics.* 2006;42(7):1917-1925.

9. White D. CFD Analysis of the HeartWare VAS Blood Pump. http://www.ansys.com/events/conference2008/downloads/biomedical-computational-fluid-dynamics-heartwave-device.pdf. 2008 International ANSYS Conference: Inspiring Engineering, Pittsburgh, PA, August 26-28, 2008.

10. Chen C, Antaki JF, Ludlow J, Paden B, Long JW. Design optimization of the HeartQuest MagLev VAD. *ASAIO J.* 2001 Mar/Apr;47(2):135.

11. Yoshida K, Tobe S, Kawata M, Yamaguchi M. Acquired and reversible von Willebrand disease with high shear stress aortic valve stenosis. *Ann Thoracic Surg.* 2006;81:490-494.

12. Geisen U, Heilman C, Beyersdorf F, et al. Non-surgical bleeding in patients with ventricular assist devices could be explained by acquired von Willebrand disease. *Eur J Cardiothoracic Surg.* 2008;33:679-684.

13. Federico P, Patrizia DV, Giuseppe C, et al. Phosphorylcholine coating may limit thrombin formation during high-risk cardiac surgery: a randomized controlled trial. *Ann Thoracic Surg.* 2006;81(3):886-889.

14. Yamazaki K, Saito S, Nishinaka T, et al. Japanese clinical trial results of an implantable centrifugal blood pump "EVAHEART." *J Heart Lung Transplant.* 2008;27(2):S246.

15. LaRose JA, Tamez D, Ashenuga M, Reyes C. Design concepts and principle of operation of the HeartWare ventricular assist system. *ASAIO J.* 2010 Jul/Aug;56(4):285-289.

16. Frazier OH, Shah NA, Myers TJ, Robertson KD, Gregoric ID, Delgado R. Use of the Flowmaker (Jarvik 2000) left ventricular assist device for destination therapy and bridging to transplantation. *Cardiology.* 2004;101(1-3):111-116.

17. Antonis A, Pitsis AN, Visouli VV, et al. First human implantation of a new rotary blood pump: design of the clinical feasibility study. *Hellenic J Cardiol.* 2006;47:368-376.

18. Antonis A, Pitsis AN, Visouli VN, et al. Elective bridging to recovery after repair: the surgical approach to ventricular reverse remodeling. *Artif Organs.* 2008;32(9):730-734.

CHAPTER 39

EVAHEART LEFT VENTRICULAR ASSIST SYSTEM

The Durable And High Flow Performance Centrifugal Blood Pump

Tomohiro Nishinaka, Kenji Yamazaki, Satoshi Saito, Hiroyuki Tsukui, and Tomoya Kitano

Donor shortage is an international limitation for heart transplantation, and Japan is no exception. In Japan, only 23 heart transplants were conducted in 2010.[1] Even for bridge-to-transplant (BTT) use in general, left ventricular assist devices, LVADs must be able to support patients for at least 2 years reliably.

EVAHEART Left Ventricular Assist System (LVAS) is an implantable LVAD developed by Sun Medical Technology Research Corp. (Nagano, Japan) (Fig. 39–1). In order to adopt the Japanese social situations as well as aiming at destination therapy (DT), EVAHEART LVAS is designed to have long-term durability, which is supported by the original fluid-lubricating hydrodynamic journal bearing and high fluid dynamical performance.[2,3]

DEVICE DESCRIPTION

■ SYSTEM CONFIGURATION OVERVIEW

EVAHEART LVAS consists of the internal component which includes the blood pump, and the external components which include the controller and power sources (Fig. 39–2).

The EVAHEART LVAS has an implantable centrifugal pump. It has a high fluid dynamic performance capable of fully replacing the dysfunctional left ventricle cardiac output.

The blood pump is connected via a percutaneous driveline to the controller which provides the electric power to drive and control the pump motor.

Additionally, the fluid lubricating hydrodynamic journal bearing rotates without making contact with other parts in a way that enables an unlimited bearing life. Water is circulated from the controller in which a water circulation loop is housed to the blood pump through the driveline. The controller has a small diaphragm pump, filter, and water reservoir.

■ IMPLANTED COMPONENTS

There are three components that are implanted into the patient's body:

1. Blood pump
2. Inflow cannula
3. Outflow graft

The blood pump is implanted into the left abdominal wall, preperitoneal, toward the rectus sheath. The inflow cannula is inserted and affixed to the left ventricular apex, and the outflow graft is affixed to the ascending aorta to create the LV-aorta bypass that works in parallel with the patient's natural heart.

The blood pump consists of a centrifugal pump with a percutaneous driveline. The centrifugal pump consists of an impeller, blood pump chamber, and motor. The volume of the centrifugal pump is 132 mL and weighs 420 g (Table 39–1). The open-type impeller rotates continuously in the blood chamber, and the motor drives the impeller by a shaft which is held by the journal bearing. A mechanical seal prevents the blood leakage from blood chamber to motor along the shaft.

The motor is driven by electric power provided by the controller through the percutaneous driveline. Two tubes are molded into the driveline along with one electric cable. The other tubes are the pathway for water circulation loop (Fig. 39–3).

■ EXTERNAL COMPONENTS

The external components consist of the controller and the power sources. The controller drives and controls the EVAHEART LVAS. It consists of the electronic circuit boards, an emergency battery, and the unit, which contains a reservoir filled with sterile water, a diaphragm pump, a filter, pressure sensors, and electronic circuit boards. Two external batteries and an outside power source, the AC/DC adapter, can provide the power to the controller directly. A replaceable emergency battery (inside the controller) is available to provide power when the patient fails to manage power sources or when all external power sources are disconnected. The battery of the EVAHEART LVAS consists of rechargeable lithium ion batteries that are charged by the dedicated battery charger.

The display panel on the top surface of the controller indicates the pump speed, electric power consumption, and event code by liquid crystal display (LCD) and indicates system alarm, connection to outside power sources, and the remaining battery life by light-emitting diode (LED).

Its system alarms include a pump alarm (automatic pump restart, etc), a fluid-lubricating hydrodynamic journal bearing alarm (abnormal pressure, etc), and controller alarm (no external battery, etc). An external monitor can be connected to the controller. The external monitor displays a graph of the pump speed, electric power consumption, estimated flow rate, and fluid pressure. It downloads the trend data and event data, which are stored in the controller. Trend data include parameters that indicate the operation condition of blood pump, and event data include the record of operation and alarms.

The principal dimensions of external components are indicated in Table 39–2. Sun Medical Technology Research Corp is

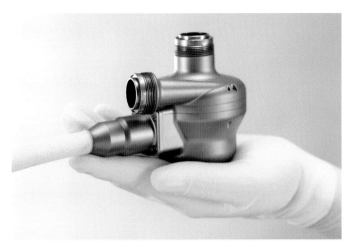

FIGURE 39-1. EVAHEART LVAS blood pump. (Reproduced with permission from Sun Medical Technology Research Corp.)

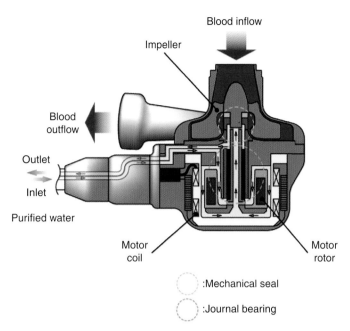

FIGURE 39-3. EVAHEART LVAS blood pump mechanisms. (Reproduced with permission from Sun Medical Technology Research Corp.)

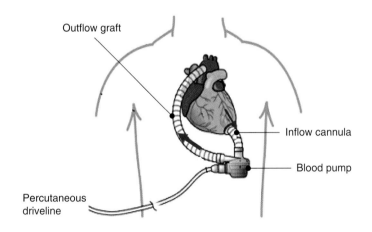

FIGURE 39-2. Implanted components. (Reproduced with permission from Sun Medical Technology Research Corp.)

developing the smaller controller, which is about half the present controller size.

UNIQUE FEATURES

The most distinctive features of EVAHEART LVAS are its fluid dynamic characteristics and reliability. Its blood compatibility is supported by the 2-methacryloyloxyethyl phosphorylcholine (MPC) polymer coating and textured surface on the inflow cannula.[5]

TABLE 39-1. Principal Dimension of Implanted Components

Unit	Principal Dimension
Pump	420 g weight, 132 mL volume
	58 mm outer diameter
Inflow cannula	110 mm total length, 16 mm in diameter
Outflow graft	400 mm total length, 16 mm in diameter

TABLE 39-2. Principal Dimension of External Components

Unit	Principal Dimension
Controller	241 × 304 × 81 mm
	1.97 kg (excluding water circulation unit, emergency battery)
	AC/DC adapter, external monitor can connect
External battery	78 × 44 × 172 mm, 810 g
	4-5 h support for each
Emergency battery	104 × 80 × 22 mm, 225 g
	30 min support
	Stored in the controller
Water circulation unit	145 × 80 × 22 mm, 1.1 kg
	Stored in the controller

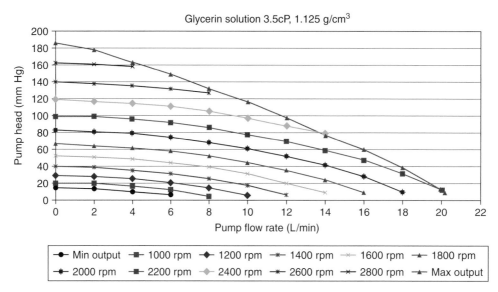

FIGURE 39-4. Fluid dynamical characteristics of EVAHEART LVAS blood pump. (Reproduced with permission from Sun Medical Technology Research Corp.)

■ FLUID DYNAMIC CHARACTERISTICS

The flow rate of centrifugal pump is set by its rotational speed and the head pressure, which is pressure difference between pump inlet and outlet. Even when pump rotational speed is kept as constant, allowing pump flow rate changes with the pressure head change, it causes the blood pressure change.

The fluid dynamic characteristics of the EVAHEART LVAS blood pump are indicated in the pressure-flow curve shown in Fig. 39–4.[4] Its pressure-flow curve is extremely flat, and EVAHEART can generate a significantly high pump flow rate of 20 L/min at a low pressure of 10 to 30 mm Hg. When the head pressure (defined as the pressure difference between pump inlet and pump outlet) decreases during systole, an instant high peak flow is achieved, which results in a higher peak pressure in the aorta (systolic pressure). During the diastolic phase, the left ventricle-aorta pressure difference increases to maximum in one cardiac cycle, and the pump flow rate decreases to minimum. Thus, the pump flow rate becomes pulsatile, and the high peak flow provides a higher mean pump flow rate.[5] For example, the curve of 2200 rpm (rotations per minute) shows the flow rate is almost 0 L/min at 100 mm Hg head pressure, but it increases to almost 20 L/min at close to 0 mm Hg head pressure. In summary, if the natural failing heart can still provide some contractility, the pump can generate pulsatile flow even though its rotational speed is kept as constant. The flat pressure-flow curve characteristic enables this pulsatile pump flow in the cardiac cycle. In the clinical trial in Japan, some pulsatility was observed on the blood pressure and blood flow when cardiac contraction remained, even though the rotational speed of blood pump was kept as constant.[4]

■ DURABILITY

EVAHEART LVAS has demonstrated good durability. In-vitro durability test of 18 devices shows no crucial failure at 2 years operation, and it has not experienced any pump failures in the initial durability test, as well as the continuation of the durability test.

An unlimited bearing life is achieved by the fluid-lubricating hydrodynamic journal bearing which rotates without contact between the parts. The water lubrication on sliding ceramic surfaces provides a low friction coefficient.

■ BLOOD COMPATIBILITY

The blood-contacting surface is covered with a molecular layer of MPC polymer that is well balanced between hydrophilicity and hydrophobicity.[5] The hydrophilic part is bonded with the titanium surface of blood pump and generates a layer which has high water-resistant properties. The phosphorylcholine group provides a hydrophobic characteristic to the biomembrane which prevents adhesion of protein or cells.

■ TEXTURED SURFACE ON INFLOW CANNULA

The inflow cannula is inserted into the apex of the left ventricle. The outside surface has a textured surface structure. It is expected that this surface induces endothelial cell growth on it and prevents the so-called wedge thrombus that might form around the junction of the cannula and myocardium in the left ventricle. The textured surface consists of titanium mesh structure.

CLINICAL TRIALS

A clinical trial was started in Japan in 2005. The product marketing approval was approved by Japanese Pharmaceuticals and Medical Devices Agency (PMDA) in 2010. Following this, a US clinical trial is due to start.

■ BRIDGE-TO-TRANSPLANT PIVOTAL TRIAL

EVAHEART MEDICAL USA, Inc received unconditional approval for a prospective, multicenter pivotal study in December, 2009. The purpose of the study is to assess the safety and efficacy of the EVAHEART LVAS as a bridge-to-transplant (BTT) for subjects with end-stage heart failure. The first implant is anticipated to occur in 2011.

Endpoints

The primary endpoint is survival to cardiac transplant or survival to device explant for recovery or survival to 180 days after implantation on the originally implanted EVAHEART LVAS. The primary endpoint will be compared to a concurrent INTERMACS (Interagency Registry for Mechanically Assisted Circulatory Systems) control group.

Secondary endpoints include survival to transplant, New York Heart Association (NYHA) functional class, 6-minute walk, quality-of-life assessments, including the Kansas City Cardiomyopathy Questionnaire (KCCQ) and the EuroQoL, neurocognitive function, and the incidence of INTERMACS-defined adverse events (unanticipated adverse device effects, and device failure, and malfunctions).

Inclusion/Exclusion Criteria

To be enrolled in the EVAHEART LVAS BTT study, patients must be older than 18 years, listed for cardiac transplant as status 1A or 1B within 72 hours of implant, NYHA class IV heart failure, hemodynamically unstable despite optimal medication regimen for heart failure with inotropic therapy, unless not tolerated by the patient, and able to provide written informed consent. Left atrial pressure or pulmonary capillary wedge pressure 20 mm Hg with either a systolic pressure 90 mm Hg or a Cardiac Index 2.2 L/min/m². Exclusion criteria for the trial include items such as infection, irreversible organ failure, body surface area less than 1.4 m², pregnancy, coagulation disorders, and the inability of the patient to manage the device or their medical regimen.

■ FUTURE PLANS

EVAHEART MEDICAL USA, Inc plans to submit an investigational device exemption application for a DT trial. Additional plans include product development focused on improving the external components, such as the controller and driveline.

REFERENCES

1. Japan Organ Transplant Network Homepage. http://www.jotnw.or.jp/datafile/offer_brain.html
2. Yamazaki K, Litwak P, Tagusari O, et al. An implantable centrifugal blood pump with a recirculating purge system (Cool-Seal system). *Artificial Organs.* 1998;22:466-474.
3. Yamazaki K, Kihara S, Akimoto T, et al. EVAHEART LVAS: an implantable centrifugal blood pump for long-term circulatory support. *Jap J Thorac Cardiovasc Surg.* 2002;50:461-465.
4. Yamazaki K, Saito S, Kihara S, Tagusari O, Kurosawa H. Completely pulsatile high flow circulatory support with a constant-speed centrifugal blood pump: mechanisms and early clinical observations. *Gen Thorac Cardiovasc Surg.* 2007;55:158-162.
5. Ishihara K, Tanaka S, Furukawa N, et al. Improved blood compatibility of segmented polyurethanes by polymeric additives having a phospholipid polar group. I. Molecular design of polymeric additives and their functions. *J Biomed Mater Res.* 1996;32:391-399.

INDEX

Note: Page numbers followed by *f* indicate figures, and those followed by *t* indicate tables.